Preparing to Pass the Medical Assisting Exam

Preparing to Pass the Medical Assisting Exam

CARLENE HARRISON, EdD, CMA (AAMA)
Dean, School of Allied Health
Hodges University

VALERIE WEISS, MD, MS
Program Chair, Health Studies
Hodges University

JONES AND BARTLETT PUBLISHERS
Sudbury, Massachusetts
BOSTON   TORONTO   LONDON   SINGAPORE

World Headquarters

Jones and Bartlett Publishers
40 Tall Pine Drive
Sudbury, MA 01776
978-443-5000
info@jbpub.com
www.jbpub.com

Jones and Bartlett Publishers
Canada
6339 Ormindale Way
Mississauga, Ontario L5V 1J2
Canada

Jones and Bartlett Publishers
International
Barb House, Barb Mews
London W6 7PA
United Kingdom

Jones and Bartlett's books and products are available through most bookstores and online booksellers. To contact Jones and Bartlett Publishers directly, call 800-832-0034, fax 978-443-8000, or visit our website, www.jbpub.com.

Substantial discounts on bulk quantities of Jones and Bartlett's publications are available to corporations, professional associations, and other qualified organizations. For details and specific discount information, contact the special sales department at Jones and Bartlett via the above contact information or send an email to specialsales@jbpub.com.

The authors, editor, and publisher have made every effort to provide accurate information. However, they are not responsible for errors, omissions, or for any outcomes related to the use of the contents of this book and take no responsibility for the use of the products and procedures described. Treatments and side effects described in this book may not be applicable to all people; likewise, some people may require a dose or experience a side effect that is not described herein. Drugs and medical devices are discussed that may have limited availability controlled by the Food and Drug Administration (FDA) for use only in a research study or clinical trial. Research, clinical practice, and government regulations often change the accepted standard in this field. When consideration is being given to use of any drug in the clinical setting, the health care provider or reader is responsible for determining FDA status of the drug, reading the package insert, and reviewing prescribing information for the most up-to-date recommendations on dose, precautions, and contraindications, and determining the appropriate usage for the product. This is especially important in the case of drugs that are new or seldom used.

Production Credits

Publisher: David Cella
Associate Editor: Maro Gartside
Editorial Assistant: Teresa Reilly
Production Manager: Julie Champagne Bolduc
Associate Production Editor: Jessica Steele Newfell
Marketing Manager: Grace Richards
Manufacturing and Inventory Control Supervisor: Amy Bacus
Composition: Glyph International
Cover Design: Kristin E. Parker
Cover Image: © Photodisc
Chapter-Opening Images: © Kimberly Ann Reinick/ShutterStock, Inc.
Printing and Binding: Courier Stoughton
Cover Printing: Courier Stoughton

Library of Congress Cataloging-in-Publication Data

Harrison, Carlene.
    Preparing to pass the medical assisting exam / Carlene Harrison and Valerie Weiss.
        p. ; cm.
    Includes index.
    ISBN 978-0-7637-5402-0 (alk. paper)
    1. Medical assistants—Examinations, questions, etc. 2. Medical assistants—Examinations—United States—Study guides. I. Weiss, Valerie, 1975– II. Title.
    [DNLM: 1. Physician Assistants—Examination Questions. 2. Practice Management, Medical—Examination Questions. W 18.2 H318p 2011]
    R728.8.H383 2011
    610.76—dc22

                                                                                2009039397
6048
Printed in the United States of America
13 12 11 10 09   10 9 8 7 6 5 4 3 2 1

Brief Contents

Contents

Contents

Chapter 5

Common Diseases and Pathology   89

Chapter 14
Coding Systems   197

SECTION IV
Clinical Knowledge   213

Chapter 15
Asepsis and Infection Control   215

Chapter 16
Patient Preparation and Assisting the Physician   227

Contents

Chapter 17

Specimen Collection, Diagnostic Testing, and Medical Equipment   **237**

Chapter 18

Pharmacology and Medication Administration   **261**

Chapter 19

Medical Emergencies and First Aid   285

Chapter 20

Nutrition   301

Acknowledgments

Every textbook is completed because of the support and help from a variety of people. The authors wish to offer a big thank you to Christine Sanders, CMA(AAMA), an Instructor at Hodges University's Medical Assisting program, who provided valuable feedback as we developed this text. We never would have completed the text without the typing and error-checking skills of Amy Mulligan, a Hodges University student who has gone on to graduate school to become a Physician Assistant.

Our families were an important part of the process. During previous projects, Bill Harrison spent lonely hours as Carlene worked. This time, however, he contributed by reviewing and reading as if he were a student to help this text be as clear as possible.

Valerie could not have accomplished writing the text without the much-needed support and encouragement of her husband, Shad White. He spent every weekend for months taking their two young children, Harrison and Kyra, on fieldtrips away from the house so Valerie could write. Valerie's parents, who are affectionately known as Gramsy and Pal, also were fabulous babysitters during those intense months of writing and teaching.

Preparing to Take the Certification Exam

The Certification Process and the Exam

If you are reading this book, you are getting ready to take either the American Association of Medical Assistants (AAMA) Certified Medical Assisting (CMA) Exam or the American Medical Technologists (AMT) Registered Medical Assisting (RMA) Exam. If you are a recent graduate of a medical assisting program, taking the exam as soon after graduation as possible is important. If you are a practicing CMA who is taking the exam, the likelihood is that you are taking the exam again because you did not keep up on your continuing education units. Why take the exam at all? There are several reasons:

- Passing a national certification exam demonstrates to patients, employers, and others that you have learned a standardized body of knowledge. Many physicians will only hire individuals who have passed one of the two exams.
- If you move, you do not have to apply for a separate certification—both the CMA and the RMA are recognized by employers throughout the United States.
- Larger medical group practices may be affiliated with local hospitals and may be required to meet Joint Commission standards. The credentials of all staff are inspected. Although the Joint Commission does not currently require that all medical assistants be certified, having certified staff is looked upon favorably.
- Because passing the certification exam(s) requires that you study and are up-to-date on current standards, you can take pride in your certification.

THE NATIONAL EXAMS

As mentioned earlier, two organizations offer nationally recognized medical assisting examinations. Both are highly respected professional organizations. The exam format is similar, using only multiple choice questions, and the content covered on the exams is similar. The difference is the eligibility criteria for each exam. Whether you take from the AAMA or the AMT depends on whether you meet the admission criteria. It also may be that one credential is better recognized in your area.

American Association of Medical Assistants (AAMA) Certification Exam

The American Association of Medical Assistants (AAMA) is the professional organization representing medical assistants throughout the country. Individuals who pass the AAMA exam earn a CMA (AAMA). This credential is recognized throughout the United States. Once they have earned the credential, individuals must be recertified every five years by continuing education or reexamination. This recertification is to demonstrate competency and knowledge in the field. All CMA (AAMA)'s must either take the exam again after five years or provide proof of 60 continuing education units to the AAMA. The specific information about recertifying by continuing education is available on the AAMA website (http://www.aama-ntl.org).

To be eligible to take the AAMA exam, candidates must meet one of the following conditions:

- *Category 1:* This is for the graduating student or recent graduate of a medical assisting program accredited by the Commission on Accreditation of Allied Health Education Programs (CAAHEP) or by the Accrediting Bureau of Health Education Schools (ABHES). Students must be within 30 days of completing their education and externship to take the exam.
- *Category 2:* This category is for the individual who is not a recent graduate of a CAAHEP or ABHES accredited program. If you graduated more than 12 months prior to the exam date, you are considered a nonrecent graduate. The fee for the examination may be higher if you are not a member of the AAMA. You must submit a transcript with proof of graduation.
- *Category 3:* The last category is for individuals who are already CMA (AAMA)s and are applying to recertify the credential. You must submit a copy of a current provider-level CPR and a copy of your current CMA (AAMA) certificate.

The AAMA certification exam is offered in a variety of locations throughout the year. It is very important that you review the current *Candidate Application and Handbook* in detail. This handbook provides the latest information on the steps you need to follow to take the exam as well as the application that must be completed. The timing of your application to take the exam is important. If you are planning to take the exam soon after graduation, you must apply no less than five months in advance of the date you will complete your medical assisting program.

The exam consists of 200 multiple choice questions. The content of the exam is outlined in the *Handbook* in detail. You should be prepared to answer questions on all of the topics outlined.

The current exam is administered in two 80-minute segments, with an optional 20-minute break between segments. The entire exam is taken on a computer, so you must be comfortable with test taking on a computer. You can use the CD that accompanies this book for practice, but the actual computerized format for the test will probably be different than the format on the CD.

American Medical Technologists (AMT) Certification Exam

The American Medical Technologists (AMT) is a nonprofit certification agency and professional membership association representing a variety of healthcare professionals. AMT's mission is to issue certification credentials to medical and dental assistants, clinical laboratory personnel, laboratory consultants, and allied health instructors. AMT is recognized throughout the country, as is its Registered Medical Assistant (RMA (AMT)) credential. Once they have passed the exam, RMA (AMT)s must maintain their credential by providing proof of 30 points of continuing education every 3 years. Check the AMT website (http://www.amt1.com) for more information about maintaining continuing education credits.

There are three different categories of eligibility to be considered for the AMT examination:

- *Category 1:* The applicant must be a graduate of, or scheduled to graduate from, a medical assistant program that is accredited by CAAHEP or ABHES *or* a medical assistant program in a postsecondary school or college that has institutional accreditation by a regional accrediting commission, or by a national accrediting organization approved by the U.S. Department of Education. The program must include a minimum of 720 hours (or equivalent) of training in medical assisting skills (including a clinical externship). If you graduated within the last three years, proof of work experience is *not required*. If you graduated over three years ago, you will be required to show proof of current work experience. Your program chair will know if you are graduating from an appropriately accredited program.
- *Category 2:* If you are a graduate of a formal medical services training program of the U.S. Armed Forces, you are eligible to take the exam.

- *Category 3:* You may register for the exam if you have been employed in the profession of medical assisting for a minimum of five years, no more than two years of which may have been as an instructor in the postsecondary medical assistant program. Proof of current work experience and high school education or equivalent is needed. Employment dates must be within the last five years.

The areas covered in the RMA examination differ slightly from the CMA exam. The examination is usually 200 questions. The AMT offers both a pencil and paper test and a computerized version of the exam. It is important that you check the AMT website for specific information about the exam.

SUMMARY

Congratulations for taking the next step in your professional career by taking a certification exam. You must begin preparing for the exam long before the actual date. Chapter 2 provides you with some study tips. It is also important that you carefully review the candidate handbook and instructions for either exam. The exam process is clearly outlined in the individual handbook.

Study Techniques and Exam-Taking Strategies

PREPARING FOR THE EXAM

The RMA and CMA exams are not like a final exam in a course. You cannot study for several days before, or cram the night before, and expect to do well. You must begin your preparation several months before the planned exam date.

Step 1: Set Up a Study Area

Find space in your home to set aside that is your special study place. In this space you should have this review book and your textbooks from your courses, as well as some other supplies listed in Step 2. People learn in different ways, but for this exam, you should have a quiet place where you can study and memorize the facts and information. The majority of the questions are knowledge based (i.e., facts and information) and you will be doing a lot of memorizing.

If you do not have a quiet space at home and must go to the library or another place to study, use a bookbag to carry all your essentials for memorizing. You can even create three or four book-bags and divide their contents by the sections of the exam (one each for general, administrative, and clinical, and one for supplies).

Depending on how much room you have, you should also have access to a computer. Both the RMA and CMA exams are computerized, so you must feel comfortable taking exams on a computer. You may also take the RMA test as a pencil and paper test at certain times of the year. Check the AMT website for more details. This textbook provides you with a CD-ROM with some 1600 questions. If you are going to study at the library, then bring the CD along and practice taking the exam over and over again. The CD will mix up the questions for you.

Step 2: Define Your Study Style

Think about your most successful study habits. Did you do better if you created flash cards on 3" × 5" cards? Did you outline material using a systematic set of headings and subheadings? Some students do well with a concept called mind mapping to help them understand and memorize material (see Figure 2-1).

Hopefully you saved all your notes from your various classes in medical assisting; however, using your notes from class and your textbooks may not be the best way to study for this type of exam. Because the exam covers so much material, if you go back and review every chapter of every text and every set of notes you had from each and every class, you may become overwhelmed. In this book, we have attempted to outline the major areas of the exam. You should create your own set of notes, either by outline or flashcards, that reflects the major points in each area.

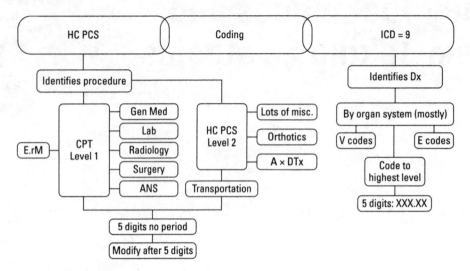

Figure 2-1 Mind Mapping

Whatever you create as study notes, try to make them portable. That way, you can take them with you and study while stuck in traffic, waiting to be seen by a doctor or dentist, or standing in line at the grocery store or bus stop.

Remember that just reading material is not enough. You must drill yourself on the material in whatever way works for you. That is why study outlines, flash cards, or some other set of review tools is so important.

Step 3: Create a Schedule

Develop a study schedule. This may be the most difficult thing you do because it requires that you maintain discipline. But once you set a schedule, follow it.

Your schedule should reflect what you are going to study when. Begin by studying difficult and/or boring subjects first. For example, many students find the administrative areas of medical assisting uninteresting; however, there are many questions on administrative topics, so it is important that you begin working on this area if it is your least favorite. If you found pharmacology difficult during your classes, add that to your study early list.

Start approximately three months before the scheduled exam date. Organize your material. Talk with the other people in your life and explain to them the importance of this study time. You may need to negotiate with them, but you must be able to say no when someone wants to interfere with your study time.

The time you set aside should be the time when you function at your best. Are you a morning person? Maybe you study best late at night. By now, you probably know when you best study time is, so use that information to your advantage.

A POSSIBLE SCHEDULE

Everyone is different, and the following schedule may not be best for you. The important thing is that you create a schedule that gives you increased study time as you get closer to the exam. Let's assume that you are going to take the exam the last day of June. Here is a possible schedule:

April 1–15: Establish your study area and your study times for the next three months. Organize what you will study in what order. Get the supplies you need. Set aside time during these first two weeks—maybe two hours—to start studying. You can do this in one 2-hour increment or two 1-hour increments. Take practice exams.

April 16–30: During this 2-week period you should put in at least four hours of study time in whatever way works best for you. At least one of the boring or difficult areas should be memorized at this point. Take practice exams.

May 1–15: Every week you should be studying approximately three hours. That means that during this period of time you have put in at least six hours studying and memorizing. Take practice exams.

May 16–31: Find a study friend from school. Set up study sessions that begin during this time where you can quiz each other. If no one is available, continue to study at least three hours each week. It is also time to review your schedule at this point. Are you more comfortable with the boring and difficult areas? Do you need to revise the schedule now that you have maintained a strict schedule? Take practice exams.

June 1–15: You should be devoting time every day to studying—even if it is only 30 minutes a day. You should be feeling comfortable with the boring and difficult areas by now, but if you are not, keep working on those areas, along with those areas with which you are more comfortable. Take practice exams.

June 16–28: Try to put in at least one hour every day reviewing material and taking practice exams. At this point, you are probably getting really tired of the material and becoming apprehensive. You may need to take a day off from studying.

Repetition, repetition, repetition. Using your flash cards or outlines and taking practice exams will help your recall facts and information. Be careful *not* to memorize practice questions, however. You are memorizing the information, not the question itself.

June 29: Don't study the day before the exam. Give yourself time to relax. Try to avoid being anxious. Make sure you know where you are going to take the exam and how long it is going to take you to get to your destination. Be sure you have your exam admission documentation and photo identification. Try to get a good night's sleep!

EXAM-TAKING STRATEGIES

The CMA and RMA exams are multiple choice exams. Both exams are 200 questions. The questions consist of the stem and either four or five lettered response choices. Only one of these choices is correct; the other three or four are called distractors. Here are some suggestions:

- Read the question carefully. Remember that you are selecting the one best answer.
- Do not read into the question by assuming information that is not provided.
- Eliminate those answers you know to be wrong.
- If you are taking the computerized version of the exam, you can write out choices (A, B, C, D, E) on your scratch paper and then cross off the ones you know aren't correct. You can repeat this technique for each question.
- If you do not see a "right" answer, choose the best answer available.
- If the possible answers cover a wide range of quantities and you don't know the correct answer, choose the one in the middle of the range.
- Pay attention to those words that are underlined, in **bold**, CAPITALIZED, or *italicized*.
- Be careful with questions that have the word *except* as part of the question. The correct answer is the opposite of what is asked in the question.
- If you really don't know the answer at all:
  - Choose the answer that uses the same language that appears in the stem.
  - Choose the answer that appears to be the most complex.
  - Choose from two answers that are possible—pick one and move on.
  - For all questions for which you simply do not know the answer, pick the same letter every time.

Every question should be answered. An unanswered question always is wrong, but you might guess correctly.

The exams are timed, so it is important that you do not linger over a question. Unless you make an obvious mistake, do not change the answer. Answer the questions you are certain about first. Then you can go back and answer the remaining questions.

Pay attention to the time. Depending on the exam, the proctor may announce how much time is left. If you are running out of time, just go through and quickly select answers to those questions you have not answered.

The exam preparation process is a difficult one. You must be prepared to sacrifice time and energy to be successful on the day of the exam.

General Knowledge

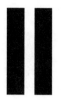

Medical Terminology

Throughout the exam there will be questions that require knowledge of medical terminology. This chapter outlines some of the main terms.

A medical term may have three parts—the prefix, the word root, and the suffix. Knowing the meaning of each will help to you to understand a variety of terms. Prefixes are found at the beginning of the word and modify the word's meaning. Table 3-1 lists some common prefixes. The suffix of a word occurs at the end of the word. The suffix also modifies the word's meaning. Table 3-2 lists some common suffixes.

The word root of a medical term is the foundation of a word that gives it meaning. Word roots typically describe the part of the body involved. Word roots are usually combined with a vowel at the end (often an "o") so that a suffix beginning with a consonant can be added. When word roots are written in this way, they are called *combining forms.*

The following pages (Tables 3-3 through 3-14) look at each of the organ systems separately. Memorizing every single medical term is not the best approach to studying for the medical terminology portion of the exam. Memorizing basic prefixes and suffixes as well as some of the major terms for each organ system is a better approach.

Body planes are imaginary vertical and horizontal lines that are used to divide the body for descriptive purposes. When using body planes, the person is assumed to be in the anatomic position, which means standing erect, facing forward, arms at the sides with palms toward the front. Questions about body planes are common on the exam. Table 3-15 identifies the various body plane terms.

It is possible that there may be several questions about abbreviations and their use. Table 3-16 lists common approved abbreviations that might appear on the exam.

Table 3-1 Common Prefixes

Prefix	Meaning	Example
a-, an-	without	*Aphasia* is the loss of ability to speak, write, and/or comprehend the written or spoken word.
ab-	from, away from	*Abduct* means to be move away from the midline of the body.
ad-	toward, in the direction of	*Adduct* means to move toward the midline of the body.
albin-	white	*Albinism* is an inherited deficiency in which there is absence of pigment (melanin) in the skin, hair, and irises.
ambi-	both	*Ambidextrous* is the ability to use both hands with equal dexterity.
ante-, pre-, pro-	before	*Prenatal* means the time and events before birth. *Antecubital* refers to the region in front of the elbow.
anti-, contra-	against	*Antibiotic* means to act against microorganisms.
auto-	self	*Autologous* means relating to self.
bi-, diplo-	two	*Bilateral* means pertaining to two sides; *diplopia* means double vision.
bio-	life	*Biology* means the study of life.
brady-	slow	*Bradycardia* means an abnormally slow heartbeat.
circum-	around	*Circumcision* means the removal of the skin around the tip of the penis.
con-	together, with	*Congenital* means present at birth.
de-	away from	*Delusion* is a false personal belief that is maintained despite obvious proof to the contrary. Delusion is a thought that strays away from the norm.
dia-	through	*Diarrhea* is the rapid movement of fecal matter through the intestines.
dys-	abnormal, difficult, painful, bad	*Dyspnea* is difficult or labored breathing.
ecto-	outside	An *ectopic pregnancy* is when the ovum becomes fertilized outside the uterus.
endo-	within	*Endoscopy* is a procedure in which an instrument is placed within the body.
epi-	upon, over	*Epidermis* is the outermost layer of skin.
eu-	normal, good	*Euphoria* is a state of well-being.
ex-, exo-, extra-	out of, away from, outside	*Exophthalmus* is an abnormal protrusion of the eyes.
hemi-, semi-	half	*Hemiplegia* is total paralysis of half of the body; *semicircular* means shaped like a half-circle.
hyper-, poly-	above normal, excessive	*Hyperhidrosis* is a condition of excess sweating; *polymyalgia* means pain in several muscle groups.
hypo-, sub-	below normal, below, underneath	*Hypocalcemia* is a condition characterized by abnormally low calcium levels in the blood; *subcutaneous injection* is the administration of medicine by injection into the fatty layer just below the skin.

(continues)

Table 3-1 Common Prefixes (Continued)

Prefix	Meaning	Example
inter-	between	*Interstitial* means between tissue.
intra-	within	*Intracranial pressure* means the amount of pressure within the skull.
iso-	same	*Isotope* is a chemical element having the same atomic number as another chemical element.
macro-, megalo-	big, large	A *macrocyte* is an abnormally large cell; *megalocephaly* is an abnormally large head.
mal-	bad, not adequate	*Malnutrition* is a lack of proper food or nutrition.
meta-	change, transformation	*Metastasize* describes the process by which cancer spreads.
micro-	small	*Microbiology* is the study of microorganisms. *Microcephaly* refers to a small head.
mono-	one	*Monochromatism* is also known as color blindness or the inability to distinguish certain colors.
multi-, pluri-	many	*Multiparous* is a term used to describe a woman who has given birth two or more times; *pluripotent stem cells* have the ability to differentiate into any of the three germ layers.
neo-	new, recent	*Neoplasm* describes new and abnormal tissue formation; also known as a tumor.
non-	not	*Noninvasive* is a term used to describe therapeutic and diagnostic procedures that do not involve the puncturing of the skin.
oligo-	few, scanty, sparse	*Oligospermia* is a low sperm count.
pan-	all	*Pandemic* is a widespread epidemic, usually worldwide.
para-	near, beside, beyond, opposite, abnormal	*Paradoxical drug reaction* describes the effect caused by a medication that is the exact opposite of what is therapeutically intended.
per-	through	*Percutaneous* means through the skin.
peri-	around	*Periosteum* describes the dense connective tissue around the bone.
poly-	many	*Polydipsia* means excessive thirst; *polyphagia* means excessive hunger.
post-	after, following	*Postmortem* means after death.
pre-	before	*Premature infant* means a neonate born before 37 weeks gestation.
primi-	first	*Primigravida* is a woman during her first pregnancy.
quadra-, quadri-	four	*Quadriplegia* is paralysis of all four extremities.
re-	again, backward	*Relapse* is the return of a disease.
rube-	red	*Rubella* is a viral disease that produces red skin rashes.
semi-	half	*Semiconscious* means half-conscious.
sub-	under, below	*Subcostal* means below the rib(s).
super-, supra-	above, superior	*Superinfection* is a new infection above and beyond the original infection which results in a serious condition.

(continues)

Table 3-1 Common Prefixes (Continued)

Prefix	Meaning	Example
syn-, sym-	together	*Symphysis pubis* is the area in front of the pelvis where the pubic bones meet.
tachy-	fast, abnormally fast	*Tachypnea* is fast breathing.
tri-	three	The *triceps brachii muscle* is the muscle of the posterior upper arm that has three divisions.
ultra-	beyond	*Ultrasound* is a procedure where high-frequency sound waves are used to visualize internal organs.
uni-	one, single	*Unilateral* means relating to one side.

Table 3-2 Common Suffixes

Suffixes	Meaning	Example
-ac, -al, -ar, -ary	pertaining to	*Cardiac* means pertaining to the heart; *congenital* means pertaining to the presence at birth; *muscular* means pertaining to the muscles; *integumentary* means pertaining to the skin.
-algia	pain	*Neuralgia* means pain in the nerves.
-ase	enzyme	*Amylase* is an enzyme that breaks down starch.
-blast	baby, immature	*Osteoblast* refers to an immature bone cell.
-cele	abnormal protrusions	*Myocele* is an abnormal protrusion of muscle; hernia.
-centesis	surgical puncture	*Abdominocentesis* is a surgical puncture of the abdominal cavity to remove fluid.
-cide	destroying	*Germicide* is a solution that kills germs.
-cyte	cell	*Erythrocyte* is a red blood cell.
-derma	skin	*Scleroderma* is the hardening of connective tissues, including the skin.
-desis	binding	*Arthrodesis* is the binding of a joint.
-dipsia	thirst	*Polydipsia* means excessive thirst, as occurs in diabetes.
-dynia	pain	*Gastrodynia* means pain in the stomach.
-ectasis	dilation	*Ureterectasis* is dilation of a ureter.
-ectomy	surgical removal	*Tonsillectomy* is surgical removal of the tonsils.
-edema	fluid accumulation, swelling	*Lymphedema* is swelling due to abnormal accumulation of lymph within the tissues.
-emesis	vomiting	*Hyperemesis* is excessive vomiting.
-emia	blood	*Uremia* is a toxic condition caused by excessive amounts of urea and other wastes in the blood.
-esthesia	sensation, feeling	*Anesthesia* refers to the absence of normal sensation.
-gen, -genesis, -genic	producing, formation	A *carcinogen* is something that produces cancer; *carcinogenesis* is the formation of the cancer; *carcinogenic* refers to an agent that produces cancer.
-gram	record	An *electrocardiogram* is a recording of the heartbeat.

(continues)

Table 3-2 Common Suffixes (Continued)

Suffixes	Meaning	Example
-graph	instrument to record	An *electrocardiograph* is the instrument used to produce electrocardiograms.
-graphy	the process of recording	*Coronary angiography* refers to the process of making a radiographic study of the coronary arteries after inserting contrast medium.
-gravida	pregnant	*Nulligravida* refers to a woman who has never been pregnant; *primigravida* refers to a woman during her first pregnancy.
-iasis	condition, formation of	*Lithiasis* is the formation of stones.
-iatric	pertaining to medical treatment	*Pediatric* is pertaining to the treatment of children.
-ic, -ical	pertaining to	*Gastric* is pertaining to the stomach.
-ism	condition	*Hypothyroidism* refers to low production of thyroid hormone.
-itis	inflammation	*Laryngitis* is inflammation of the larynx.
-logist	someone who studies a specific area	A *neurologist* is a physician who specializes in diagnosing and treating disorders of the nervous system.
-logy	the study of	*Cardiology* is the study of the heart.
-lysis	destruction	*Hemolysis* refers to the destruction of red blood cells.
-malacia	softening	*Osteomalacia* is the softening of bone due to defective bone mineralization.
-mania	abnormal preoccupation	*Pyromania* is defined as a pattern of deliberate setting of fires for pleasure.
-megaly	enlargement	*Cardiomegaly* is the enlargement of the heart.
-meter, metry	measuring device, the process of measuring	*Spirometry* is a noninvasive test in which a person breathes into a device that measures airflow, volume, and time of each breath.
-oma	tumor	*Carcinoma* is a malignant tumor that arises from epithelial tissue; *sarcoma* is a malignant tumor that arises from connective tissue.
-otomy	the process of cutting, an incision	*Phlebotomy* is the puncture of a vein for the purpose of drawing blood.
-para, -parous	to have a child, to bring forth	*Nullipara* refers to a woman who has never borne a viable child; *primipara* refers to a woman who has had one viable child; multiparous refers to a woman who has had two or more children.
-pathy, -pathic	disease	*Idiopathic disease* is a disease of unknown origin.
-penia	deficiency	*Leukopenia* is the decrease in the number of circulating white blood cells.
-pepsia	digestion	*Dyspepsia* is an upset stomach.
-pexy	surgical fixation	*Cystopexy* is the surgical fixation of the bladder to the abdominal wall.
-phagia	eating	*Polyphagia* means excessive hunger, as occurs in diabetes.

(*continues*)

Table 3-2 Common Suffixes (Continued)

Suffixes	Meaning	Example
-phobia	fear of	*Agoraphobia* is anxiety about being in outdoor, open, or public places.
-plasty	surgical repair	*Valvoplasty* is the surgical repair or replacement of a heart valve; also known as *valvuloplasty*.
-pnea	breath or breathing	*Apnea* is the cessation of breathing.
-prandial	meal	*Postprandial* is after a meal.
-ptosis	sagging or drooping	*Cystoptosis* is the prolapse of the bladder.
-rrhage, -rrhagia	heavy discharge	*Hemorrhage* is a heavy discharge of blood in a short amount of time.
-rrhaphy	surgical suturing (to close a wound)	*Myorrhaphy* is the surgical suturing of muscle.
-rrhea	discharge	*Amenorrhea* is the absence of menstrual flow.
-rrhexis	rupture	*Myorrhexis* is the rupture of muscle.
-scope	an instrument used to view	A *laparoscope* is an instrument through which structures in the abdomen and pelvis can be seen.
-scopy	visual examination	*Laparoscopy* is the visual examination of the interior of the abdomen with a laparoscope.
-stasis	stopping	*Hemostasis* means to stop or control bleeding.
-stenosis	narrowing	*Arteriostenosis* is the abnormal narrowing of an artery or arteries.
-stomy	opening	*Colostomy* is the creation of an artificial opening between the colon and the surface of the body for excretion of wastes.
-tropic	having an affinity for	A *vasotropic agent* acts on blood vessels.
-uria	urine	*Dysuria* is difficult or painful urination.

Table 3-3 Integumentary System

Combining Form	Meaning	Example
alopec/i	baldness	*Alopecia* is the partial of complete loss of hair.
cry/o	cold	*Cryosurgery* is surgery that uses liquid nitrogen to freeze the tissue.
cutane/o	skin	*Subcutaneous* means beneath the skin.
cyan/o	blue	*Cyanosis* is a bluish discoloration of the skin.
dermat/o	skin	*Dermatoplasty* is the surgical repair of the skin with a skin graft.
erythr/o, erythem/o	red	*Erythroderma* is widespread redness accompanied by scaling of the skin.
hidr/o	sweat	*Hyperhidrosis* is a condition of excess sweating.
hist/o	tissue	*Histology* is the study of tissues.
leuk/o	white	*Leukopenia* is a reduction of the number of leukocytes in the blood.
lip/o	fat	*Lipoma* is a benign fatty deposit under the skin.
melan/o	black	*Melanosis* is any condition of unusual deposits of black pigment in different parts of the body.
onych/o	nail	*Onychomycosis* is a fungal infection of a nail.
pil/i	hair	*Arrector pili* are tiny muscle fibers attached to the hair follicles that respond to cold or fright.
scler/o	hard, hardening	*Scleroderma* is a condition of hardened skin and other connective tissues.
seb/o	sebum (oil)	*Seborrhea* is a condition in which there is an overproduction of sebum.
trich/o	hair	*Trichotillomania* is a behavior in which one has a compulsion for hair pulling.
xanth/o	yellow	*Xanthoderma* is any yellow discoloration of the skin.
xer/o	dry	*Xeroderma* is excessive dryness of the skin.

Table 3-4 Musculoskeletal System

Combining Form	Meaning	Example
ankyl/o	to make crooked; stiff	*Ankylosis* is stiffness in a joint due to disease, injury, or surgery.
arth/o	joint	*Arthralgia* is pain in a joint or joints.
burs/o	bursa	*Bursitis* is inflammation of a bursa.
carp/o	wrist	*Carpals* are bones of the wrist.
cervic/o	neck	*Cervical* means pertaining to a neck.
chir/o	hand	*Chiropractors* are specialists who manipulate the spine with their hands to realign the vertebrae.
chondr/o	cartilage	*Chondroma* is a slow-growing tumor derived from cartilage.
cost/o	rib	*Costal* means between the ribs.
crani/o	skull, head	*Craniotomy* is a surgical incision or opening into the skull.
dors/o	back	*Dorsal* means pertaining to the back.
kyph/o	hump	*Kyphosis* is abnormal outward curvature of the thoracic spine; humpback.
lamin/o	posterior portion of a vertebra	*Laminectomy* is the surgical removal of the lamina.
lei/o	smooth muscle	*Leiomyoma* is a benign tumor of the smooth muscle.
lord/o	bent backward	*Lordosis* is abnormal forward curvature of the lumbar spine; swayback.
myel/o	bone marrow (or spinal cord—depends on context)	*Myeloma* is a tumor of the bone marrow.
myo, myos/o	muscle	*Myomalacia* is abnormal softening of muscle tissue.
orth/o	straight	An *orthopedist* is a surgeon that specializes in straightening/treating injuries of bones.
osteo/o	bone	*Osteoplasty* is the surgical repair of bone(s).
scoli/o	curved	*Scoliosis* is abnormal lateral curvature of the spine.
synovi/o, synov/o	synovial fluid or membrane	*Synovitis* is inflammation of the synovial membrane.
ten/o	tendon	*Tenodynia* is pain in a tendon.

Table 3-5 Cardiovascular System

Combining Form	Meaning	Example
angi/o	vessel	*Angiostenosis* is the narrowing of a blood vessel.
aort/o	aorta; main vessel of the heart	The *aortic semilunar valve* is located between the left ventricle and the aorta.
arteri/o	artery	*Arterionecrosis* is death of an artery.
atri/o	atrium	*Atriomegaly* is the abnormal enlargement of the atrium.
cardi/o	heart	A *cardiologist* is a physician who specializes in treatment of heart diseases.
cyt/o	cell	*Cytology* is the study of the cell.
erythr/o	red	*Erythrocytes* are red blood cells.
hem/o, hemat/o	blood	*Hemorrhage* is a heavy discharge of blood in a short amount of time.
leuc/o, leuk/o	white	*Leukocytes* are white blood cells.
lymph/o	lymph	*Lymphadenopathy* is enlargement of the lymph nodes.
phleb/o	vein	*Phleborrhexis* is the rupture of a vein.
plasm/o	plasma	*Plasmapheresis* is the removal of whole blood from the body, separation of the cellular elements, and return of those blood cells to the body's circulation.
thromb/o	clot	*Thrombus* is a blood clot attached to the interior of an artery or a vein.
valv/o, valvul/o	valve	*Valvuloplasty* is the surgical repair or replacement of a heart valve; also known as *valvoplasty*.
vas/o	vessel	A *vasodilator* is a medication that dilates the blood vessels.
ven/o	vein	*Venography* is an x-ray image of veins after the injection of contrast medium.
ventricul/o	ventricular	*Ventricular fibrillation* refers to the rapid, irregular, and useless contractions of the ventricle(s) that are usually fatal; also known as *V-fib*.

Table 3-6 Lymphatic and Immune Systems

Combining Form	Meaning	Example
immun/o	immune system	*Immunology* is the study of the immune system.
lymph/o	lymph	*Lymphedema* is swelling due to abnormal accumulation of lymph within the tissues.
lymphaden/o	lymph nodes	*Lymphadenectomy* is the surgical removal of a lymph node.
lymphangi/o	lymph vessels	*Lymphangiography* is the radiographic examination of the lymphatic vessels.
onc/o	tumor	An *oncologist* is a physician who specializes in the treatment of tumors.
splen/o	spleen	*Splenomegaly* is an abnormal enlargement of the spleen.
thym/o	thymus	*Thymoma* means a tumor originating in the thymus.
tonsill/o	tonsils	*Tonsillitis* refers to inflammation of the tonsils.

Table 3-7 Respiratory System

Combining Form	Meaning	Example
alveol/o	air sac	*Alveoli* are the small grape-like clusters found at the end of each bronchiole.
bronch/o	bronchus or bronchi	*Bronchopneumonia* is the form of pneumonia that affects patches of the bronchioles throughout both lungs.
epiglott/o	epiglottis	*Epiglottitis* refers to inflammation of the epiglottis.
laryng/o	larynx	*Laryngitis* is inflammation of the mucous membrane in the larynx.
lob/o	lobes	*Lobar pneumonia* affects one or more lobes of a lung.
muc/o	mucus	*Mucolytic* is an agent that destroys mucus.
nas/o, rhin/o	nose	The *nasal septum* is a wall of cartilage that divides the nose into two equal sections.
ox/o	oxygen	*Anoxia* is the absence of oxygen in the body's tissues.
pharyng/o	pharynx	*Pharyngoplasty* is the surgical repair of the pharynx.
phon/o	voice or sound	*Dysphonia* means any voice impairment.
pleur/o	pleura	*Pleurisy* or *pleuritis* is an inflammation of the pleura that produces sharp chest pain.
pneum/o	lung, air	A *pneumothorax* is the accumulation of air in the pleural space causing a pressure imbalance and potentially a collapsed lung.
pulmon/o	lung	*Pulmonary fibrosis* is the formation of scar tissue in the lung, resulting in difficulty breathing.
sinus/o	sinus	*Sinusitis* is the inflammation of the sinuses.
spir/o	to breathe	*Spirometry* is a noninvasive test in which a patient breathes into a device that measures airflow, the length of time of each breath, and air volume.
tonsil/o	tonsils	*Tonsillectomy* is the removal of the tonsils.
trache/o	trachea	*Tracheotomy* is an emergency procedure in which an incision is made into the trachea to gain access to the airway; this is usually intended to be temporary.

Table 3-8 Gastrointestinal System

Combining Form	Meaning	Example
aer/o	air	*Aerophagia* is the excessive swallowing of air while eating or drinking.
ailment/o	nourishment or food	*Alimentary* canal is another name for the digestive tract.
amyl/o	starch	*Amylase* describes the enzyme that digests starch.
bil/i	bile	*Biliary cirrhosis* is a liver disorder due to the obstruction of bile ducts.
chol/e	gall, bile	*Cholelithiasis* is the presence of stones in the gallbladder or bile ducts.
cholecyst/o	gall bladder	*Cholecystalgia* is pain in the gallbladder; *cholelithotripsy* is the procedure for crushing gallstones.
col/o	colon	*Colonoscopy* is the visual examination of the colon.
dent/o	tooth	*Edentulous* means without natural teeth.
duoden/o	duodenum	*Gastroduodenostomy* is the establishment of a connection between the upper portion of the stomach and the duodenum.
enter/o	intestine	*Enteritis* is inflammation of the small intestine.
esophag/o	esophagus	*Esophagogastroduodenoscopy* (EGD) is the endoscopic examination of the esophagus, stomach, and duodenum.
gastr/o	stomach	*Gastroesophageal reflux disease* (GERD) is a syndrome of chronic epigastric pain, accompanied by belching and nausea.
gingiv/o	gums	*Gingivitis* is inflammation of the gums.
gloss/o	tongue	*Glossoplegia* is paralysis of the tongue.
hepat/o	liver	*Hepatectomy* is the surgical removal of all or part of the liver.
intest/o	intestines	*Intestinal adhesions* are fibrous bands of tissues in the intestines.
lapar/o	abdomen	*Laparoscopy* is the visualization of the interior of the abdomen with a small camera.
lith/o	stone	*Lithotripsy* is a non-invasive medical treatment that uses shock waves to break up stones in the kidneys, bladder, ureters, or gallbladder.
pancreat/o	pancreas	*Pancreatotomy* is a surgical incision into the pancreas.
peritone/o	peritoneum	*Peritoneum* is the serous membrane that lines the abdominal cavity.
phag/o	eat	A *phagocyte* is a cell that ingests bacteria, foreign particles, and other cells.
pharyng/o	pharynx	*Pharyngoplasty* is the surgical repair of the pharynx.
proct/o	rectum	*Proctopexy* is the surgical fixation of a prolapsed rectum to an adjacent organ.
rect/o	rectum	*Rectal* means relating to the rectum.
sigmoid/o	sigmoid colon	*Sigmoidectomy* is surgical removal of all or part of the sigmoid colon.
stomat/o	mouth	*Stomatitis* is inflammation of the mucous tissue of the mouth.

Table 3-9 Urinary System

Combining Form	Meaning	Example
albumin/o	protein (called albumin)	*Albuminuria* refers to protein in the urine.
bacteri/o	bacteria	*Bacteriuria* refers to bacteria in the urine.
cyst/o	urinary bladder	A *cystocele* is the hernia of the bladder through the vaginal wall; *cystotomy* refers to surgical incision into the bladder wall.
lith/o	stone	*Nephrolithiasis* is the presence of a renal stone.
nephr/o	kidney	*Nephrectomy* is the removal of a kidney.
pyel/o	renal pelvis	*Pyelolithotomy* is the surgical removal of stones from the renal pelvis.
ren/i, ren/o	kidney	*Renography* is radiography of the kidney.
ur/o, urin/o	urine	*Urinalysis* is the analysis of urine to help in the diagnosis of diseases.
ureter/o	ureters	*Ureterectasis* is distention of a ureter.
urethr/o	urethra	*Urethrorrhagia* is bleeding from the urethra.

Table 3-10 Nervous System

Combining Form	Meaning	Example
cerebell/o	cerebellum	*Cerebellitis* is inflammation of the cerebellum.
cerebr/o	cerebrum	*Cerebropathy* refers to any disorder of the cerebrum.
crani/o	skull	*Cranioplasty* refers to surgical repair of the skull.
encephal/o	brain	An *encephalocele* is the congenital herniation of brain substance through a gap in the skull.
mening/o	the membranes covering the brain and spinal cord	*Meningitis* is an inflammation of the membranes covering the brain and/or spinal cord.
myel/o	spinal cord (or bone marrow—depends on context)	*Myelitis* is inflammation of the spinal cord; also could be inflammation of the bone marrow.
neur/o	nerve	A *neurologist* is a physician who specializes in diagnosing and treating diseases and disorders of the nervous system.
psych/o	mind	A *psychiatrist* is a physician who specializes in diagnosing and treating chemical dependencies, emotional problems, and mental illnesses.

Table 3-11 Endocrine System

Combining Form	Meaning	Example
aden/o	gland	*Adenopathy* refers to large, swollen lymph node glands.
adrenal/o	adrenal gland	*Adrenalectomy* is the surgical remove of one or both of the adrenal glands.
andr/o	male	*Androgen* is a hormone produced in the male testes.
cortic/o	cortex	A *corticosteroid* is a steroid produced by the adrenal cortex.
gluc/o, glyc/o	sugar	*Glucosuria* is sugar in the urine; *hypoglycemia* is low blood sugar.
gonad/o	sex gland	*Gonadopathy* is any disease of the gonads.
pancreat/o	pancreatic islets	*Pancreatitis* is any inflammation of the pancreas.
parathyroid/o	parathyroid gland	*Hypoparathyroidism* is insufficient or absent secretion from the parathyroid glands.
pineal/o	pineal gland	*Pinealectomy* is the surgical removal of the pineal gland.
pituitar/o, pituit/o	pituitary gland	*Hyperpituitarism* is pathology that results in excessive secretion by the hormones of the anterior pituitary.
thym/o	thymus gland	*Thymoma* is a benign tumor of the thymus.
thyr/o	thyroid gland	*Thyrotoxicosis* is a life-threatening condition resulting from the release of excessive quantities of thyroid hormone into the bloodstream.

Table 3-12 Reproductive System

Combining Form	Meaning	Example
amni/o	amnion	*Amniocentesis* is a surgical puncture of the amnion for diagnostic testing.
cervic/o	cervix	*Endocervicitis* is inflammation of the mucous membrane lining the cervix.
colp/o	vagina	*Colporrhaphy* is the surgical suturing of a tear in the vagina.
crypt/o	concealed, hidden	*Cryptorchidism* is a developmental defect in which one or both of the testes fail to descend into the scrotum.
galact/o	milk	*Galactorrhea* is the spontaneous flow of milk from the breasts unassociated with nursing.
gyn/o	woman, female	*Gynecomastia* is the excessive development of mammary glands in the male.
hyster/o	uterus	*Hysterectomy* is surgical removal of the uterus.
mamm/o, mast/o	breast	*Mammalgia* and *mastalgia* both mean pain in the breast.
meno/o	menstruation	*Dysmenorrhea* is painful menstruation caused by uterine cramps; *polymenorrhea* refers to excessive menstrual flow.
nat/o	birth	*Neonatal* means the first month of life.
oophor/o	ovary	*Oophorectomy* is the surgical removal of an ovary.
orchid/o	testes, testicle	*Orchidectomy* is the removal of one or both testes.
salping/o	fallopian tube	*Salpingectomy* is the surgical removal of a fallopian tube.
vas/o	vessel, duct	*Vasectomy* is the removal of a section of the vas deferens for male sterilization.

Table 3-13 The Eye

Combining Form	Meaning	Example
blephar/o	eyelid	*Blepharoptosis* is drooping of the upper eyelid.
conjunctiv/o	conjunctiva	*Conjunctivitis* is inflammation of the conjunctiva, better known as pink eye.
dacry/o	tear duct	*Dacryorrhea* is the excessive flow of tears.
dipl/o	double	*Diplopia* is the perception of two images of one object, better known as double vision.
ir/i, ir/o, irid/o	iris	*Iritis* is any inflammation of the iris.
nyct/o	night	*Nyctalopia* is poor night vision.
ocul/o	eye	*Oculomycosis* is any fungal disease of the eye.
phac/o, phak/o	lens	*Phacoemulsification* is the use of ultrasound to break up a cataract in order to make it easier to remove.
phot/o	light	*Photoretinitis* is retinitis due to exposure to intense light.
presby/o	old	*Presbyopia* refers to the common changes in the eye that occur with aging.
retin/o	retina	*Retinopexy* refers to the treatment to reattach a detached area of the retina.

Table 3-14 The Ear

Combining Form	Meaning	Example
acous/o, acoust/o	hearing	*Acoustic* is pertaining to hearing.
audi/o	hearing	An *audiometer* is an instrument to measure hearing.
labyrinth/o	inner ear	*Labyrinthitis* is an inflammation of the inner ear that can result in vertigo and/or deafness.
ot/o	ear	*Otitis media* is inflammation of the middle ear.
pinn/i	outer ear	The *pinna* is also known as the auricle, and is the external portion of the ear.
presby/o	old	*Presbycusis* refers to a gradual sensorineural hearing loss that occurs with aging.
tympan/o, myring/o	tympanic membrane	*Tympanostomy tubes* are also known as pediatric ear tubes that are placed through the tympanic membrane to provide on-going drainage of fluids; *myringotomy* is the surgical incision of the tympanic membrane to create an opening for tympanostomy tubes.

Table 3-15 Body Planes

Body Plane	Meaning
Coronal plane	Divides the body into anterior and posterior portions; also known as the frontal plane (hint: think of placing a crown on your head)
Frontal plane	Divides the body into anterior and posterior portions; also known as the coronal plane
Horizontal plane	Divides the body into superior (upper) and inferior (lower) portions; also known as the transverse plane (hint: think of the horizon)
Transverse plane	Divides the body into superior (upper) and inferior (lower) portions; also known as the horizontal plane
Sagittal plane	Divides the body into left and right portions; a vertical plane
Midsagittal plane	Divides the body into *equal* left and right halves; a vertical plane

Table 3-16 Commonly Used Medical Abbreviations

Abbreviation	Meaning
a	before
a.c.	before meals
AD	right ear
ad lib	as desired, as needed
AS	left ear
AU	each ear or both ears
bid or b.i.d.	twice a day
BP	blood pressure
bpm	beats per minute
c̄	with
CA, ca	cancer
CBC	complete blood count
CNS	central nervous system
C/O	complains of
COPD	chronic obstructive pulmonary disease
CVA	cerebrovascular accident (stroke)
D5W	dextrose, 5% in water
D&C	dilation and curettage
DC	discontinue
DX	diagnosis
ECG, EKG	electrocardiogram
EEG	electroencephalogram
EGD	esophagogastroduodenoscopy
Fe	iron
FH	family history
g	gram
GERD	gastroesophageal reflux disease
GI	gastrointestinal
gtt	drop
GU	genitourinary
GYN	gynecology
H&P	history and physical
HEENT	head, ears, eyes, nose, and throat
h.s.	at bedtime (hour of sleep)
HX	history
I&D	incision and drainage
ICU	intensive care unit

(continues)

Table 3-16 Commonly Used Medical Abbreviations (Continued)

Abbreviation	Meaning
IM	intramuscular
IV	intravenous
K	potassium
KCl	potassium chloride
kg	kilogram
L	liter
mcg	microgram
mg	milligram
MI	myocardial infarction
mL or ml	milliliter
mm	millimeter
Na	sodium
NaCl	sodium chloride
NPO, npo	nothing by mouth
OD	right eye
oint	ointment
OR	operating room
OS	left eye
OTC	over the counter
OU	each eye (or both eyes)
$\bar{p}$	after
p.c.	after meals
PE	physical exam
PMH	past medical history
p.o., PO	by mouth, orally
POSTOP; postop	postoperative
PREOP; preop	preoperative
PRN, prn	whenever necessary
q	every
qd or q.d.	every day
qh or q.h.	every hour
q2h or q.2h	every 2 hours
q4h or q.4h	every 4 hours
qid or q.i.d.	four times a day
RE√	recheck
R/O	rule out
ROS/SR	review of systems/systems review

(continues)

Table 3-16 Commonly Used Medical Abbreviations (Continued)

Abbreviation	Meaning
Rx	prescription
s̄	without
sig	write
SOB	shortness of breath
sol	solution
stat	immediately and once only
subq, SubQ, subcu	subcutaneous
susp	suspension
tab	tablet
tid or t.i.d.	three times a day
TX	treatment
U/A	urinalysis
URI	upper respiratory infection
US	ultrasound
UTI	urinary tract infection

QUESTIONS

3-1. The prefix "dys-" means

    A. a pathologic tissue change.
    B. good, benign, or harmless.
    C. bad, difficult, or painful.
    D. abnormal narrowing.
    E. abnormal softening.

3-2. The suffix meaning "to rupture" is

    A. -rrhage.
    B. -rrhagia.
    C. -rrhea.
    D. -rrhexis.
    E. -rrhaphy.

3-3. The combining form meaning "blue" is

    A. cyan/o-.
    B. erythr/o-.
    C. leuk/o-.
    D. poli/o-.
    E. melan/o-.

3-4. The suffix that means "abnormal softening" is

    A. -necrosis.
    B. -malacia.
    C. -maegaly.
    D. -sclerosis.
    E. -stenosis.

3-5. Which term means the direction toward or nearer the midline?

    A. Distal
    B. Medial
    C. Lateral
    D. Ventral
    E. Dorsal

3-6. Which term means the death of bone tissue?

    A. Osteoporosis
    B. Osteomyelitis
    C. Osteitis deformans
    D. Osteonecrosis
    E. Osteoclasis

3-7. Which term refers to an outbreak of a disease occurring over a large geographic area, possibly worldwide?

    A. Endemic
    B. Epidemic
    C. Pandemic
    D. All of the above
    E. None of the above

3-8. What word means an abnormal increase in the outward curvature of the thoracic spine, also known as humpback?

    A. Scoliosis
    B. Lordosis
    C. Swayback
    D. Kyphosis
    E. Spondylosis

3-9. The correct spelling for a fracture in which the bone is broken into many pieces is

    A. conmitted.
    B. cominnuted.
    C. cominuted.
    D. conminuted.
    E. comminuted.

3-10. Which term means the breakdown of muscle tissue?

    A. Myocele
    B. Myorrhaphy
    C. Myoclonus
    D. Myotomy
    E. Myolysis

3-11. Which term means the condition commonly known as hiccups?

    A. Myasthenia
    B. Singultus
    C. Contracture
    D. Torticollis
    E. Aponeurosis

3-12. Which term means the paralysis of both legs and the lower part of the body?

    A. Myoparesis
    B. Hemiparesis
    C. Hemiplegia
    D. Paraplegia
    E. Quadriplegia

3-13. Which term means bending the foot upward at the ankle?

    A. Abduction
    B. Dorsiflexion
    C. Elevation
    D. Plantar flexion
    E. Pronation

3-14. Which term describes the abnormal hardening of an artery?

    A. Arthrosclerosis
    B. Atherosclerosis
    C. Ischemia
    D. Arrhythmia
    E. Aneurysm

3-15. An abnormally fast heartbeat is referred to as

    A. bradycardia.
    B. palpitation.
    C. tachycardia.
    D. prolapse.
    E. stenosis.

3-16. Which of the following refers to an abnormally high white blood cell count?

    A. Hypochromia
    B. Anemia
    C. Leukopenia
    D. Leukocytosis
    E. Leukoplakia

3-17. Which of the following words is misspelled?

    A. Easinophil
    B. Thrombocyte
    C. Basophil
    D. Erythrocyte
    E. Neutrophil

3-18. The condition commonly known as chickenpox is caused by which virus?

    A. *West Nile*
    B. *Rubeola*
    C. *Varicella zoster*
    D. *Rubella*
    E. *Epstein-Barr*

3-19. A person might experience dyspnea with which of the following conditions?

    A. Heart failure
    B. Liver failure
    C. Rheumatoid arthritis
    D. Benign prostatic hypertrophy
    E. Otitis media

3-20. The emergency procedure in which an incision is made into the trachea in order to gain access to the airway is called a

    A. tracheoplasty.
    B. lobectomy.
    C. pleurectomy.
    D. thoracotomy.
    E. tracheotomy.

3-21. The medical term for runny nose is

    A. epistaxis.
    B. pertussis.
    C. croup.
    D. sinusitis.
    E. rhinorrhea.

3-22. Another term for heartburn is

    A. melena.
    B. pyrosis.
    C. hemoptysis.
    D. colostomy.
    E. halitosis.

3-23. A colonoscopy would be performed by a(n)

    A. urologist.
    B. endocrinologist.
    C. gastroenterologist.
    D. oncologist.
    E. neonatologist.

3-24. A stone in the urinary bladder is known as a

    A. uretorolith.
    B. nephrolith.
    C. cystolith.
    D. cholecystolith.
    E. urinarolith.

3-25. Which of the following refers to a congenital abnormality in the male in which the urethral opening is located on the upper surface of the penis?

    A. Epispadius
    B. Hypospadius
    C. Paraspadius
    D. All of the above
    E. None of the above

3-26. Which term refers to an irrational fear of going out in public?

    A. Acrophobia
    B. Agoraphobia
    C. Claustrophobia
    D. Hypochondrias
    E. Conversion disorder

3-27. An abbreviation that refers to the right ear is

    A. OD.
    B. OS.
    C. OU.
    D. AD.
    E. AS.

3-28. A doctor who treats disorders of the eyes is called a(n)

    A. ophthalmologist.
    B. urologist.
    C. otolaryngologist.
    D. endocrinologist.
    E. oncologist.

3-29. _____ is also known as itching.

    A. Purulent
    B. Pruritis
    C. Granuloma
    D. Gangrene
    E. Ichthyosis

3-30. Which of the following is written in its plural form?

    A. Cicatrices
    B. Nevus
    C. Fungus
    D. Epidermis
    E. Keratosis

3-31. With regards to menstrual disorders, menorrhagia refers to

    A. painful menstrual flow.
    B. absence of menstrual flow.
    C. excessive menstrual flow.
    D. light menstrual flow.
    E. premature menopause.

3-32. Which term refers to excessive thirst?

    A. Polyuria
    B. Polyphagia
    C. Polydipsia
    D. Polyglycia
    E. Polythirstia

3-33. An unexpected reaction to a drug is called a(n) _____ reaction.

    A. palliative
    B. agglutination
    C. radiopaque
    D. idiosyncratic
    E. speculum

3-34. A(n) _____ is a set of signs and symptoms that occur together as part of a specific disease process.

    A. syndrome
    B. iatrogenic genome
    C. idiopathic epidemic
    D. nosocomial eponym
    E. organic dyskinesia

3-35. Olfaction refers to which of the following sensations?

    A. Smell
    B. Sight
    C. Hearing
    D. Taste
    E. Touch

3-36. Which of the following is a neural tube defect?

    A. Tetanus
    B. Hydrocephalus
    C. Spina bifida
    D. Meninigitis
    E. Reye's syndrome

3-37. The term to describe an inflammation of the brain would be:

    A. cephalalgia.
    B. myelitis.
    C. meningitis.
    D. hydrocephalus.
    E. encephalitis.

3-38. Which of the following organs separates the thoracic cavity from the abdominal cavity?

    A. Colon
    B. Spleen
    C. Diaphragm
    D. Pancreas
    E. Liver

3-39. Which term refers to shortness of breath or difficult, labored breathing?

    A. Apnea
    B. Tachypnea
    C. Dyspnea
    D. Bradypnea
    E. Hyperventilation

ANSWERS

3-1. The correct answer is C. The prefix "dys-" means bad, difficult, or painful. Examples include dysfunctional (not working properly) and dysphagia (difficulty in swallowing).

3-2. The correct answer is D. The suffixes beginning with two R's are often referred to as the "double r's" and are often confused. The suffix "-rrhexis" means to rupture. Myorrhexis is the rupture of a muscle. The suffixes "-rrhagia" and "-rrhage" mean bleeding, bursting forth, or abnormal or excessive flow. A hemorrhage is the loss of a large amount of blood in a short time. The suffix "-rrhaphy" means surgical suturing to close a wound. Myorrhaphy is the surgical suturing of a muscle wound. The suffix "-rrhea" means flow or discharge. Diarrhea is the flow of frequent loose or watery stools.

3-3. The correct answer is A. Some combining forms indicate color. "Cyan/o-" refers to the color blue. Cyanosis is a blue discoloration of the skin caused by a lack of adequate oxygen. "Erythr/o-" means red, "leuk/o-" means white, "melan/o-" means black, and "poli/o-" means gray.

3-4. The correct answer is B. "-malacia" means abnormal softening, as in arteriomalacia, which is the abnormal softening of the walls of the arteries. The opposite suffix, in terms of meaning, is "-stenosis," which means abnormal hardening.

3-5. The correct answer is B. Medial means the direction toward or nearer the midline. Lateral is the exact opposite and means the direction away from the midline. Distal means situated farthest from the midline. Ventral refers to the front or belly side of the body. Dorsal refers to the back of the body.

3-6. The correct answer is D. "Osteo-" means bone and "-necrosis" means tissue death. Thus, osteonecrosis is the destruction and death of bone tissue caused by an insufficient blood supply, infection, malignancy, or trauma.

3-7. The correct answer is C. Pandemic refers to an outbreak of a disease occurring over a large geographic area, possibly worldwide. AIDS is considered a pandemic. Endemic refers to the ongoing presence of a disease within a population, group, or area. The common cold may be considered endemic because it is always present within a given population. An epidemic is a sudden, widespread outbreak of a disease within a population or area. An example is the bird flu epidemic in Thailand and Cambodia.

3-8. The correct answer is D. Kyphosis is an abnormal increase in the *outward* curvature of the thoracic spine (as viewed from the side). This condition is also known as humpback or dowager's hump.

3-9. The correct answer is E. Comminuted means crushed into small pieces.

3-10. The correct answer is E. "My/o-" means muscle and "-lysis" refers to the breakdown or destruction of something. Therefore, myolysis means the breakdown of muscle tissue.

3-11. The correct answer is B. Hiccups is also known as singultus. A spasm of the diaphragm causes the characteristic hiccup sound. This term needs to be memorized because it does not follow the typical medical term with the three parts—the prefix, the word root, and the suffix.

3-12. The correct answer is D. Paraplegia is the paralysis of both legs and the lower part of the body. In contrast, quadriplegia is the paralysis of all four extremities. The suffix "-plegia" means paralysis. The suffix "-paresis" means partial or incomplete paralysis. Myoparesis is a weakness or slight paralysis of a muscle. Hemiparesis is a slight paralysis of one side of the body. Hemiplegia is the total paralysis of one side of the body. This form of paralysis is usually associated with a stroke.

3-13. The correct answer is B. Dorsiflexion means bending the foot upward at the ankle. Plantar flexion is the opposite: bending the foot downward at the ankle. (Mnemonic: Plant your foot on the ground with plantar flexion.)

3-14. The correct answer is B. Abnormal hardening of an artery is called atherosclerosis and is caused by a buildup of cholesterol plaques. "Ather/o-" means plaque or fatty substance and "-sclerosis" means abnormal hardening.

3-15. The correct answer is C. An abnormally fast heartbeat is also known as tachycardia. "Tachy-" means rapid, "card" means heart, and "-ia" means abnormal condition. Tachycardia typically refers to a rate greater than 100 beats per minute.

3-16. The correct answer is D. An abnormally high white blood cell count is known as leukocytosis. "Leuk/o-" means white, "cyt/o" means cell, and "-osis" means abnormal condition.

3-17. The correct answer is A. Eosinophil is spelled with an "o." These cells destroy parasites and play a major role in allergic reactions.

3-18. The correct answer is C. Chickenpox is caused by the *Varicella zoster* virus. The *Epstein-Barr* virus causes infectious mononucleosis. *Rubella* is caused by the rubella virus. The *West Nile* virus causes flu-like symptoms. If untreated, the *West Nile* virus can cause inflammation of the spinal cord and brain. The *Rubeola* virus causes measles.

3-19. The correct answer is A. Dyspnea is also known as shortness of breath. A person with heart failure would have difficulty breathing. Dyspnea may also be caused by extreme physical exertion or lung damage.

3-20. The correct answer is E. The emergency procedure in which an incision is made into the trachea is called a tracheotomy. "Trache-" means trachea and "-otomy" means surgical incision. This opening is usually temporary.

3-21. The correct answer is E. Rhinorrhea is the medical term for a runny nose. "Rhin/o-" means nose and "-rrhea" means abnormal discharge. Epistaxis is the medical term for a bloody nose.

3-22. The correct answer is B. Another term for heartburn is pyrosis. "Pyr/o-" means fire and "-osis" refers to an abnormal condition. Pyrosis, or heartburn, refers to the burning sensation caused by the reflux of stomach acid into the esophagus.

3-23. The correct answer is C. "Gastr/o-" means stomach, "enter" means small intestine, and "-ologist" means specialist. Thus, a gastroenterologist is a specialist in treating diseases and disorders of the stomach and intestines. A colonoscopy examines the inner surface of the colon and rectum.

3-24. The correct answer is C. A stone in the urinary bladder is known as a cystolith. "Cyst/o-" means urinary bladder and "-lith" means stone.

3-25. The correct answer is A. The congenital abnormality in the male in which the urethral opening is located on the upper surface of the penis is called epispadius. Hypospadius is a congenital abnormality in which the urethral opening is on the undersurface of the penis. Paraspadius is a congenital abnormality in which the urethral opening is on the side surface of the penis.

3-26. The correct answer is B. Agoraphobia refers to a fear of leaving a familiar setting like home and going out in public. "Agor/a-" refers to the marketplace and comes from the Greek word for marketplace, *agora*.

3-27. The correct answer is D. The abbreviation for the right ear is AD. The abbreviation for the left ear is AS. The abbreviation used for both ears is AU.

3-28. The correct answer is A. An ophthalmologist is a physician who specializes in diagnosing and treating disorders of the eye as well as performing surgeries of the eye. In contrast, an optometrist is not a medical doctor but is licensed and has earned a Doctor of Optometry degree. An optometrist specializes in vision problems and corrective lenses.

3-29. The correct answer is B. Pruritis is also known as itching and is associated with inflammation of the skin.

3-30. The correct answer is A. Cicatrices is the plural form of cicatrix, which means a scar. If a term ends in "-ix" or "-ex," the plural is usually formed by changing the ending to "-ices." All of the other terms are written in their singular forms.

3-31. The correct answer is C. Menorrhagia is also known as hypermenorrhea because the term refers to an excessive amount of menstrual flow over a period of more than 7 days. Dysmenorrhea refers to abdominal pain caused by a menstrual period. Hypomenorrhea is a small amount of menstrual flow during a shortened period of time. Menometrorrhagia is excessive uterine bleeding occurring both during menses and at irregular intervals between periods.

3-32. The correct answer is C. Polydipsia refers to excessive thirst, as in the case of diabetics. Polyuria is excessive urination. Polyphagia is excessive hunger. Polyglycia and polythirstia are not real words.

3-33. The correct answer is D. An idiosyncratic reaction to a drug is unexpected. For example, if you expect a drug to induce sleep and instead it causes excitement, this is an idiosyncratic reaction.

3-34. The correct answer is A. A syndrome is a set of signs and symptoms that occur as a disease process; for example, Down's syndrome or acquired immune deficiency syndrome (AIDS).

3-35. The correct answer is A. Olfaction refers to one's sense of smell.

3-36. The correct answer is C. Neural tube defects are birth defects of the brain and spinal cord. The two most common neural tube defects are spina bifida and anencephaly. In spina bifida, the fetal spinal column doesn't close completely during the first month of pregnancy. In anencephaly, much of the brain does not develop. Getting enough folic acid, a B vitamin, before and during pregnancy prevents most neural tube defects.

3-37. The correct answer is E. The term to describe an inflammation of the brain would be encephalitis. "Encephal/o-" is the word root referring to brain and "-itis" is the suffix meaning inflammation.

3-38. The correct answer is C. The diaphragm separates the thoracic cavity from the abdominal cavity. The diaphragm is the large muscle that aids in breathing. The thoracic cavity contains the heart and lungs. The abdominal cavity contains the major organs of digestion.

3-39. The correct answer is C. Dyspnea is also known as shortness of breath. "Dys-" means painful and "-pnea" means breathing. Apnea is the absence of spontaneous respiration. Tachypnea is an abnormally rapid rate of respiration. Bradypnea is an abnormally slow rate of respiration.

Anatomy and Physiology

Anatomy is the study of the structure of the human body, and physiology is the study of the body's functions. The exam will contain a variety of questions about basic anatomy and physiology. This chapter provides a review of the basic structure and function of the human body.

STRUCTURAL UNITS

The body can be organized into different structural units. Table 4-1 illustrates the different structural units of the body from smallest to largest.

Table 4-1 Structural Units of the Body

Structural Unit	Description
Chemical	Refers to the millions of molecules that contribute to our body's make-up.
Cell	The most basic unit of life.
Tissue	Many cells organized together form tissues.
Organ	Tissues form larger structural units known as organs.
Organ system	Groups of organs that work together to perform a specific function are organisms.
Organism	Organ systems combine to form the organism, also known as the human body.

ANATOMIC DIVISIONS

The study of anatomy requires the visualization of internal organs. Anatomic divisions include the body planes, body cavities, and abdominal quadrants and regions. The exam will include questions from all areas.

Body Planes

Body planes use cross-sectional imaginary surfaces to organize the body for anatomical reference. The use of such planes has application in medical imaging studies such as computerized tomography (CT) and magnetic resonance imaging (MRI). Table 4-2 describes these planes.

Table 4-2 Body Planes

Body Plane	Description
Coronal	Divides the body into anterior and posterior portions; also known as the frontal plane. (Hint: think of placing a crown on your head.)
Frontal	Divides the body into anterior and posterior portions; also known as the coronal plane.
Horizontal	Divides the body into superior (upper) and inferior (lower) portions; also known as the transverse plane. (Hint: think of the horizon.)
Transverse	Divides the body into superior (upper) and inferior (lower) portions; also known as the horizontal plane.
Sagittal	Divides the body into left and right portions; a vertical plane.
Midsagittal	Divides the body into *equal* left and right halves; a vertical plane.

Body Cavities

Body cavities are hollow body spaces that house the internal organs. Figure 4-1 shows the various cavities in the human body. The *dorsal cavity* is located posteriorly and consists of the cranial cavity, which houses the brain, and the spinal cavity, which houses the spinal cord. The *ventral cavity* is located ventrally and is made up of the thoracic cavity and the abdominopelvic cavity. The *thoracic cavity* contains organs of the thorax (heart, lungs, and large vessels). The mediastinum is the central compartment of the thoracic cavity and is clinically important. Organs located in the mediastinum include the heart, the aorta, the thymus gland, the trachea, the esophagus, lymph nodes, and some important nerves. The left and right lungs lie on either side of the mediastinum. The thoracic cavity is separated from the abdominal cavity by the diaphragm. The abdominopelvic cavity can be further divided into the abdominal cavity and the pelvic cavity. The abdominal cavity houses the stomach, most of the intestines, kidneys, liver, gallbladder, pancreas, and spleen. The pelvic cavity contains the urinary bladder, rectum, and internal organs of the male and female reproductive system.

Abdominal Quadrants and Regions

In order to describe the location of injuries and/or pain more easily, medical assistants and others in the healthcare field have two methods of dividing the abdominal area. It can be divided into either four quadrants or nine regions. Both methods are illustrated in Figure 4-2.

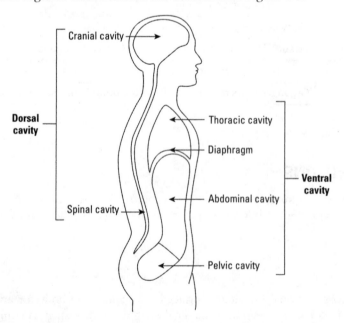

Figure 4-1 Body Cavities

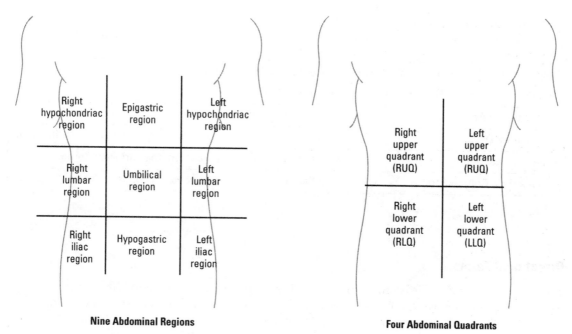

Nine Abdominal Regions

Four Abdominal Quadrants

Figure 4-2 Abdominal Quadrants and Regions

POSITIONS AND DIRECTIONS

Anatomic Position

The anatomic position is used as a standard anatomical reference in medicine. In this position, the body is erect, limbs are extended, arms are at the sides, and palms are forward. Figure 4-3 illustrates this important position.

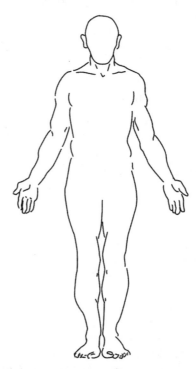

Figure 4-3 Anatomical Position

Table 4-3 Directional Terms

Directional Term	Definition
Superior or cranial *vs.* Inferior or caudal	Toward the head *vs.* Away from the head
Anterior or ventral *vs.* Posterior or dorsal	Front *vs.* Back
Medial *vs.* Lateral	Toward the midline *vs.* Away from the midline
Proximal *vs.* Distal	Toward or nearest the trunk *vs.* Away or farthest from the trunk
Superficial *vs.* Deep	Close to the surface *vs.* Far from the surface; internal
Ipsilateral *vs.* Contralateral	On the same side of the body *vs.* On opposite sides of the body

Directional Terms

The language of anatomy is essential to a medical assistant's ability to communicate in the healthcare world. Directional terms describe the position of structures relative to other structures of the body while in the anatomic position. Table 4-3 defines directional terms as oppositional pairs.

Common Anatomic Descriptors

In clinical medicine, the common names of body parts are given more precise anatomic descriptors. The exam may contain questions related to the location of specific organs using this more specific terminology, which is described in Table 4-4.

HOMEOSTASIS

Homeostasis refers to the body being in a state of equilibrium. Homeostasis is continuously disturbed by external or internal changes. In most cases, the body responds quickly to these changes by using both negative and positive feedback. Table 4-5 describes both types of feedback and gives examples of each.

TISSUES

As outlined in Table 4-1, the most basic unit of life is the cell. Cells make up tissues, and tissues make up organs. There are four basic tissues of the body: epithelial, connective, muscle, and nervous.

Epithelial Tissue

Epithelial tissue forms the body's surfaces, the surfaces of the body's cavities, and their contained viscera, glands, and all ducts and vessels. The function of this tissue is diverse, including filtration, diffusion, secretion, and absorption.

Epithelial tissue can be arranged into simple (single layer) or stratified (several) layers, or it can be classified by shape:

- *Squamous (flat):* Simple squamous epithelial tissue lines the alveoli of the lungs and capillary walls for easy passage of cells; stratified squamous lines the skin, vagina, and anus for protection.
- *Cuboidal (cube-like):* Simple cuboidal epithelial tissue lines the kidney tubules and smaller ducts of many glands.
- *Columnar (column-like):* Nonciliated simple columnar epithelial tissue lines the gastrointestinal tract.
- *Pseudostratified columnar (irregularly placed nuclei give the appearance of many layers, but all cells do lie on basement membrane):* Pseudostratified columnar epithelial tissue typically exhibits cilia and goblet cells and lines ducts of reproductive tract and air conduction pathways.
- *Transitional (transitions from flat to cube-like):* Transitional epithelial tissue lines the bladder.

Table 4-4 Common Anatomic Descriptors

Term	Definition
Antebrachial	Forearm
Antecubital	Anterior to the elbow
Axillary	Armpit
Brachial	Upper arm
Buccal	Cheek
Carpal	Wrist
Cervical	Neck
Costal	Ribs
Cranial	Skull
Cutaneous	Skin
Femoral	Thigh
Gluteal	Butt
Inguinal	Groin
Lumbar	Lower back
Mammary	Breast
Occipital	Posterior, lower part of skull
Ophthalmic	Eyes
Otic	Ears
Patellar	Kneecap
Pectoral	Chest
Pedal	Foot
Plantar	Sole of foot
Popliteal	Back of knee
Sacral	Lowest area of spine (sacrum)
Tarsal	Ankle
Umbilical	Navel

Table 4-5 Homeostasis: Negative and Positive Feedback Systems

Feedback	Definition	Examples
Negative	The response diminishes the original stimulus. This is the most common homeostatic feedback mechanism.	Body temperature; Heart rate
Positive	The response enhances the original stimulus.	Hemorrhage (blood-clotting cascade); Childbirth (oxytocin); Lactation (prolactin)

Connective Tissue

Connective tissue connects, binds, and supports body structures. This tissue consists of various numbers of cells, fibers, and ground substance (fluid, viscous, or mineralized).

Among the various types are loose areolar, adipose, dense regular, dense irregular, hyaline cartilage, elastic cartilage, fibrocartilage, blood, and bone.

Muscle Tissue

Muscle tissue shortens (contracts) in response to stimulation. There are three types of muscle tissue:

- *Skeletal:* Moves bones at the joints—under voluntary control
- *Cardiac:* Compresses heart muscle to orchestrate blood flow through the heart—under involuntary control
- *Smooth:* Moves the contents of internal body cavities—under involuntary control

Nervous Tissue

Nervous tissue is composed of neurons and neuroglia. Neurons are the basic cells of the nervous system and function to carry the nerve impulses throughout the body via electrochemical signals. The body has billions of neurons. Neuroglia are supporting cells and have various functions, among them are insulation, support, nutrition, and anchorage.

MEMBRANES

Membranes are thin sheets of tissue that line and protect body surfaces and organs. There are two different types of membranes: epithelial and connective tissue.

Epithelial Membranes

Epithelial membranes consist of an epithelial layer and an underlying connective tissue component. There are three types of epithelial membranes:

- *Serous membranes:* These secrete watery fluid and line organs on the interior; they are composed of an outer parietal layer and an inner visceral layer.
  - *Pericardial membrane:* Surrounds the heart
  - *Pleural membrane:* Surrounds the lungs
  - *Peritoneum:* Surrounds the abdomen
- *Mucous membranes:* These secrete mucus and line the passages leading to the exterior (e.g., nostrils, lips, genital area, and anus).
- *Cutaneous membranes:* This is another name for the skin; it is composed of stratified squamous epithelium.

Connective Tissue Membranes

Another type of membrane is classified as a connective tissue membrane because it is made up of only connective tissue, with no epithelium. Some different types include:

- *Synovial membranes:* Line joint cavities interiorly
- *Meninges:* Line the brain and spinal cord
- *Fascia:* Lines and separates muscles
- *Periosteum:* Lines bone
- *Perichondrium:* Lines cartilage

ORGAN SYSTEMS

The organ systems govern all of your physiologic activities. They are as follows:

- Integumentary system
- Muscular system
- Skeletal system
- Nervous system
- Cardiovascular system
- Hematopoietic system
- Lymphatic and immune system
- Respiratory system
- Digestive system

- Urinary system
- Reproductive system
- Endocrine system
- Special senses

Each of your organ systems consists of groups of organs that work together to carry out specific duties in your body. For example, your digestive system is an organ system that requires contributions from a number of organs, including your stomach, small intestine, large intestine, liver, pancreas, and gall bladder; all of these organs work together to digest the foods you eat and transfer the nutrients in the foods you eat from your small intestine to your cells.

The following sections provide some key facts about each body system. These are high-yield facts commonly seen in questions on the exam. The best way to study for the exam is by doing practice questions. If you feel weak in a certain area, please reference a more detailed anatomy and physiology textbook.

Integumentary (Skin) System

The integument is a vital organ of the body. It measures approximately 16–20 square feet, and is extremely helpful in revealing general health conditions in relation to other organ systems. For example, in liver disease, the skin turns yellow or becomes jaundiced. Many autoimmune diseases cause skin changes such as rash, irritation, and other signs of inflammation.

The integument has an epidermal layer made of keratinized stratified squamous epithelium. The epidermis is four to five layers thick and is mainly composed of keratinocytes. These cells contain the protein keratin, which allows the skin to be waterproof and resistant to bacteria and viruses. Another cell type of the epidermis is the melanocyte, which is responsible for making the pigment melanin and contributes to the color of our skin. The layers of the integument are described in more detail in Table 4-6. (A mnemonic for the layers of the epidermis is Californians like Girls that are Strong and Buff.)

Muscular System

The main function of the muscular system is to produce body movement. Other functions include maintenance of body posture, protection of bones and internal organs, and generation of heat.

Table 4-6 Layers of the Integument

Layer	Description
Epidermis: stratum corneum	Top layer of integument; contains dead, keratinized cells 25–30 rows thick. These cells are continuously shed and replaced by cells from deeper layers. (The entire process takes about 4 weeks.)
Epidermis: stratum lucidum	Present only in thick skin (palms of hands and soles of feet).
Epidermis: stratum granulosum	Organelles in keratinocytes that are beginning to degenerate as they move up to the stratum corneum.
Epidermis: stratum spinosum	Eight to ten layers of spiny keratinocytes; this layer contains Langerhans cells of the immune system.
Epidermis: stratum basalis	The bottom layer of the epidermis; also called stratum germinativum because it contains stem cells that produce new keratinocytes. Melanocytes are located in this layer.
Dermis	Composed of connective tissue, blood, lymphatic vessels, nerve fibers and sensory receptors, glands, and hair follicles. The dermis binds the epidermis to the hypodermis.
Subcutaneous tissue (hypodermis)	Mostly adipose tissue with blood vessels and nerves distributed throughout.

Table 4-7 Skeletal Muscles and Their Actions

Skeletal Muscle	Action
Frontalis	Raises eyebrows
Orbicularis oris	Allows lips to pucker
Orbicularis oculi	Allows eyes to close
Zygomaticus	Smiling muscle: pulls corners of mouth up
Platysma	Pulls corners of mouth down
Masseter	Closes the jaw as in chewing
Temporalis	Closes the jaw as in chewing
Sternocleidomastoid	Pulls the head to one side and also pulls the head to the chest
Trapezius	Raises the arm and pull the shoulders downward
Pectoralis major	Pulls the arm across the chest; rotates and adducts the arm
Latissimus dorsi	Extends, adducts, and rotates the arm inward
Deltoid	Abducts and extends the arm at the shoulder
Subscapularis	Rotates the arm medially
Infraspinatus	Rotates the arm laterally
Biceps brachii	Flexes the arm at the elbow and rotates the hand laterally
Triceps brachii	Extends the arm at the elbow
Brachioradialis	Flexes the forearm at the elbow
Brachialis	Flexes the arm at the elbow
Supinator	Supinates the forearm by rotating it laterally
Pronator teres	Pronates the forearm by rotating it medially
Gluteus maximus	Extends the thigh
Iliopsoas	Flexes the thigh
Gluteus medius and minimus	Abduct the thigh; rotate the thigh medially
Quadriceps femoris (rectus femoris, vastus lateralis, vastus medialis, and vastus intermedius)	Extend the leg at the knee
Sartorius	Multiple movements; allows you to sit cross-legged
Hamstrings (biceps femoris, semitendinosus, and semimembranosus)	Flex the leg at the knee and extend the thigh
Adductor longus and magnus	Adduct the thigh and rotate the thigh laterally
Gastrocnemius	Plantar flexes the foot
Soleus	Plantar flexes the foot
Tibialis anterior	Dorsiflexes the foot (points foot up) and inverts the foot
Diaphragm	Allows inspiration
External and internal intercostals	Expand and lower ribs during breathing
External and internal obliques	Compress abdominal wall
Transversus abdominis	Compresses abdominal wall
Rectus abdominis	Compresses abdominal wall and flexes the vertebral column

Skeletal muscles attach to bones at tendons, and must cross a joint in order to cause movement. Skeletal muscle cells are long, striated, and multi-nucleated. Many mitochondria are found within the skeletal muscle to produce energy.

Muscle tissue shortens (contracts) in response to stimulation. Myofibrils are the contractile units of the muscle cell and consist of thick myofilaments (namely myosin) and thin myofilaments (namely actin). These two filaments are arranged in contractile units called sarcomeres. At the end of each sarcomere, the thin filaments are permanently attached to the Z line (also called Z disc), which separates one sarcomere from the next. The arrangement of the thick and thin myofilaments creates the appearance of striations in skeletal (and cardiac) muscles. Muscle contraction occurs when the thin filaments slide toward the center, bringing the Z lines closer together in each sarcomere. This sliding motion is aided by cross-bridge formation from the thick myofilaments as they draw the thin filaments toward them.

The name of a skeletal muscle often describes it in some way—by location, action, shape, size, or number of attachments. When you study the muscular system, remember that you may be asked about the action of some of the more common muscles. Table 4-7 lists some of the skeletal muscles and their actions. You should be familiar with the major skeletal muscles, which can be found in any anatomy book.

Skeletal System

Bone is a living, vascular structure composed of cells and an extracellular matrix. The matrix consists of water, collagen, and crystallized mineral salts (calcium and phosphate). Collagen contributes to bones' flexibility, and the mineral salts give bones their rigidity.

Four types of cells are present in bone: osteoprogenitor cells, osteoblasts, osteocytes, and osteoclasts. They are described in Table 4-8.

Bone tissue can be either compact or spongy. Compact bone contains few spaces and is the strongest form of bone tissue. It is made of repeating structural units called osteons (or Haversian systems) aligned along the bone's shaft to resist fracturing. Compact bone is mostly found in the diaphyses of long bones. In contrast, spongy bone does not contain osteons but is made up of trabeculae. Trabeculae help to make bone lighter and may be filled with red bone marrow. Spongy bone is found in the interiors of short, flat, and irregular bones as well as in the epiphyses of long bones.

Bones are classified by their shape: long, short, flat, or irregular. The femur, radius, and humerus are long bones. The structure of a long bone includes various components, as described in Table 4-9.

You should be familiar with the bones of the body, including the bones that make up the skull, vertebral column, bony thorax (sternum and ribs), pectoral girdle (clavicle, scapula, and humerus), pelvic girdle (coxal bones and sacrum), and appendicular skeleton. These bones can be found in any anatomy book.

Nervous System

The nervous system is complex and coordinates body functions and responses throughout the body. The central nervous system (CNS) is made up of the brain and spinal cord. The brain can be divided into four major areas: the cerebrum, diencephalon, brainstem, and cerebellum. The cerebrum is the

Table 4-8 Bone Cells

Bone Cell	Function
Osteoprogenitor cells	Bone stem cells
Osteoblasts	Bone building cells; synthesize and secrete collagen fibers needed to build the extracellular matrix; become osteocytes
Osteocytes	Mature bone cells; maintain exchange of nutrients and wastes
Osteoclasts	Release lysosomal enzymes and acids that break down the bone matrix for reabsorption

Table 4-9 Structure of a Long Bone

Structure	Description
Diaphysis	Bone shaft (main portion of the bone)
Epiphyses	Distal and proximal ends of the bone
Metaphyses	Where the diaphysis and epiphyses meet; in growing bone the epiphyseal plate allows for elongation; becomes the epiphyseal line
Articular cartilage	Hyaline cartilage covering the epiphyses
Periosteum	Dense irregular connective tissue covering bone that is not covered by articular cartilage; attached to bone by Sharpey's fibers
Medullary (marrow) cavity	Contains fatty yellow bone marrow
Endosteum	Lines the medullary cavity

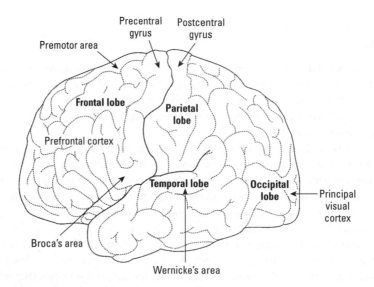

Figure 4-4 Areas of the Central Nervous System

largest part of the brain and is composed of the outer cerebral cortex made up of grey matter and inner tracts composed of white matter. Figure 4-4 illustrates the areas of the cerebrum and labels important areas of the cerebral cortex. Table 4-10 describes various areas of the CNS that you should be familiar with for the exam.

You should also be familiar with the connective tissue coverings of the brain and spinal cord. Collectively, these layers are called the meninges. The three layers from most superficial to deepest are the dura mater, arachnoid, and pia mater. The subarachnoid space contains the cerebrospinal fluid (CSF) that circulates around the brain and spinal cord to provide cushioning. Table 4-11 describes each layer.

The peripheral nervous system (PNS) is composed of nerves that extend out from the CNS in order to transmit information to and from the CNS. Peripheral nerves can be furthered classified as cranial nerves or spinal nerves. There are 31 pairs of spinal nerves that originate from the corresponding region of the spinal cord (cervical, C1–C8; thoracic, T1–T12; lumbar, L1–L5; sacral, S1–S5; and coccyx, Co). Cranial nerves originate from the brain. For the exam, you should be familiar with the name, number, and function of all the cranial nerves, as outlined in Table 4-12.

The peripheral nervous system can be further divided into the somatic nervous system and the autonomic nervous system. The somatic nervous system is also called the voluntary nervous system because it controls skeletal muscles that are under voluntary control. For example, when you lift

Table 4-10 Areas of the Central Nervous System

CNS Structure	Description
Premotor area	Area of the cortex (frontal lobe) responsible for generating a plan for movement, which is transferred to the principal motor cortex for execution ("mental rehearsal").
Precentral gyrus (also called primary motor cortex)	Area of the cortex (frontal lobe) responsible for the execution of movement. Excitation of neurons in this area is transferred to the brainstem and spinal cord, where neurons are activated and cause voluntary movement. A somato-topically organized cortex exists called the motor homunculus. This means that different muscles are represented unequally in the primary motor area.
Postcentral gyrus (also called sensory motor cortex)	Area of the cortex (parietal lobe) directly posterior to the precentral gyrus that is responsible for the sense of touch. A somato-topically organized cortex exists called the sensory homunculus.
Prefrontal cortex	Area of the cortex (frontal lobe) responsible for executive function, which relates to abilities to differentiate among conflicting thoughts, determine good and bad, better and best, same and different, future consequences of current activities, working toward a defined goal, prediction of outcomes, expectation based on actions, and social "control" (the ability to suppress urges that, if not suppressed, could lead to socially unacceptable outcomes).
Limbic system (emotional brain)	Plays a role in emotions such as pain, pleasure, docility, affection, anger, and fear; also plays a role in motivation and in emotional association with memory. It is composed of various structures including the hippocampus and amygdala. A person whose amygdala is damaged fails to recognize fearful situations and respond appropriately.
Hippocampus	The hippocampus is a paired structure located deep inside the temporal lobes and is involved in the formation of long-term memories.
Basal ganglia	Three nuclei deep within each cerebral hemisphere: globus pallidus, putamen, and caudate nucleus. The basal ganglia receive input from the cerebral cortex and provide output back to motor areas of the cortex via nuclei of the thalamus. A major function is to help regulate initiation and termination of movements. The basal ganglia control subconscious contractions of skeletal muscles (e.g., arm swing while walking and true laughter). Damage to basal ganglia results in resting tremor, muscular rigidity, and involuntary muscle movements (e.g., Parkinson's disease is caused by destruction of dopaminergic neurons that extend from the substantia nigra to the putamen and caudate; Huntington's disease (HD) is an inherited disorder in which the caudate nucleus and putamen degenerate. A key sign of HD is chorea in which rapid, jerky movements occur involuntarily and without purpose.
Blood–brain barrier (BBB)	Protects brain cells from harmful substances and pathogens by preventing passage of many substances from blood into brain tissue, while supplying the brain with the required nutrients for proper function. The BBB consists mainly of tight junctions that seal together the endothelial cells of brain capillaries along with a thick basement membrane.
Corpus callosum	Information is transferred between the two hemispheres of the cerebral cortex through the corpus callosum.
Right hemisphere	Dominant in facial expression, intonation, body language, and spatial tasks.

(continues)

Table 4-10 Areas of the Central Nervous System (Continued)

CNS Structure	Description
Left hemisphere	Dominant with respect to language. Lesions of the left hemisphere cause aphasia. Damage to Wernicke's area causes sensory aphasia (difficulty understanding written or spoken language). Damage to Broca's area causes motor aphasia (expressive aphasia) (speech and writing are affected but understanding is intact). Mnemonic: *BROca's is BROKEN speech. Wernicke's is Wordy but makes no sense.*
Diencephalon	Area of the brain that includes the thalamus and hypothalamus—both areas perform a variety of functions because of their broad connections with other parts of the brain. The thalamus is a relay station for sensory tracts traveling from the body to the cortex. It integrates sensory experiences resulting in appropriate motor and emotional responses and maintains the conscious state. The hypothalamus maintains homeostasis by regulating a variety of important functions including control of the autonomic nervous system; body temperature; hunger, thirst, and satiety; circadian rhythms; hormones of the pituitary; and emotional and behavioral patterns (along with the limbic system).
Brainstem	The brainstem connects the cerebrum with the spinal cord and consists of the midbrain, pons, and medulla oblongata. The midbrain controls visual and auditory reflexes; the pons helps to regulate breathing and is the main connection of the cerebellum to the cerebrum; the medulla oblongata is directly connected to the spinal cord and controls many vital activities like heart rate, blood pressure, breathing, and reflexes associated with coughing, sneezing, and vomiting.
Cerebellum	The primary function of the cerebellum is to evaluate how well movements initiated by motor areas in the cerebrum are actually being carried out. When movements initiated by the cerebral cortex are not being carried out correctly, the cerebellum detects discrepancies and helps correct errors. The cerebellum also regulates posture and balance. It contributes over longer periods of time to the learning of new motor skills, such as how to ride a bike or serve a tennis ball. Damage to the cerebellum results in ataxia: lack of coordination and inability to perform rapid alternating movements. Intention tremor occurs during attempts to perform voluntary movements. People who consume too much alcohol show signs of ataxia because alcohol inhibits the activity of the cerebellum.

Table 4-11 Meninges

Layer of Meninges	Description
Dura mater	Most superficial, toughest layer of the meninges. Dura mater translates to tough mother.
Arachnoid	Middle layer; resembles a spider web. Arachnoid translates to spider.
Subarachnoid space	Space between the arachnoid and pia mater that contains the CSF.
Pia mater	Innermost, delicate layer of the meninges that sits directly on top of brain and spinal cord. Pia mater translates to soft mother.

weights, you tell your brain that you want to move a muscle and then you move it. In contrast, the autonomic nervous system controls organs such as the bladder, small intestine, and kidneys that are not under voluntary control. Hence, this system is often referred to as the involuntary nervous system. The autonomic nervous system has two divisions—the sympathetic division and the parasympathetic division. For the exam, it is important that you know the difference between these two divisions. The sympathetic division is sometimes referred to as the "fight or flight" division because it prepares the body for stressful situations and emergencies. The parasympathetic division is sometimes referred to as the "rest and digest" division because it allows the body to relax. Both divisions compliment each other. Table 4-13 compares the two divisions.

Table 4-12 Cranial Nerves

Cranial Nerve	Number	Function
Olfactory	I	Smell
Optic	II	Sight
Oculomotor	III	Eye movement, pupil constriction, accommodation, eyelid opening
Trochlear	IV	Eye movement
Trigeminal	V	Mastication muscles, facial sensation
Abducens	VI	Eye movement
Facial	VII	Facial movement (expression), taste in anterior two thirds of tongue, lacrimation, salivation (submaxillary and submandibular glands)
Vestibulocochlear	VIII	Hearing, balance
Glossopharyngeal	IX	Taste in posterior one third of tongue, swallowing, salivation (parotid gland), monitoring carotid body and sinus
Vagus	X	"Wandering" nerve: visceral organs—thorax and abdomen; also taste, swallowing, palate elevation, talking
Accessory	XI	Head turning, shoulder shrugging
Hypoglossal	XII	Tongue movements

Table 4-13 The Autonomic Nervous System

Structure	Sympathetic Nervous System	Parasympathetic Nervous System
Iris	Pupil dilation	Pupil constriction
Salivary glands	Saliva production reduced	Saliva production increased
Oral and nasal mucosa	Mucus production reduced	Mucus production increased
Heart	Heart rate increased	Heart rate decreased
Lungs	Airway relaxation (easier to breathe in emergency state)	Airway constriction
Stomach	Peristalsis decreased	Peristalsis increased; gastric juices secreted
Small intestine	Peristalsis decreased	Peristalsis increased
Large intestine	Peristalsis decreased	Peristalsis increased
Liver	Breakdown of glycogen stores—makes glucose	Glycogen synthesis
Kidney	Decreased urine secretion	Increased urine secretion
Adrenal medulla	Norepinephrine and epinephrine secreted	No effect
Bladder	Bladder wall relaxed; sphincter closed (no bathroom stops)	Bladder wall contracted; sphincter open

Cardiovascular System

The heart, also known as the myocardium, is a hollow, muscular, four-chamber pump made of cardiac muscle. There are two upper atria and two lower ventricles. The left ventricle is larger and thicker than the other chambers because it needs to pump blood to the entire body. A double layer of connective tissue, the pericardium, surrounds the heart and provides protection. The pericardium

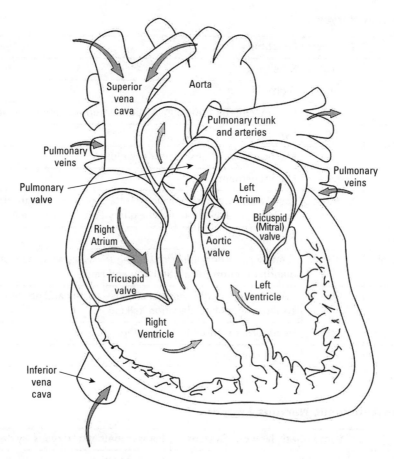

Figure 4-5 Structure of the Heart

consists of the parietal and visceral layers. The space between these two layers is called the pericardial cavity, and it contains serous fluid that reduces friction when the heart contracts. Four valves help blood to flow correctly through the heart: tricuspid valve, bicuspid valve, pulmonary valve, and aortic valve. The endocardium is a smooth, inner lining that covers the valves. Figure 4-5 illustrates the structures of the heart.

Blood Circulation

Blood leaves the heart through arteries and returns to the heart from veins. Arteries typically carry oxygenated blood and veins carry deoxygenated (venous) blood. Capillaries are the smallest blood vessel and provide the connection between the arteries (or arterioles—smaller arteries) and veins (or venules—smaller veins). The general (systemic) circulation carries blood throughout the body. Cardiopulmonary circulation carries blood from the heart to the lungs and back.

Blood that is low in oxygen and rich in the waste product carbon dioxide travels from the tissues through the superior vena cava or inferior vena cava (or the coronary sinus from the coronary circulation) to the right atrium. From the right atrium, blood flows through the tricuspid valve to the right ventricle. When the right ventricle contracts, blood moves through the pulmonary valve into a large artery called the pulmonary trunk. The pulmonary trunk branches into the pulmonary arteries. These arteries are unique because they are the only arteries in the body carrying deoxygenated (venous) blood. In the pulmonary capillaries of the lung, blood loses the carbon dioxide and picks up oxygen. The pulmonary veins return this oxygenated blood to the heart. Again, the pulmonary veins are unique because they are carrying oxygenated blood whereas normally veins carry venous blood. Blood from the pulmonary veins empties into the left atrium and then travels through the bicuspid valve (also known as the mitral valve) into the left ventricle. When the left ventricle contracts, blood travels through the aortic valve into the aorta. The aorta is the largest artery in the body. The aorta

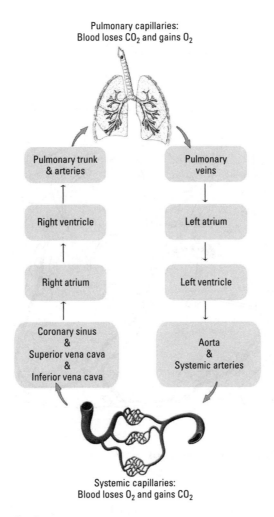

Pulmonary capillaries:
Blood loses CO_2 and gains O_2

Pulmonary trunk & arteries	Pulmonary veins
Right ventricle	Left atrium
Right atrium	Left ventricle
Coronary sinus & Superior vena cava & Inferior vena cava	Aorta & Systemic arteries

Systemic capillaries:
Blood loses O_2 and gains CO_2

Figure 4-6 Blood Circulation

and its branches distribute blood throughout the body. At the tissue level, blood gives oxygen to the cells and picks up carbon dioxide waste, and the circuit continues. Figure 4-6 illustrates this important circuit by which blood flows from the tissue, through all the chambers and valves of the heart, and then back to the tissue.

Cardiac Cycle and Heart Sounds

A cardiac cycle consists of the systole (contraction) and diastole (relaxation) of both atria, rapidly followed by the systole and diastole of both ventricles. During a cardiac cycle, atria and ventricles alternately contract and relax, forcing blood from areas of high pressure to areas of lower pressure. The cardiac cycle corresponds to the sounds heard when you listen to the heart with a stethoscope—the lubb and dupp.

Lubb (lub): The sound made when the tricuspid and bicuspid valves close between the atria and ventricles (ventricular systole has begun; the ventricles are contracting so there is no backwards flow into the atria).

Dupp (dub): The sound made when the aortic and the pulmonic valves close (end of ventricular systole; the ventricles are relaxing and the heart is filling with blood).

Conduction System of the Heart

The conduction system of the heart coordinates the contraction of heart muscle. Cardiac muscle cells are *autorhythmic* because they are self-excitable. They repeatedly generate spontaneous action potentials that then trigger heart contractions. The sinoatrial (SA) node is a group of cells in the right

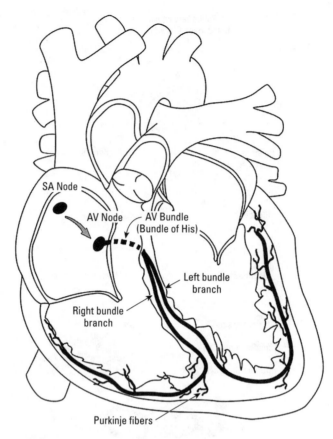

SA Node

AV Node — AV Bundle
(Bundle of His)

Left bundle
branch

Right bundle
branch

Purkinje fibers

Figure 4-7 Cardiac Conduction System

atrium that acts as a *pacemaker* to set the rhythm for the entire heart at approximately 70–90 beats/minute. Signals from the autonomic nervous system and hormones, such as epinephrine, modify the heartbeat (in terms of rate and strength of contraction), but do not establish the fundamental rhythm. Caffeine and nicotine can also increase the activity of the SA node. The action potential from the SA node travels to both atria to allow them to contract together. Next, the action potential travels to the atrioventricular (AV) node, located in the interatrial septum. From the AV node, the action potential enters the AV bundle (also known as the bundle of His). The AV bundle allows the signal to conduct from the atria to the ventricles. After propagation of the action potential through the AV bundle, the action potential enters the right and left bundle branches that extend through the interventricular septum out to the ventricles. The final step is to carry the action potential to the Purkinje fibers, which allow the ventricles to contract. The cycle then starts over again with the SA node firing. Figure 4-7 shows an illustration of the cardiac conduction system.

Hematopoietic System

The hematopoietic system involves the blood and the formation of blood cells. Blood cells are formed from pluripotent hematopoietic stem cells by a process called either hematopoiesis or hemopoiesis. In the embryo, hematopoiesis occurs in the yolk sac, liver, spleen, thymus, and lymph nodes. In the adult, hematopoiesis occurs only in the red marrow of flat bones like the sternum, ribs, skull, and pelvis, and in the ends of long bones.

Blood is composed of plasma and formed elements.

Blood plasma: 55%; the liquid portion of blood

Formed elements: 45%; cells, of which a large portion is red blood cells

Table 4-14 gives a detailed description of the formed elements of the blood.

Table 4-14 Formed Elements of Blood

Cell Type	Appearance	Function
Erythrocyte (red blood cell [RBC])	Biconcave disc for larger surface area; easy gas exchange; no nucleus or other organelles; survives for only 120 days and then is recycled	Gas exchange of O_2 and CO_2. Eryth = red; cyte = cell
Reticulocyte	Slightly larger than a mature RBC with some organelles	Immature red blood cell that escapes from the bone marrow into the blood and in 1–2 days ejects remaining organelles to become a mature RBC. Production of new red blood cells is called erythropoiesis. The main stimulus for erythropoiesis is hypoxia and the hormone erythropoietin (EPO).
Leukocyte (white blood cell)	Either granular: • Neutrophils • Eosinophils • Basophils Or agranular: • Lymphocytes (T cells, B cells, and natural killer cells) • Monocytes	Responsible for defense against infections. Leuk = white; cyte = cell
Basophil	Bilobate nucleus obscured by densely staining basophilic granules containing heparin (anticoagulant) and histamine (vasodilator); <1% of all leukocytes	Mediates allergic reactions. Mnemonic: Basophilic = staining readily with *basic* stains
Mast cell	*Found in the tissue (not blood)* Resembles basophils structurally and functionally, but is not the same cell type	Mediates allergic reactions
Eosinophil	Bilobate nucleus packed with large granules of uniform size; 1–6% of all leukocytes	Eosinophil count rises with: • Neoplasms • Asthma • Allergic responses • Collagen vascular diseases (autoimmune diseases) • Parasites
Neutrophil	Multilobed nucleus (3–5 lobes); contains granules composed of phagocytic enzymes; 40–75% of all leukocytes	Mediates acute inflammatory response; phagocytes.
Monocyte	Large cell with a kidney-shaped nucleus; differentiates into macrophages in the tissue	Monocytes move to sites of infection to become macrophages. Mono = one; cyte = cell
Macrophage	Found in the tissue (differentiate from circulating blood monocytes); may have a long life in tissues	Scavenger; phagocytizes bacteria, cell debris, and old red blood cells. Macro = big; phage = eater
Lymphocyte	Small, round cell with a densely staining nucleus and a small amount of cytoplasm—two major types: B and T cells	Participates in the immune response.

(continues)

Table 4-14 Formed Elements of Blood (Continued)

Cell Type	Appearance	Function
B lymphocyte	Small, round cells with a densely staining nucleus and a small amount of cytoplasm	Part of humoral immune response: when an antigen is encountered, B cells differentiate into plasma cells and produce antibodies; B cells have memory *B* = arise from *Bone* marrow
Plasma cell	Large cell with an off-center nucleus; B cells differentiate into plasma cells	Produces large amounts of antibody specific to a particular antigen.
T lymphocyte	Small, round cell with a densely staining nucleus and a small amount of cytoplasm	Part of cellular immune response; helps to regulate B lymphocytes and macrophages. T cells can differentiate into cytotoxic T cells (MHC I, CD8) or helper T cells (MHC II, CD4). They originate from bone marrow cells, but *T* cells mature in the *Thymus*.
Thrombocyte (platelet)	Very small fragment broken off from a large megakaryocyte cell	Helps with clotting.

Table 4-15 Blood Proteins

Blood Protein	Functions
Albumins	Very important protein for maintaining blood pressure (oncotic pressure); produced by the liver
Fibrinogen	Important in blood clotting; produced by the liver
Globulins	Transport lipids and some vitamins; some globulins are antibodies (made from plasma cells)

The blood plasma is the liquid portion of the blood. A huge percentage (about 90%) of the plasma is water, but it also contains an assortment of blood proteins that serve a wide array of functions. Table 4-15 describes the functions of these major proteins. Other components of plasma include electrolytes, nutrients, gases, enzymes, and waste products.

There are four blood types: A, B, AB, and O. Table 4-16 explains the distinctions. Understanding blood types is important in establishing compatibility for blood transfusions.

Lymphatic and Immune System

The lymphatic and immune system functions in defense against microorganisms entering the body as well as in the destruction of cells no longer recognizable to the body. Lymphoid tissues and organs are predominantly collections of lymphocytes and related cells supported by a network of connective tissue. Primary lymphoid organs include the red bone marrow and thymus. Secondary lymphoid organs include the spleen, lymph nodes, mucosal-associated lymphoid tissue (MALT), tonsils, and appendix. These organs (and tissues) are further described in Table 4-17. Cells involved in the immune system include B lymphocytes, plasma cells, T lymphocytes, and macrophages, which also are described in Table 4-17. These lymphocytes circulate continuously through lymph fluid in order to achieve maximum exposure to foreign antigens.

Lymph fluid forms when fluid leaks out of the blood capillaries and collects in the spaces between cells (interstitial space). Most of this nutrient-rich fluid is picked up by the body's cells; however, some of this fluid persists and the body picks up the remaining fluid through the lymphatic vessels. Lymphatic vessels accompany and are similar to veins. They are in almost all tissues and organs that have blood vessels. The lymphatic system differs from the circulatory system in that lymph

Table 4-16 Blood Types

Blood Type	Surface Antigen on Red Blood Cell	Plasma Antibodies	May Donate to Blood Type(s) . . .	May Receive from Blood Type(s) . . .
A	A antigens	Anti-B antibodies	A and AB	A and O
B	B antigens	Anti-A antibodies	B and AB	B and O
AB	A and B antigens	None	AB	A, B, AB, and O *Universal recipient*
O	No antigens	Anti-A and anti-B antibodies	O, AB, A, and B *Universal donor*	O

Table 4-17 Structures of the Lymphatic and Immune System

Structure	Description
Lymphocyte	Two major types: B and T cells; participate in the immune response.
B lymphocyte	Part of the humoral immune response: when an antigen is encountered, B cells differentiate into plasma cells and produce antibodies; B cells have memory. Mnemonic: *B* = arises from *B*one marrow
Plasma cell	B cells differentiate into (become) plasma cells. They produce large amounts of antibody specific to a particular antigen.
T lymphocyte	Part of cellular immune response; helps to regulate B lymphocytes and macrophages. T cells can differentiate into cytotoxic T cells (MHC I, CD8) or helper T cells (MHC II, CD4). They originate from bone marrow cells but *T* cells mature in the *T*hymus.
Macrophage	Scavenger; phagocytizes bacteria, cell debris, and old red blood cells. Macro = big; phage = eater
Lymph nodes	Lymph nodes are located along lymphatic vessels and filter and trap foreign material. Knowledge of the location of the lymph nodes and the direction of lymph flow is important in the diagnosis and prognosis of the spread of cancer and disease. Lymph nodes are tissues surrounded by a connective tissue capsule. The nodes consist of an outer cortex, which contains spherical clusters of cells (primarily B lymphocytes) called lymphatic nodules. The area of the cortex deep in the nodules houses mostly T lymphocytes. The innermost region of the node, the medulla, houses macrophages, which are highly active phagocytes. Examples: cervical, axillary, inguinal.
Red bone marrow	Primary lymphatic organ that provides the environment for stem cells to divide and mature into B and T lymphocytes. Red bone marrow gives rise to mature B cells; T cells will circulate to the thymus and mature there.
Spleen	The spleen consists of two types of tissue: 1. Red pulp, which is involved in the destruction of old, worn-out red blood cells. 2. White pulp, which contains phagocytes and lymphocytes and plays a large role in the immune system by filtering foreign material.
Thymus	A large organ in infants that atrophies in the adult; the main function of the thymus is to "mature" and develop the T cells that migrate from the red bone marrow.
Mucosal-associated lymphoid tissue (MALT)	Concentrations of lymphatic tissue *not* surrounded by a capsule in the mucosa of the body. Peyer's patches in the ileum of the small intestine are one specific example of MALT.
Tonsils	Lymphatic nodules in the pharyngeal region that participate in the immune response against inhaled or ingested foreign material. There are two palatine tonsils, one pharyngeal tonsil (adenoid), and two lingual tonsils.

fluid travels in only one direction—from the body organs to the heart. There are two large main lymphatic vessels, also known as lymphatic ducts.

- *Thoracic duct (left lymphatic duct):* The thoracic duct receives lymph from the left side of the head, neck, and chest; the left upper extremity; and the entire body below the diaphragm. It begins as a dilation called the cisterna chyli and is the main collecting duct of the lymphatic system.
- *Right lymphatic duct:* This duct receives lymph from the upper right side of the body.

Respiratory System

The respiratory system works with the cardiovascular system to allow our bodies to deliver oxygen to the tissues and remove carbon dioxide. External respiration refers to the exchange of gases between alveoli in the lungs and blood in the pulmonary capillaries. Internal respiration refers to the exchange of gases between systemic capillaries and tissue cells. The organs of the respiratory system include the upper respiratory organs (the nose and pharynx) and the lower respiratory organs (the larynx, trachea, bronchi, and lungs). Air passes from the upper respiratory organs to the lower respiratory organs. In the lungs, gas exchange occurs at the level of the alveoli. Each organ is described in more detail in Table 4-18. Figure 4-8 illustrates the organs of the respiratory system.

Table 4-18 Organs of the Respiratory System

Structure	Description
Nose	The nose filters, warms, moistens, smells, and modifies vibration of sounds. It contains various structures: shelves called nasal conchae, the nasal septum, cilia, mucous membranes, mucus, and olfactory receptors.
Sinuses	The sinuses are air-filled spaces within the bones of the skull. They are lined with tissue called mucosa that secretes a viscous fluid called mucus that lubricates the sinuses. As the mucus drains from the sinuses, it travels down the throat and is dissolved by the stomach's acid. The sinuses are the frontal sinus, ethmoid sinus, maxillary sinus, and sphenoid sinus.
Pharynx	The pharynx is made up of three divisions: • *Nasopharynx:* Only used for the passage of air. • *Oropharynx:* Shared by the respiratory and digestive systems. • *Laryngopharynx:* Air, fluid, and food continue through here and go to the trachea *or* the esophagus.
Larynx	Makes speech possible; made up of cartilages: thyroid cartilage, epiglottis, and cricoid cartilage. The vocal cords stretch between the thyroid cartilage and the cricoid cartilage. When the vocal cords vibrate (stretch), sound is produced.
Trachea	Also known as the windpipe; its primary function is to transport air to and from the pharynx to the bronchi. The trachea is lined with pseudostratified ciliated columnar cells and goblet cells and has 16–20 C-shaped cartilage rings to hold it open.
Bronchi and bronchioles	The bronchial tree is a series of branches off the trachea in which cartilage decreases and smooth muscle increases. The primary (main stem) bronchi are the first branches off the trachea. They're followed by: Secondary bronchi Tertiary bronchi Terminal bronchiole Respiratory bronchiole
Alveoli	Very thin sacs made up of simple squamous epithelium and surrounded by capillaries. Gas exchange occurs at the alveoli. Red blood cells in the capillaries release carbon dioxide into the alveoli to breathe out and new air in the alveoli transfers oxygen into the red blood cells of the capillaries. Surfactant is fluid produced in the alveoli that reduces the tendency of the alveoli to collapse.

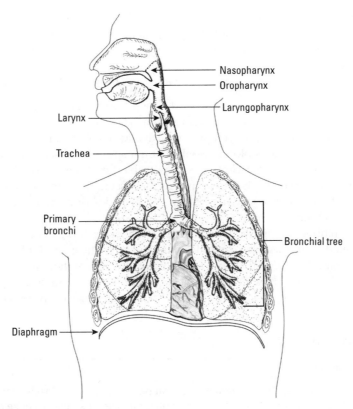

Figure 4-8 Organs of the Respiratory System

The Mechanics of Breathing

Breathing consists of inhalation or inspiration and exhalation or expiration. Inhalation allows oxygen-rich air to enter the lungs from the atmosphere whereas exhalation is the process of breathing out carbon-dioxide rich air. Air flows between the atmosphere and the lungs due to a difference in pressure caused by the respiratory muscles. During inspiration, the diaphragm contracts and the intercostal muscles raise the rib cage. Hence, lung volume increases. The atmospheric pressure outside the body is now greater than the pressure inside the cavity so air is able to flow in. Exhalation is normally a passive process that is due to muscle relaxation. The diaphragm relaxes (rises) and the internal intercostal muscles relax (the ribs fall). Air now flows out of the thoracic cavity because the pressure is higher than atmospheric pressure.

During normal inspiration, tidal volume refers to the amount of air that moves into and out of the lungs. Residual volume refers to the volume of air that remains in the lungs and can never be exhaled because the lungs would collapse.

Breathing is controlled by the respiratory center, a group of neurons in the pons and medulla oblongata. The medulla oblongata controls the rhythm and depth of breathing whereas the pons controls the rate of breathing.

Digestive System

Digestion includes the following basic processes:

- *Ingestion* is taking food into the mouth (eating).
- *Secretion* is the release, by cells within the walls of the GI tract and accessory organs, of water, acid, buffers, and enzymes into the lumen of the tract.
- *Mixing* and *propulsion* result from the alternating contraction and relaxation of the smooth muscles within the walls of the GI tract.
- *Mechanical digestion* consists of movements of the GI tract that aid chemical digestion.

- *Chemical digestion* is a series of catabolic (hydrolysis) reactions that break down large carbohydrate, lipid, and protein food molecules into smaller molecules that are usable by body cells.
- *Absorption* is the passage of end products of digestion from the GI tract into blood or lymph for distribution to cells.
- *Defecation* is emptying of the rectum, eliminating indigestible substances from the GI tract.

Organs of the digestive system extend from the mouth to the anus. Each organ consists of four layers—the mucosa, submucosa, muscularis, and serosa. The mucosa is the innermost layer that secretes enzymes and mucus into the lumen. It is very active in absorbing nutrients. The submucosa lies just beneath the mucosa. It contains blood vessels that transport the absorbed nutrients. The muscularis layer is composed of smooth muscle and is responsible for mixing, propulsion, and mechanical digestion. The final layer, the serosa, is also known as the visceral peritoneum. It secretes serous fluid to keep the outside of the canal moist. The serosa also provides protection for all the organs along with the parietal peritoneum.

Many organs contribute to digestion. Table 4-19 describes each organ of the gastrointestinal tract and the role it plays in digestion as food passes from the mouth to the anus. Table 4-20 describes the accessory organs and their role in digestion. The accessory organs of digestion include the salivary glands, pancreas, liver, and gallbladder. These organs produce secretions that aid in digestion, although the food never travels directly through these structures. Figure 4-9 illustrates the organs of the digestive system.

Table 4-19 Organs of Digestion

Structure	Description
Mouth	Includes the lips, cheeks, hard palate, soft palate, and uvula. Mechanically starts to break down food. Chemical digestion of carbohydrates begins here because saliva contains salivary amylase.
Pharynx	Food passes through the oropharynx and laryngopharynx. The epiglottis covers the opening of the larynx so food cannot enter.
Esophagus	The esophagus is a muscular tube beginning at the lower end of the pharynx, passing through the diaphragm, and connecting to the upper portion of the stomach. The esophagus passes through a hole in the diaphragm in order to connect to the stomach. This hole is called the esophageal hiatus. Food is pushed through the esophagus by peristalsis.
Stomach	Parts of the stomach include the cardioesophageal sphincter (upper esophageal sphincter), cardia, fundus, body, antrum, and pyloric sphincter (lower esophageal sphincter). The stomach lies in folds called rugae that allow for its expansion. Mechanical digestion occurs with mixing waves via peristalsis. This mixing turns the food into chyme. Chyme triggers hormones in the small intestine to be released (CCK and secretin). Chemical digestion occurs as well when the stomach's hydrochloric acid from the parietal cells converts pepsinogen to pepsin and protein digestion begins. Parietal cells also secrete intrinsic factor, which is necessary for Vitamin B$_{12}$ absorption.
Small intestine	The small intestine is made up of the duodenum, jejunum, and ileum. Most absorption of nutrients occurs here. Absorption in the small intestine is accomplished through specially adapted structures that provide a large surface area—circular folds, villi, and microvilli. The indigestible portion is passed through to the large intestine. Major enzymes secreted by the small intestine are peptidases, sucrase, maltase, lactase, and lipase. Proteins, carbohydrates, and fats are broken down in response to these enzymes.
Large intestine	Parts of the large intestine include the cecum with vermiform appendix, ascending colon, hepatic flexure, transverse colon, splenic flexure, descending colon, and sigmoid colon. The large intestine is responsible for completion of absorption, production of certain vitamins (vitamin K and some B vitamins), and formation of feces.
Rectum and anal canal	Feces is composed of water, inorganic salts, epithelial cells, bacteria, products of bacteria decomposition, and unabsorbed digested parts of food, which are pushed out through the rectum and anal canal. Mass movements of feces from the large intestine trigger the defecation reflex, which allows anal sphincters to relax.

Table 4-20 Accessory Organs of Digestion

Accessory Structure	Description
Teeth	Mechanically help to break down food particles.
Tongue	Contains filiform papillae, fungiform papillae, and circumvallate papillae for taste receptors.
Salivary glands	Include the parotid gland, submandibular gland, and sublingual gland that make saliva. Saliva wets and dissolves food for tasting. It also contains bicarbonate ions (which buffer acidic foods), salivary amylase (which begins chemical digestion of starch), and lysozyme (which destroys bacteria). The parotid gland is located below the ear and over the masseter. The submandibular gland is located under the lower edge of the mandible. The sublingual gland is deep below the tongue in the floor of the mouth. All have ducts that empty into the oral cavity.
Pancreas	The acinar cells of the pancreas are the exocrine portion of the pancreas. These cells secrete enzymes, bicarbonate, and water into ducts that merge to form the main pancreatic duct, which empties into the duodenum. The islets of Langerhans (alpha and beta cells) make up the endocrine portion and release insulin and glucagons.
Liver	Cells of the liver are called hepatocytes. The liver has many functions: carbohydrate metabolism, lipid metabolism, protein metabolism (prepares urea), processing of drugs and hormones, excretion of bilirubin and its formation into bile, storage of fat-soluble vitamins, and activation of vitamin D.
Gallbladder	The gallbladder stores and concentrates bile until it is needed. Bile is secreted into the small intestine where bile salts break large fat globules into smaller ones so they can be more easily digested by enzymes.

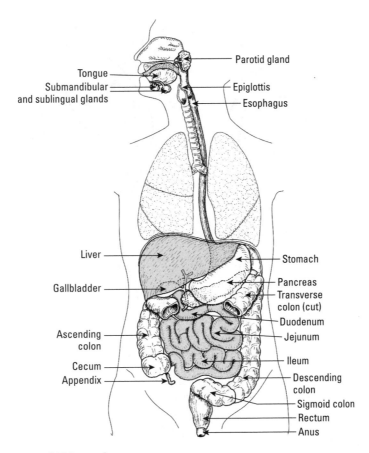

Figure 4-9 Organs of Digestion

Urinary System

The urinary system consists of two kidneys, two ureters, the bladder, and the urethra. Urine flows from each kidney, down its ureter to the bladder, and to the outside via the urethra. In general terms, the function of the urinary system is to filter the blood and remove waste products via formation and secretion of urine. More specifically, the kidneys help to regulate the blood's ionic composition (concentration of Na^+, K^+, Ca^{+2}, Cl^-, and phosphate ions in the blood), assist in maintaining pH balance, regulate blood volume by conserving or eliminating water, help to regulate blood pressure by secreting the enzyme renin (used in the renin-angiotensin-aldosterone system), and contribute to the release of erythropoietin, which stimulates red blood cell production, and calcitriol (active vitamin D).

The functional unit of the kidney is the nephron, which can be seen only under a microscope. Each kidney has over 1 million nephrons. The nephron is composed of a corpuscle and tubule. The renal corpuscle is the site of plasma filtration and is composed of the glomerulus and the glomerular capsule, also called Bowman's capsule. The glomerulus is a capillary bed where filtration from the blood occurs. The glomerular capsule is a double-walled epithelial cup that surrounds the glomerulus and collects the filtrate.

The renal tubule is composed of the proximal convoluted tubule, the loop of Henle, and the distal convoluted tubule. Distal convoluted tubules from several nephrons merge together to form collecting ducts. These collecting ducts drain urine and deliver it to the renal pelvis, which empties into the ureter and eventually the bladder. Figure 4-10 illustrates the organs of the urinary system; Figure 4-11 illustrates the structure of a nephron.

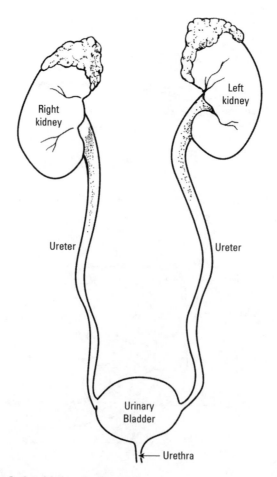

Figure 4-10 Organs of the Urinary System

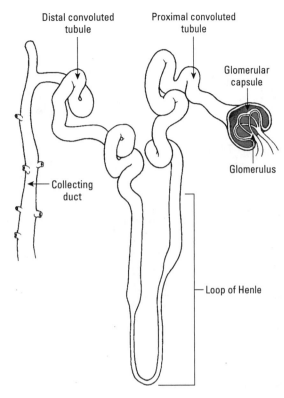

Distal convoluted tubule

Proximal convoluted tubule

Glomerular capsule

Glomerulus

Collecting duct

Loop of Henle

Figure 4-11 Structure of a Nephron

Urine Formation

There are three processes or steps in urine formation. They are:

1. Filtration by the glomerulus
2. Tubular reabsorption (from filtrate into blood)
3. Tubular secretion (from blood into filtrate)

The first step, glomerular filtration, occurs in the renal corpuscle. Blood flows from the glomerulus into Bowman's capsule. The amount of blood filtered depends greatly on the blood pressure in the glomerulus. The rate at which blood flows is called glomerular filtration rate (GFR). If blood pressure and/or blood volume drops, GFR decreases, which leads to less glomerular filtrate and ultimately less urine formed. The second step is tubular reabsorption, in which the peritubular capillaries reabsorb many of the substances (nutrients, water, and ions) that were originally filtered at the glomerulus. Water reabsorption is largely under the influence of two hormones—antidiuretic hormone and aldosterone. The third step is tubular secretion, in which ions and waste products move from the peritubular capillaries into the renal tubules to be added to the urine. Figure 4-12 shows the process of urine formation.

Reproductive System

The reproductive system includes the necessary organs capable of creating offspring. In the male, these organs include the scrotum, two testes, the seminal duct, glands (prostate, seminal vesicle, and bulbourethral), and penis. Each of these organs is further described in Table 4-21. In the female, these organs include two ovaries, the uterus, two fallopian tubes, and the vagina. Each of these organs is further described in Table 4-22. Figure 4-13 illustrates the male reproductive organs; Figure 4-14 illustrates the female reproductive organs.

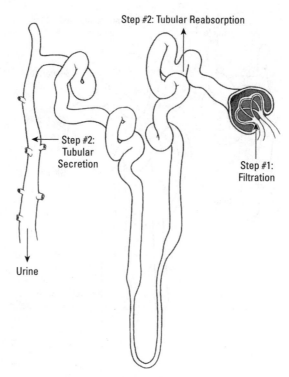

Step #2: Tubular Reabsorption

Step #2:
Tubular
Secretion

Step #1:
Filtration

Urine

Figure 4-12 Process of Urine Formation

Table 4-21 Male Reproductive Organs

Organ	Description
Scrotum	The scrotum is a pouch that supports the testes. The production and survival of the sperm requires a temperature lower than body temperature. The temperature of the testes is regulated by skeletal muscles, which elevate them and bring them closer to the pelvic cavity or relax them to move them away from the pelvic cavity.
Testes	The testes develop in the embryo's posterior abdominal wall and usually begin their descent to the scrotum during the latter half of the seventh month of development. The testes contain seminiferous tubules, Sertoli cells, and Leydig cells. Sperm are produced by the process of spermatogenesis in the seminiferous tubules. The Sertoli cells support, protect, and nourish sperm cells. The Leydig cells secrete the male hormone, testosterone.
Seminal vesicles	The seminal vesicles secrete an alkaline (acid-neutralizing), viscous fluid that contains fructose (to make ATP or Adenosine Triphosphate), prostaglandins (for motility), and clotting proteins (for coagulation). The fluid secreted constitutes about 60% of the volume of semen and contributes to sperm viability.
Prostate	The prostate secretes a milky, slightly acidic fluid that contains citric acid (used in the ATP-Krebs cycle), acid phosphotase (which serves an unknown function), and protein-digesting enzymes (prostate-specific antigen). The fluid secreted constitutes about 25% of the volume of semen.
Bulbourethral (Cowper's) gland	The bulbourethral (Cowper's) gland secretes an alkaline substance into the urethra to neutralize acids from the urine and a mucus to lubricate the end of the penis during sexual intercourse.
Penis	The penis consists of a root, the body, and the glans penis. It is used to introduce sperm into the vagina. Expansion of its blood sinuses under the influence of sexual excitation causes an erection.

Table 4-22 Female Reproductive Organs

Organ	Description
Ovaries	The ovaries are female gonads located in the upper pelvic cavity, on either side of the uterus. They are maintained in position by a series of ligaments.
Uterus	The uterus (womb) is an inverted pear-shaped organ that functions in transporting sperm, menstruation, implantation of a fertilized ovum, development of the fetus during pregnancy, and labor. Parts of the uterus include the fundus, body, and cervix. Two important layers of the uterus are the myometrium and endometrium.
Fallopian tubes	The uterine (fallopian) tubes transport the secondary oocytes from the ovaries to the uterus, and are the normal site of fertilization. Ciliated cells and peristaltic contractions help move the secondary oocyte through the uterine tubes towards the uterus. Fertilization takes place in the fallopian tube up to 24 hours after ovulation. The zygote then descends and implants in the uterus within 7 days.
Perineum	The perineum is a diamond-shaped area between the thighs and buttocks of both females and males. It is of clinical importance in females because it is sometimes incised during vaginal deliveries to accommodate the fetal head in a procedure called an episiotomy.
Vulva	The vulva, or pudendum, is a collective term for the external genitals of the female. The vulva consists of the mons pubis, labia majora and minora, clitoris, vestibule, vaginal and external urethral orifices, and paraurethral and greater vestibular glands.
Vagina	The vagina is a tubular canal that acts as an outlet for menstrual flow. It also is the receptacle for the penis during sexual intercourse, and the lower portion of the birth canal. The vagina has an acid environment that retards microbial growth.
Mammary glands	The mammary glands, located in the breasts, are modified sudoriferous glands, which produce milk. Mammary gland development is dependent upon estrogens and progesterone produced by the ovaries. The essential function of the mammary glands is lactation, the secretion and ejection of milk. Milk production is stimulated by the hormone prolactin (PRL), and milk ejection is stimulated by oxytocin (OT), which is released by the posterior pituitary gland in response to sucking.

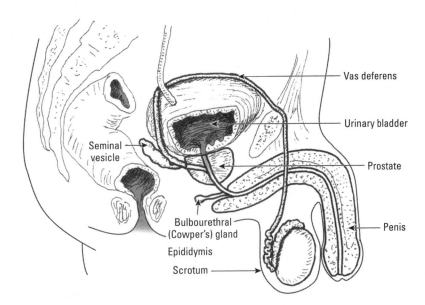

Figure 4-13 Male Reproductive Organs

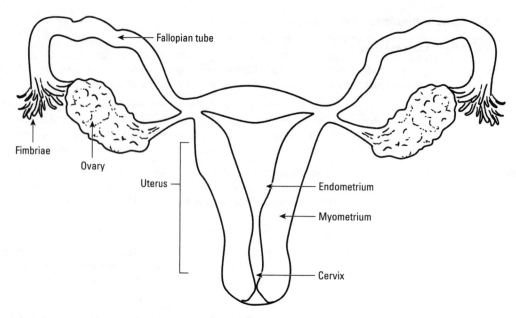

Figure 4-14 Female Reproductive Organs

Spermatogenesis and Sperm Movement

Spermatogenesis refers to the production of sperm cells that begins in males during puberty and continues throughout life. The process is complex and occurs in the seminiferous tubules of the testes. There are many steps involved. The most immature of the sperm-developing cells are called spermatogonia and contain 46 chromosomes. These divide by mitosis, and the daughter cells are pushed out towards the lumen. These cells become primary spermatocytes. Primary spermatocytes undergo meiosis I and become secondary spermatocytes, now containing 23 chromosomes. Secondary spermatocytes undergo meiosis II and become spermatids. In the last step, called spermiogenesis, each spermatid develops a head and a tail. Sperm are produced at the rate of 300 million per day. They may live up to 48 hours in the female reproductive tract.

Following spermatogenesis, the sperm move from the seminiferous tubules into the epididymis, which is the site for sperm maturation and storage. The ductus (vas) deferens stores sperm and propels them toward the urethra during ejaculation. The spermatic cord is a supporting structure of the male reproductive system and consists of the ductus (vas) deferens, blood vessels, autonomic nerves, and lymphatic vessels.

Semen is a mixture of sperm and secretions of the accessory sex glands. These secretions provide nutrients and the fluid in which the sperm are transported. Semen neutralizes the acidity of the male urethra and female vagina and also contains an antibiotic for destroying bacteria within the vagina. The volume of semen in a typical ejaculation is 2.5–5 milliliters, with 50–150 million sperm per milliliter.

Oogenesis and the Menstrual Cycle

Oogensesis is the process of egg cell formation. The mature egg will contain 23 chromosomes. In contrast to the male, the process of oogenesis actually begins before a female is born and is completed only if a secondary oocyte is fertilized. Prebirth in the fetus, the ovary contains approximately 7 million oocytes. These oocytes begin meiosis I. At birth, the number of oocytes has already decreased and is between 200,000 and 2 million. These oocytes are arrested in prophase of meiosis I. At puberty 40,000 remain, but only about 400 go on to mature. With each menstrual cycle, a group of primary oocytes begins to mature under follicle-stimulating hormone (FSH). Six or more follicles may begin growth and maturation in any cycle, but only one follicle fully develops into a graafian follicle. With a luteinizing hormone (LH) surge, it ruptures. Under the influence

Table 4-23 The Menstrual Cycle

Organ	Days	Description
Menstrual phase	1–5	Endometrium is sloughed off (50–150 ml of blood, tissue fluid, and epithelial cells). Occurs because of declining levels of progesterone and estrogen. The thickness of the endometrium is 2–5 mm.
Follicular phase/ preovulatory phase/proliferative phase	6–13, most variable part of cycle	A primordial follicle develops into the mature (graafian) follicle with atresia of the neighboring follicles. Estrogen levels produced by the growing follicles steadily increase, which stimulate the repair of (proliferation of) the uterus. The thickness of the endometrium doubles to approximately 4–10 mm.
Ovulation	14 (or 14 days prior to menses)	Rupture of the graafian follicle (secondary oocyte). The high levels of estrogen during the last part of the preovulatory phase exert a positive feedback effect on the cells that secrete gonadotropin-releasing hormone (GnRh) and LH.
Luteal phase/ postovulatory phase/secretory phase	15–28	Development of the corpus luteum, which synthesizes estrogen and progesterone (lives about 2 weeks). There is increased vascularity and secretory activity of the endometrium to prepare for receipt of the fertilized egg. Basal body temperature increases because of progesterone's effect on the hypothalmic regulatory center.

of the LH surge, a primary oocyte becomes a secondary oocyte (and a first polar body). Meiosis II does not continue unless fertilization takes place.

The menstrual cycle has four stages or phases: the menstrual stage, preovulatory stage, ovulation, and postovulatory stage. Each is described in Table 4-23.

Reproductive Hormones

The reproductive hormones are necessary for the development of reproductive organs and secondary sex characteristics. In the male, testosterone is the dominant hormone. The Leydig cells of the testes make testosterone under the influence of LH. In the female, estrogen and progesterone are both important and vital hormones. Estrogen and progesterone are produced in the ovary under the influence of FSH and LH. In general terms, FSH causes follicle development (egg) and LH causes ovulation and development of the corpus luteum. Both FSH and LH are secreted by the anterior pituitary, which is under the influence of GnRH (gonadotropin-releasing hormone) secreted from the hypothalamus. The detailed functions of testosterone, estrogen, and progesterone are described in Table 4-24.

Pregnancy

Pregnancy results when a sperm containing 23 chromosomes unites with an egg that also contains 23 chromosomes. Fertilization takes place in the fallopian tube up to 24 hours after ovulation of the egg. A zygote forms, which undergoes cell division called cleavage. A blastocyst then forms, which implants into the wall of the uterus within 7 days after fertilization. The embryonic period extends from the second week to the eighth week of pregnancy. The fetal period spans from week 9 to delivery.

Many hormonal changes take place when a woman is pregnant. Pregnancy is characterized by steadily increasing levels of estrogen and progesterone. Both hormones maintain the endometrium for the fetus, suppress FSH and LH secretion (to prevent ovulation), and stimulate development of the breast. Human chorionic gonadotropin (hCG) is the hormone made by the embryo (about 8 days after fertilization) and then the placenta in the second and third trimester. It is used to detect pregnancy

Table 4-24 Reproductive Hormones and Their Functions

Reproductive Hormone	Function
Testosterone	• Causes prenatal differentiation of the Wolffian ducts and external genitalia • Causes development of male secondary sex characteristics at puberty (distribution of male hair, growth of external genitalia, laryngeal enlargement, increased muscle mass) • Causes pubertal growth spurt • Maintains spermatogenesis (along with help from Sertoli cells) • Stimulates anabolism: protein synthesis • Increases libido
Estrogen	• Feedback inhibition of FSH; LH surge (estrogen feedback on LH is positive) • Causes maturation and development of fallopian tubes, uterus, cervix, and vagina • Responsible for the development of female secondary sex characteristics at puberty such as development of breasts • Increases fat deposition • Causes growth of ovarian follicle • Causes endometrial proliferation
Progesterone	• Prepares endometrium for implantation/secretory activity of uterus during the luteal phase • Maintains pregnancy • Increases body temperature (0.5 degree) • Has negative feedback effects on LH and FSH • Causes uterine smooth muscle relaxation • Aids in development of breasts/mammary glands

because it appears in the urine and blood 8 days after successful fertilization. This hormone is important because it maintains the corpus luteum in the ovary for the first trimester so that it will continue to secrete estrogen and progesterone. When the corpus luteum degenerates, the placenta takes over producing estrogen and progesterone.

Endocrine System

The endocrine system is complex and regulates various reactions in the body via hormones. Hormones are chemicals released directly into the blood that have an effect on target organs some distance from their source. Most hormones are regulated via negative feedback. When there is a drop in the level of a hormone, a chain reaction of responses occurs, which causes an increase in the level of that hormone. Table 4-25 organizes the endocrine system by endocrine organ, the organ's location, and which hormones that endocrine organ secretes. Table 4-26 describes the major hormones, their target tissue, and their effects on that target tissue.

Special Senses

The special senses are smell, taste, vision, hearing, and equilibrium. They are housed in complex sensory organs in the head.

Table 4-25 Endocrine Organs

Endocrine Organ	Location	Hormone(s) Secreted
Hypothalamus	Brain	Releases and inhibits hormones that influence the pituitary gland
Anterior pituitary gland	Sits in the hypothalamus	hGH (Human growth hormone), TSH (Thyroid-stimulating hormone), FSH (Follicle-stimulating hormone), LH (Luteinizing hormone), PRL (Prolactin), ACTH (Adrenocorticotropic hormone), MSH (Melanocyte-stimulating hormone)
Posterior pituitary gland	Sits in the hypothalamus	Oxytocin, ADH (Antidiuretic hormone)
Pineal gland	Roof of the third ventricle of the brain at the midline	Melatonin
Thyroid gland	Below the larynx, anterior to the trachea	Thyroxine (T4), triiodothyronine (T3), calcitonin
Thymus gland	Mediastinum	Thymosin
Parathyroid glands	Partially embedded on the posterior surface of the thyroid gland	PTH (Parathyroid hormone)
Pancreas	Abdomen	Insulin, glucagon
Adrenal cortex	On the adrenal gland on kidneys	Aldosterone (salt), cortisol (sugar), androgens (sex) Mnemonic: Salt, sugar, sex: The deeper you go, the sweeter it gets!
Adrenal medulla	On the adrenal gland on kidneys	Epinephrine (stress), norepinephrine
Testes	Male gonads	Testosterone
Ovaries	Pelvic cavity	Estrogen, progesterone

Smell

Millions of smell receptors are located in the superior nasal cavity. Olfactory receptors sense an odor and convey nerve impulses to the olfactory nerve, cranial nerve I. The olfactory nerve sends the information to the cerebrum, where it is interpreted. Genetic evidence suggests there are hundreds or even thousands of primary scents. Adaptation to odors occurs quickly, and the threshold of smell is low: only a few molecules of certain substances need be present in the air to be smelled.

Taste

Taste receptors are called taste buds and are located on the tongue, soft palate, pharynx, and epiglottis. Taste is a chemical sense. To be detected, molecules must be dissolved in saliva. Five classes of taste stimuli exist—sour, bitter, sweet, salty, and umami (recognized as a new taste stimuli that takes its name from the Asian culture and is thought to be savory, tasty, or meaty). Other "tastes" are a combination of the five taste sensations plus olfaction.

Vision

Vision is an extremely important sense. More than half the sensory receptors in the human body are located in the eyes. A large part of the cerebral cortex is devoted to processing visual information. The eye is constructed of three layers or tunics. The fibrous tunic is the outer layer and is composed of the cornea and sclera. The vascular tunic is the middle layer and is composed of the choroid, ciliary body, iris, pupil,

Table 4-26 Hormones

Hormone	Target Tissue	Hormone Effects
Antidiuretic hormone	Kidneys, sweat glands, arterioles	Decreases urine production; causes kidneys to retain water; also causes decreased production of sweat and constriction of blood vessels (vasopressin), thereby retaining water
Oxytocin	Uterus and breasts	Milk ejection, uterine contraction
Thyroid-stimulating hormone	Thyroid gland	Stimulates synthesis and secretion of thyroid hormones by the thyroid gland
Adrenocorticotropic hormone	Adrenal cortex	Stimulates secretion of glucocorticoids by the adrenal cortex
Growth hormone	Cartilage, bone, skeletal muscle, liver, and other body tissues	Stimulates the liver, muscle, bone, and other tissues to synthesize and secrete insulin-like growth factors (IGFs)
Follicle-stimulating hormone	Testes and ovaries	In females, initiates development of oocytes and induces secretion of estrogens by the ovaries; in males, stimulates testes to produce sperm
Lutenizing hormone	Testes and ovaries	In females, stimulates secretion of estrogens and progesterone, ovulation, and formation of corpus luteum; in males, stimulates testes to produce testosterone
Prolactin	Mammary gland	Stimulates milk production by the mammary glands
Melatonin	Brain	Sets the body's biological clock
Thyroxine and triiodothyronine	Most body cells	Basal metabolic rate
Calcitonin	Osteoclast cells in bones (inhibits osteoclasts)	Decreases level of calcium in blood
Thymosin	T cells	Stimulates maturation of the T cells
Parathyroid hormone	Osteoclast cells in bones (stimulates osteoclasts)	Increases level of calcium in blood and decreases level of phosphate in blood Mnemonic: PTH = *Phosphate Trashing Hormone*
Cortisol	Liver, muscle, and cells involved in body defenses	Protein breakdown, glucose formation, breakdown of triglycerides, anti-inflammatory, depression of immune responses
Aldosterone	Kidneys	Regulates homeostasis of K^+ and Na^+
Estrogen	Uterus, mammary glands, and other body cells involved in female sexual characteristics	Development of female sex characteristics; regulates menstrual cycle
Testosterone	Testes, muscle, other body cells involved in male sexual characteristics	Regulates production of sperm and maintains male characteristics
Progesterone	Uterus, mammary glands, and other body cells involved in female sexual characteristics	Development of female sex characteristics; regulates menstrual cycle

(*continues*)

Table 4-26 Hormones (Continued)

Hormone	Target Tissue	Hormone Effects
Epinephrine and norepinephrine	Medulla	Fight or flight: stress response
Insulin	Various body cells	Promotes facilitated diffusion of glucose into cells; speeds synthesis of glycogen from glucose; increases uptake of amino acids and increases protein synthesis
Glucagon	Liver cells	Breaks down glycogen into glucose; forms glucose from lactic acid and certain amino acids

and suspensory ligament of the lens. The nervous tunic is the innermost layer and is composed of the retina with its photoreceptors. Each structure of the eye is described in more detail in Table 4-27.

These structures create two cavities in the eye—the anterior and posterior cavities. The anterior cavity is in front of the lens and filled with a watery fluid called aqueous humor. Aqueous humor provides nutrients to the structures found in the anterior cavity. The posterior cavity is behind the lens and is filled with a thicker fluid called vitreous humor. Vitreous humor helps to maintain the shape of the eye and keeps the retina flat.

Table 4-27 Structures of the Eye and Their Functions

Structure	Description
Cornea	Transparent and curved structure of the eye; allows light to enter and helps to focus this light on the retina.
Sclera	White, opaque, fibrous portion of the eye that provides shape, structure, and protection to the eye.
Choroid	Consists of melanocytes (absorb scattered light so image on retina is clear) and blood vessels (provide nutrients to the retina).
Ciliary body	Composed of ciliary processes (folds on ciliary body) that secrete aqueous humor fluid of the eye and the ciliary muscle that alters the shape of the lens in order to focus light on the retina.
Iris	Colored portion of the eye (amount of melanin determines color); controls the amount of light entering the eye—circular muscle fibers contract in bright light to shrink pupil and radial muscle fibers contract in dim light to enlarge pupil.
Pupil	The hole in the center of the iris through which light enters; the pupil dilates and constricts in response to the muscles of the iris.
Suspensory ligament	Suspensory ligaments attach the lens to the ciliary processes of the ciliary body; the suspensory ligaments control tension on the lens, which allows it to alter its shape in order to refract light onto the retina.
Lens	Avascular and perfectly transparent portion of the eye held in place by suspensory ligaments; functions to focus light on the retina.
Retina	Posterior three fourths of the eyeball that contains the visual receptors, rods and cones. Rods are specialized for black-and-white vision in dim light, allow us to discriminate between different shades of dark and light, and permit us to see shapes and movement. Cones are specialized for color vision and sharpness of vision (high visual acuity) in bright light. Cones are most densely concentrated in the central fovea, a small depression in the center of the macula lutea. The central fovea (fovea centralis) is the area of the retina responsible for the most acute vision. In contrast, the optic disc is the area of the retina where there is a blind spot because there are no photoreceptors. At this spot, the optic nerve (cranial nerve II) exits and travels back to the brain.

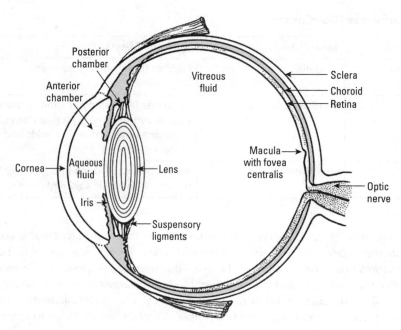

Figure 4-15 Structures of the Eye

Image formation occurs when light rays fall upon the retina. Light is able to fall on the retina because it is refracted by both the cornea and lens. The photoreceptors of the retina (rods and cones) translate the light into action potentials that are transmitted to the optic nerve, cranial nerve II. The optic nerve travels to the thalamus and then to the primary visual cortex, located in the occipital region of the brain. Parts of the optic nerve cross at the optic chiasm. This crossing means that half of the visual information detected in each eye is interpreted on the opposite side of the brain. Figure 4-15 illustrates the structures of the eye.

Hearing and Equilibrium

The ear is responsible not only for hearing, but also for balance. Structurally, the ear is divided into three parts: the external ear, middle ear, and inner ear. The external (outer) ear collects sound waves. It is composed of the auricle and external auditory canal. The middle ear (tympanic cavity) is a small, air-filled cavity in the temporal bone that contains auditory ossicles (middle ear bones: the malleus, incus, and stapes) and the eustachian tube. The inner (internal) ear is also called the labyrinth because of its complicated series of canals. The inner ear can be further divided into three portions—the semi-circular canals, vestibule, and cochlea. These three structures make up the bony labyrinth of the inner ear. The bony labyrinth contains a fluid called perilymph. This fluid, chemically similar to cerebrospinal fluid, surrounds the membranous labyrinth. The membranous labyrinth is a series of sacs and tubes lying inside the bony labyrinth and having the same general form.

The membranous labyrinth contains a fluid called endolymph, which is chemically similar to intracellular fluid. Fluid pressure waves in the perilymph cause movement of the enodlymph inside the cochlear duct to move the hair cells of the organ of Corti inside the cochlea. The bending of the hairs produces receptor potentials that lead to the generation of nerve impulses that allow us to hear. Each structure of the ear is described in more detail in Table 4-28. Figure 4-16 illustrates the structures of the ear.

The process of hearing is complex. The following steps simplify the process:

1. The auricle directs sound waves into the external auditory canal.
2. Sound waves strike the tympanic membrane, causing it to vibrate back and forth (slow vibration in response to low-pitched sounds, rapid vibration in response to high-pitched sounds).

Table 4-28 Structures of the Ear and Their Functions

Structure	Description
Auricle (pinna)	Elastic cartilage covered by skin.
External auditory canal	Curved 1-inch tube of cartilage and bone leading into temporal bone; contains ceruminous glands that produce cerumen (ear wax).
Tympanic membrane (eardrum)	Receives the sound waves from the external ear and transmits them to the middle ear ossicles.
Ossicles	The three ear ossicles—malleus, incus, and stapes—are connected by synovial joints. The malleus is attached to the tympanic membrane; the incus connects the malleus to the stapes; and the stapes fits into a small opening between the middle and inner ear called the oval window which is where the inner ear begins. Thus, the ossicles transmit sound to the inner ear.
Eustachian tube (auditory tube)	Leads to the nasopharynx and helps to equalize pressure on both sides of the eardrum (tympanic membrane).
Semicircular canals	Made up of three canals that lie at right angles to each other. Contain receptors called cristae ampullaris for equilibrium—specifically dynamic equilibrium—and maintain body position (head) during sudden movement of any type: rotation, deceleration, or acceleration.
Vestibule	Contains receptors for equilibrium—specifically static equilibrium—and maintains position of the body (head) relative to the force of gravity. The membranous labyrinth in the vestibule consists of two sacs called the utricle and saccule where the maculae receptors lie.
Cochlea	Contains receptors for hearing in the organ of Corti.

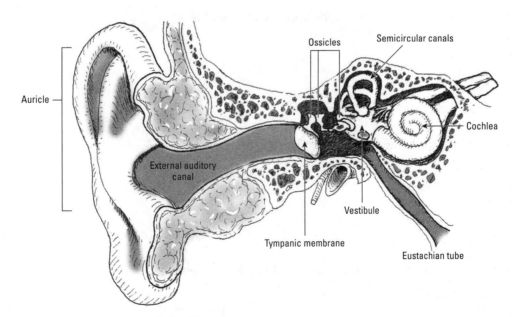

Figure 4-16 Structures of the Ear

3. The vibration conducts sound waves from the tympanic membrane through the ossicles (through the malleus to the incus and then to the stapes).
4. The ossicles vibrate because the malleus is attached to the eardrum.
5. The stapes move back and forth, pushing the membrane of the oval window in and out, which produces fluid pressure waves in the cochlea (scala vestibuli) and tympani.
6. The movement of the oval window sets up fluid pressure waves in the perilymph of the cochlea. The oval window vibration is 20 times more vigorous than the tympanic membrane, but the frequency of vibration is unchanged.
7. Pressure waves in the scala vestibuli are transmitted to the scala tympani and eventually to the round window, causing it to bulge outward into the middle ear.
8. As the pressure waves deform the walls of the scala vestibuli and scala tympani, they push the vestibular membrane back and forth, which causes pressure waves in the endolymph inside the cochlear duct.
9. Pressure fluctuations of the endolymph inside the cochlear duct move the hair cells of the organ of Corti (spiral organ) against the tectorial membrane.
10. The bending of the hairs produces receptor potentials that lead to the generation of nerve impulses in the cochlear nerve.
11. The cochlear nerve is part of cranial nerve VIII, the vestibulocochlear nerve, which is responsible for hearing and balance. The nerve sends information about the sound waves back to the auditory cortex of the temporal lobe of the brain, where it is interpreted as sound.

QUESTIONS

4-1. Which of the following is the basic unit of life?

    A. Organ
    B. Tissue
    C. Cell
    D. Organism
    E. Body system

4-2. The directional term that means the opposite of medial is

    A. posterior.
    B. anterior.
    C. proximal.
    D. lateral.
    E. distal.

4-3. Which of the following organs would be found in the thorax?

    A. Lungs
    B. Femur
    C. Spleen
    D. Pancreas
    E. Thyroid

4-4. Which of the following planes divides the body into superior and inferior portions?

    A. Midsagitttal
    B. Sagittal
    C. Frontal
    D. Transverse
    E. Costal

4-5. The maintenance of a relatively stable internal environment in the body is known as

   A. anabolism.
   B. catabolism.
   C. metabolism.
   D. homeostasis.
   E. peristalsis.

4-6. The posterior portion of the knee joint is known as the _____ region.

   A. crural
   B. digital
   C. femoral
   D. plantar
   E. popliteal

4-7. Organs found in the lower right abdominopelvic quadrant include the

   A. sigmoid colon, left ureter, and small intestine.
   B. stomach, spleen, left kidney, and small intestine.
   C. gallbladder, liver, duodenum, and small intestine.
   D. appendix, cecum, ascending colon, and small intestine.
   E. liver, gallbladder, duodenum, and head of pancreas.

4-8. Moving your arms away from your body so that the letter "T" is formed is known as

   A. adduction.
   B. abduction.
   C. inversion.
   D. eversion.
   E. dorsiflexion.

4-9. A coronal MRI would section the body into

   A. superior/inferior sections.
   B. anterior/posterior sections.
   C. medial/lateral sections.
   D. sagittal sections.
   E. proximal/distal sections.

4-10. While examining a slice of tissue, you note several characteristics. There are numerous cells packed tightly together, one side of the cells opens into a cavity, and the other is attached to a thin layer of extracellular material. Several of the cells are in some stage of mitosis. Which primary tissue type do you think this is most likely to be?

   A. Cartilage
   B. Connective
   C. Nervous
   D. Muscular
   E. Epithelial

4-11. Which of the following tissues provides the greatest protection from mechanical injury?

   A. Simple squamous epithelium
   B. Simple cuboidal epithelium
   C. Stratified squamous epithelium
   D. Simple columnar epithelium
   E. Transitional epithelium

4-12. As cells are pushed from the deeper portion of the epidermis toward the surface,

    A. they become part of the hypodermis.
    B. their supply of nutrients increases.
    C. they become dermal cells.
    D. they degenerate and die.
    E. they do not divide.

4-13. Which of the following cells would be expected to be most active in replacing bone matrix lost due to an injury?

    A. Osteoblasts
    B. Osteoclasts
    C. Osteocytes
    D. Both A and C are correct.
    E. Both B and C are correct.

4-14. The atlas bone

    A. is a lumbar vertebra.
    B. is the first cervical vertebra.
    C. has the largest spinous process.
    D. articulates with the hyoid bone.
    E. is also known as the axis.

4-15. How many vertebrae make up the cervical region of the body?

    A. 5
    B. 7
    C. 8
    D. 9
    E. 12

4-16. Which of the following bones forms the upper jaw?

    A. Maxilla
    B. Mandible
    C. Ethmoid
    D. Frontal
    E. Sphenoid

4-17. Which bone is superior to the fibula and inferior to the ischium?

    A. Tibia
    B. Humerus
    C. Ulna
    D. Radius
    E. Femur

4-18. Joints are lined by which type of membrane?

    A. Serous
    B. Mucous
    C. Meninges
    D. Filtration
    E. Synovial

4-19. Which of the following may be the basis for the name of a muscle?

    A. The direction of the muscle's fibers
    B. The size of the muscle
    C. The shape of the muscle
    D. The location of the muscle
    E. All of the above may be used to name a muscle.

4-20. Which large muscle separates the thoracic cavity from the abdominal cavity?

    A. Trapezius
    B. Pectoralis major
    C. Latissimus dorsi
    D. Diaphragm
    E. Deltoid

4-21. The type of muscle that is attached to the bone of the skeleton is called

    A. smooth.
    B. cardiac.
    C. skeletal.
    D. respiratory.
    E. involuntary.

4-22. The contractile unit of a myofibril that lies between two successive Z lines is called a

    A. sarcoplasm.
    B. sarcolemma.
    C. myofibril.
    D. sarcomere.
    E. retinaculum.

4-23. In synaptic transmission, the postsynaptic neuron is stimulated to form an impulse by a neurotransmitter released from the

    A. axon tip of the presynaptic neuron.
    B. dendrite tip of the presynaptic neuron.
    C. axon tip of the postsynaptic neuron.
    D. dendrite tip of the postsynaptic neuron.
    E. None of the above.

4-24. Cerebrospinal fluid is located in the

    A. pia mater.
    B. dura mater.
    C. arachnoid mater.
    D. subarachnoid space.
    E. cerebellum.

4-25. Interpretation of sensory impulses occurs in which part of the cerebrum?

    A. Precentral gyri in the frontal lobes
    B. Postcentral gyri in the parietal lobes
    C. Premotor areas
    D. Association areas
    E. Occipital area

4-26. Select the response that is NOT regulated by a control center in the hypothalamus.

    A. Sleep
    B. Body temperature
    C. Appetite
    D. Memory
    E. Fluid and electrolyte balance

4-27. The impulse pathway in a spinal reflex is

    A. receptor - motor neuron - interneuron - sensory neuron - effector.
    B. effector - sensory neuron - interneuron - motor neuron - receptor.
    C. receptor - sensory neuron - interneuron - motor neuron - effector.
    D. receptor - interneuron - sensory neuron - motor neuron - effector.
    E. effector - sensory neuron - interneuron - receptor - motor neuron.

4-28. Select the response that is NOT regulated by the autonomic nervous system.

    A. Heart rate
    B. Urine secretion
    C. Respiration rate
    D. Speech
    E. Digestion

4-29. The neurotransmitter released at the neuromuscular junction is

    A. epinephrine
    B. dopamine
    C. endorphins
    D. norepinephrine
    E. acetylcholine

4-30. The term that refers to areas of myelinated axons is

    A. gray matter
    B. white matter
    C. horns
    D. Nissl bodies
    E. chromatin

4-31. The area of the retina where the nerve fibers leave the eye and there is a blind spot is known as the

    A. optic disc or optic nerve
    B. pupil
    C. iris
    D. fovea centralis
    E. cornea

4-32. The hormones regulating blood calcium levels are

    A. insulin and glucagon.
    B. glycogen and PTH.
    C. inhibiting hormones.
    D. PTH and calcitonin.
    E. estrogen and progesterone.

4-33. Oxytocin:

    A. is a neurotransmitter.
    B. exerts its most important effects during menstruation.
    C. controls blood pressure.
    D. stimulates uterine contraction.
    E. is released by the pancreas.

4-34. The hormone erythropoietin increases the production of

    A. neutrophils.
    B. basophils.
    C. eosinophils.
    D. platelets.
    E. red blood cells.

4-35. Insulin is synthesized by the beta cells of the pancreas. This hormone is released

    A. in excessive amounts in obese people.
    B. in response to severe physical stress.
    C. when the body's glucose level drops.
    D. when the body's glucose level rises.
    E. without regard to glucose level in the body.

4-36. Which of the following endocrine organs is sometimes known as the "master" gland because it makes hormones that control several other endocrine glands?

    A. Thymus
    B. Spleen
    C. Thyroid
    D. Adrenal gland
    E. Pituitary gland

4-37. An individual who is blood type B

    A. has B antigens on the red blood cells and A antibodies in the plasma.
    B. has A antigens on the red blood cells and B antibodies in the plasma.
    C. has A and B antigens on the red blood cells and no antibodies in the plasma.
    D. has no antigens on the red blood cells and A and B antibodies in the plasma.
    E. can donate blood to all blood types.

4-38. Which blood cell aids in clotting?

    A. Basophil
    B. Eosinophil
    C. Lymphocyte
    D. Thrombocyte
    E. Neutrophil

4-39. The valve located between the right atrium and the right ventricle is the

    A. tricuspid valve.
    B. bicuspid valve.
    C. aortic valve.
    D. semilunar valve.

4-40. Which portion of the heart has the thickest myocardium?

    A. Left atrium
    B. Right atrium
    C. Left ventricle
    D. Right ventricle

4-41. Blood transported by the pulmonary veins returns to the

    A. left atrium.
    B. right atrium.
    C. left ventricle.
    D. right ventricle.

4-42. Parasympathetic innervation of the heart is mediated by cranial nerve

    A. V
    B. VI
    C. VIII
    D. X
    E. III

4-43. The specialized area in the heart that initiates each heartbeat and sets its pace is the

    A. SA node.
    B. AV node.
    C. bundle of His.
    D. bundle branches.
    E. Purkinje fibers.

4-44. By secreting hormones, the thymus causes what cells to become immunocompetent?

    A. Basophils
    B. Monocytes
    C. Lymphocytes
    D. Macrophages
    E. Neutrophils

4-45. The redness and heat of an inflamed area are due to a local hyperemia caused by

    A. vasoconstriction of vessels.
    B. production of complement and interferon.
    C. phagocyte mobilization.
    D. vasodilation of vessels.
    E. All of the above.

4-46. The thoracic duct:

    A. receives lymph from the left side of the head, neck, chest, left upper arm, and entire body below the ribs.
    B. receives lymph from the upper right side of the body.
    C. receives lymph from the whole right side of the body.
    D. is NOT the most important lymphatic duct.
    E. is part of the arterial system.

4-47. Worn-out and damaged red blood cells are destroyed in the

    A. thymus.
    B. tonsils.

    C. spleen.

    D. lymph nodes.

    E. bone marrow.

4-48. The exchange of gases occurs in small air sacs called

    A. trachea.

    B. terminal bronchioles.

    C. alveoli.

    D. primary bronchus.

    E. vocal cords.

4-49. Surfactant helps to prevent the alveoli from collapsing by

    A. warming the air before it enters.

    B. reducing the surface tension of alveolar fluid.

    C. humidifying the air before it enters.

    D. protecting the surface of alveoli from dehydration.

    E. stimulating the phrenic nerve.

4-50. The structure that closes off the larynx during eating is the

    A. vocal cords.

    B. thyroid.

    C. epiglottis.

    D. tongue.

    E. trachea.

4-51. Bile is produced in the liver and stored in the

    A. spleen.

    B. bone marrow.

    C. gallbladder.

    D. stomach.

    E. pancreas.

4-52. Saliva contains an enzyme that breaks down

    A. starch.

    B. fat.

    C. protein.

    D. artificial ingredients.

    E. minerals.

4-53. What is the term for movement of food through the digestive tract?

    A. Emulsification

    B. Radiation

    C. Absorption

    D. Secretion

    E. Peristalsis

4-54. The kidneys are stimulated to produce renin

    A. when the pH of the urine decreases.

    B. by a decrease in the blood pressure.

    C. when the peritubular capillaries are dilated.

D. when the calcium in the blood rises
E. in pathologic conditions only.

4-55. The first step in urine formation is

    A. tubular secretion.
    B. secretion of ADH.
    C. glomerular filtration.
    D. water reabsorption.
    E. renin secretion.

4-56. The functional and structural unit of the kidneys is

    A. the nephron.
    B. the basement membrane of the capillaries.
    C. Bowman's capsule.
    D. the loop of Henle.
    E. the hilum.

4-57. What is the cluster of blood capillaries found in each nephron called?

    A. Afferent arteriole
    B. Efferent arteriole
    C. Loop of Henle
    D. Collecting duct
    E. Glomerulus

4-58. Which of the following shows the correct order in which urine is expelled?

    A. Urethra - ureter - kidney - urethral meatus - bladder
    B. Kidney - ureter - bladder - urethral meatus - urethra
    C. Urethral meatus - urethra - bladder - kidney - ureter
    D. Kidney - ureter - bladder - urethra - urethral meatus
    E. Ureter - kidney - urethral meatus - bladder - urethra

4-59. The inner lining of the uterus that sheds every month during menstruation is known as the

    A. lining of the cervix.
    B. peritoneum.
    C. perimetrium.
    D. myometrium.
    E. endometrium.

4-60. The rupture of the mature follicle (egg) during ovulation is due to a surge in

    A. FSH.
    B. LH.
    C. progesterone.
    D. estrogen.
    E. growth hormone.

4-61. The presence of which hormone in the maternal blood or urine indicates pregnancy?

    A. hCG
    B. FSH

    C. LH
    D. GnRH
    E. Progesterone

4-62. Where is sperm produced?

    A. Seminal vesicle
    B. Prostate
    C. Vas deferens
    D. Testes
    E. Urethra

4-63. Fertilization generally occurs in the

    A. fallopian tubes.
    B. ovary.
    C. uterus.
    D. vagina.
    E. cervix.

4-64. Normally, menstruation occurs when

    A. blood levels of estrogen and progesterone decrease.
    B. the corpus luteum secretes estrogen.
    C. blood levels of estrogen and progesterone increase.
    D. blood levels of FSH fall off.
    E. blood levels of LH rise sharply.

4-65. For fertilization to occur, the sperm has to penetrate which layers surrounding the oocyte?

    A. Zona glomerulosa and corona granulose
    B. Zona pellucida and zona glomerulosa
    C. Corona radiata and zona pellucida
    D. Corona granulose and zona rapida
    E. Zona rapida and zona pellucida

ANSWERS

4-1. The correct answer is C. The cell is the basic structural unit of all organisms. Groups of cells that carry out the same function make up a tissue. A collection of tissues that serve a common function is called an organ. A group of organs that work together comprise a body system. Finally, our body is made up of many body systems.

4-2. The correct answer is D. The directional term that means the opposite of medial is lateral.

4-3. The correct answer is A. The lungs are found in the thorax or thoracic cavity.

4-4. The correct answer is D. The transverse (or horizontal) plane divides the body into superior and inferior portions. The sagittal plane divides the body into right and left portions. Finally, the frontal (or coronal) plane divides the body into ventral (anterior) and dorsal (posterior) portions.

4-5. The correct answer is D. The maintenance of a relatively stable internal environment in the body is known as homeostasis. It is important that our body maintains homeostasis.

4-6. The correct answer is E. The posterior portion of the knee joint is known as the popliteal region.

4-7. The correct answer is D. Organs found in the lower right abdominopelvic quadrant include the appendix, cecum, ascending colon, and small intestine. The appendix is the key organ that you should realize is in the right lower quadrant.

4-8. The correct answer is B. Moving your arms away from your body so that the letter "T" is formed is known as abduction. In contrast, adduction is a movement that brings a limb closer to the body.

4-9. The correct answer is B. A coronal MRI would section the body into anterior and posterior positions.

4-10. The correct answer is E. The tissue described is epithelial tissue, which commonly functions as a covering or lining for organs and other tissues. Epithelial tissue has a free surface (no contact with another cell) and is avascular (no blood vessels); it must depend on underlying tissues for the nutrients and oxygen it needs to maintain homeostasis. Another characteristic of epithelial tissue is that its cells are tightly packed together, meaning there is no intercellular matrix between the cells. Cells undergo mitosis (cell division) and eventually become keratinized and die.

4-11. The correct answer is C. Stratified squamous epithelium provides the greatest protection from mechanical injury because it has many layers that can be sequentially sloughed off and replaced before the basement membrane is exposed.

4-12. The correct answer is D. As cells are pushed from the deeper portion of the epidermis toward the surface, they degenerate and die. These superficial cells slough off.

4-13. The correct answer is A. Osteoblasts are responsible for new bone formation. In contrast, osteoclasts break down bone. Osteocytes are mature, nondividing bone cells. Bone is a dynamic tissue that is constantly being reshaped by osteoblasts, which build bone, and osteoclasts, which resorb bone.

4-14. The correct answer is B. The atlas is the first cervical vertebra. The axis is the second cervical vertebra. The atlas is named after a Greek god who supported the world on his shoulders. The joint between the two bones is a pivot joint and allows the head to turn from side to side, as in saying, "no."

4-15. The correct answer is B. The spinal column is divided into five different areas containing groups of vertebrae, as follows: 7 cervical vertebrae in the neck, 12 thoracic vertebrae in the upper back corresponding to each pair of ribs, 5 lumbar vertebrae in the lower back, 5 sacral vertebrae that are fused together to form one bone called the sacrum, and 4 coccygeal vertebrae that are fused together to form the coccyx or tailbone.

4-16. The correct answer is A. The upper jaw bone is the maxilla. The lower jaw bone is the mandible.

4-17. The correct answer is E. The femur, the thigh bone, is superior to the fibula and inferior to the ischium.

4-18. The correct answer is E. Synovial membranes line joint cavities interiorly. Synovial membranes secrete synovial fluid into the joint cavity to lubricate the cartilage on the ends of the bones so they can move freely.

4-19. The correct answer is E. Muscles are named based on many characteristics: the direction of the muscle's fibers, the size of the muscle, the shape of the muscle, the location of the muscle, the number of origins and insertions, and the muscle's action.

4-20. The correct answer is D. The diaphragm is the major muscle used in breathing. It is dome-shaped and separates the thorax from the abdomen.

4-21. The correct answer is C. Muscle tissue is classified into three types: cardiac, smooth, and skeletal. Skeletal muscle tissue is named for its location—attached to bones. Smooth muscle tissue is located in the walls of hollow internal structures such as blood vessels, the stomach, intestines, and urinary bladder. Cardiac muscle tissue forms the walls of the heart.

4-22. The correct answer is D. A sarcomere is the basic unit of a muscle's cross-striated myofibril. A sarcomere is defined as the segment between two neighboring Z discs. The sarcomeres are what give skeletal and cardiac muscles their striated appearance.

4-23. The correct answer is A. Synaptic transmission refers to the propagation of nerve impulses from one nerve cell to another. This occurs at a junction at which the axon of the presynaptic neuron communicates via neurotransmitters with the postsynaptic neuron.

4-24. The correct answer is D. CSF or cerebrospinal fluid is located in the subarachnoid space. The spinal cord is bounded by the spinal meninges. The pia mater is a delicate membrane that closely covers the surface of the spinal cord. The subarachnoid space lies between the pia mater and the arachnoid mater. The dura mater is the tough, outermost layer of the meninges. Dura mater is from the Latin meaning "tough mother." Pia mater is from the Latin meaning "delicate mother."

4-25. The correct answer is B. The postcentral gyrus is the fold of brain tissue located just posterior to the central sulcus in the parietal lobe. It is the location of the primary somatosensory cortex, the main sensory receptive area for the sense of touch.

4-26. The correct answer is D. The hypothalamus performs a variety of functions that contribute to the body's homeostasis. It helps to maintain blood pressure, body temperature, fluid and electrolyte balance, sleep, and appetite. However, the hypothalamus does not contribute to memory.

4-27. The correct answer is C. A reflex arc is the simplest pathway able to receive a stimulus, enter the central nervous system for immediate interpretation, and produce a response. The pathway travels from the receptor to the sensory neuron to the interneuron to the motor neuron to the effector.

4-28. The correct answer is D. The autonomic nervous system regulates many involuntary functions of the body including heart rate, blood pressure, pupil size, contraction of the bladder, and digestion. The response that is NOT controlled by the autonomic nervous system is speech.

4-29. The correct answer is E. The neuromuscular junction is where the axon of a motor nerve meets a muscle. The neuron communicates with the muscle via chemicals called neurotransmitters. The neurotransmitter released at the neuromuscular junction is acetylcholine.

4-30. The correct answer is B. Areas of myelinated axons are referred to as white matter because they look white to the naked eye because myelin is full of fat and surrounds the nerve fibers (axons). Gray matter is where the nerve cell bodies are located.

4-31. The correct answer is A. The optic disc is the area of the retina in which nerve fibers leave the eye to form the optic nerve (cranial nerve II). The optic nerve makes vision possible because it connects the eyes with the brain. There are no rods or cones at this part of the retina, which causes the blind spot.

4-32. The correct answer is D. The hormones regulating blood calcium levels are PTH and calcitonin. Parathyroid hormone (PTH), released by the parathyroid glands, is the most important control of calcium homeostasis. PTH regulates serum calcium by promoting bone resorption and releasing that calcium into the blood. Calcitonin is a hormone made in the thyroid that inhibits bone removal by osteoclasts (thus, promoting bone formation and decreasing serum calcium).

4-33. The correct answer is D. Oxytocin is made in the posterior pituitary to stimulate uterine contraction during labor. Oxytocin is also responsible for the milk "letdown" response during breastfeeding.

4-34. The correct answer is E. Erythropoietin (EPO) is produced by the kidneys to increase production of red blood cells in the bone marrow if necessary. Because red blood cells carry oxygen, this process is stimulated by increased tissue demand for oxygen.

4-35. The correct answer is D. Insulin is synthesized by the beta cells of the pancreas. This hormone is released when the body's glucose level rises. Insulin helps to move glucose into the cells of the body in order to use it as an energy source.

4-36. The correct answer is E. The pituitary controls the function of most other endocrine glands and is, therefore, sometimes called the master gland. In turn, the pituitary is controlled in large part by the hypothalamus.

4-37. The correct answer is A. Blood group B individuals have the B antigen on the surface of their RBCs, and blood serum containing antibodies against the A antigen.

4-38. The correct answer is D. Another name for thrombocyte is platelet. Platelets are crucial to blood clotting.

4-39. The correct answer is A. The valve located between the right atrium and the right ventricle is the tricuspid valve. The valve located between the left atrium and the left ventricle is the bicuspid or mitral valve. The other two valves in the heart are the semilunar valves—the pulmonary semilunar valve and the aortic semilunar valve.

4-40. The correct answer is C. The left ventricle has the thickest myocardium because it has to work the hardest to pump blood to the entire body.

4-41. The correct answer is A. Blood transported by the pulmonary veins returns blood from the lungs to the left atrium.

4-42. The correct answer is D. Parasympathetic innervation of the heart is mediated by cranial nerve X (the vagus). The vagus nerve is a major nerve of the parasympathetic nervous system. The nerve is well-named because vagus means wandering. It travels (wanders) down below the head, to the neck, chest, and abdomen, where it contributes to the innervation of the viscera.

4-43. The correct answer is A. The specialized area in the heart that initiates each heartbeat and sets its pace is the SA node. Located in the right atrium, this specialized bundle of neurons "fires" at regular intervals to cause the heart to beat with a regular rhythm and triggers a sequence of electrical events in the heart to control the organized sequence of muscle contractions that pumps blood through the heart.

4-44. The correct answer is C. By secreting the hormone thymosin, the thymus causes lymphocytes (specifically T cells) to become immunocompetent. Thymosin "educates" the T cells so they can recognize and distinguish foreign antigens from the body's own cells.

4-45. The correct answer is D. Inflammation is reaction of the tissue to all kinds of injury. The reaction typically causes redness, heat, edema, and pain. The redness and heat are a result of increased blood flow (hyperemia) because of vasodilation of blood vessels.

4-46. The correct answer is A. The thoracic duct is the main duct of the lymphatic system. It receives lymph from the left side of the head, neck, chest, left upper arm, and entire body below the ribs and empties into the left subclavian vein. The right lymphatic duct collects lymph from the right arm and the right side of the chest, neck, and head.

4-47. The correct answer is C. One of the main functions of the spleen is to destroy worn-out and damaged red blood cells.

4-48. The correct answer is C. The alveoli are tiny air sacs within the lungs where the exchange of oxygen and carbon dioxide takes place.

4-49. The correct answer is B. Surfactant reduces the surface tension of alveolar fluid and hence prevents the alveoli and lung from collapsing at the end of expiration.

4-50. The correct answer is C. The epiglottis is a flap of elastic cartilage, attached to the base of the tongue, that closes off the larynx during swallowing, preventing food from entering the pharynx and lungs.

4-51. The correct answer is C. Bile is produced in the liver and stored in the gallbladder. Bile aids in the digestion of fats, and is released from the gallbladder into the upper small intestine in response to fatty food.

4-52. The correct answer is A. Saliva contains an enzyme called amylase that breaks down starch. Proteins and fats are broken down later in the stomach and small intestine by other enzymes. Many enzymes used in digestion are made in the pancreas (pancreatic juice) and released into the small intestine via a duct.

4-53. The correct answer is E. Peristalsis refers to the wave-like contractions that move food through the digestive tract.

4-54. The correct answer is B. When blood pressure falls, the kidneys release the enzyme renin into the bloodstream. This stimulates the renin-angiotensin-aldosterone system. Aldosterone causes the kidneys to retain salt and excrete potassium. The sodium causes water to be retained, thus increasing blood volume and blood pressure.

4-55. The correct answer is C. Glomerular filtration is the first step in urine formation. Blood is filtered through the glomerulus into Bowman's capsule and the tubules; the filtrate consists primarily of water, excess sodium and potassium, glucose, and urea.

4-56. The correct answer is A. The nephron is the functional unit of the kidney, responsible for the filtration of the blood. About 1 million nephrons are in each kidney.

4-57. The correct answer is E. The cluster of blood capillaries found in each nephron is called the glomerulus. The glomerulus is semipermeable, allowing water and soluble wastes to pass through and be excreted as urine.

4-58. The correct answer is D. Urine flows from the kidney to the ureter to the bladder, then out the urethra through the urethral meatus (opening).

4-59. The correct answer is E. The inner lining of the uterus that sheds every month during menstruation is known as the endometrium. During the menstrual cycle, the endometrium thickens in order to prepare for implantation of the zygote. If this doesn't occur, the lining is shed.

4-60. The correct answer is B. The pituitary releases a large amount of luteinizing hormone (LH), called the LH surge, when the egg is mature. This rise in LH signals the mature follicle to release its egg.

4-61. The correct answer is A. The hormone human chorionic gonadotropin (hCG) is produced during pregnancy by cells of the placenta. Levels can first be detected by a blood test about 11 days after conception and in the urine about 12–14 days after conception. In general the hCG levels will double every 72 hours. The level will reach its peak in the first 8–11 weeks of pregnancy and then will decline and level off for the remainder of the pregnancy.

4-62. The correct answer is D. The testes are the essential male sex organs that serve to produce the male gametes, sperm, and the male sex hormone, testosterone. The testes contain interstitial Leydig cells and Sertoli cells. Sertoli cells within the testes play an active role in maturing the sperm and releasing them into the seminiferous tubules. The Leydig cells within the testes respond to hormone stimulation (FSH) and produce testosterone.

4-63. The correct answer is A. The fallopian tubes capture the egg after its release from the ovary and serve as a conduit for its travel toward the uterus. Fertilization of the egg by the sperm occurs in the fallopian tube. Following fertilization, the zygote develops into an embryo and continues to travel through the fallopian tube into the uterine cavity, where it implants in the endometrium.

4-64. The correct answer is A. In a normal cycle, menstruation occurs when estrogen and progesterone levels drop rapidly. These hormone drops cause the uterus to shed its lining in a process termed menstruation.

4-65. The correct answer is C. To reach the oocyte, the sperm must pass through the corona radiata and the zona pellucida. These two layers cover and protect the oocyte from fertilization by more than one sperm.

Common Diseases and Pathology

Chapter 4 outlined the body's anatomy and physiology and discussed the body's various systems. This chapter covers some common diseases and pathology of the body's systems.

INTEGUMENTARY SYSTEM

A burn is an injury caused by heat, sun, a chemical, or radiation. Burns are classified according to the depth or layers involved. Table 5-1 illustrates the types of burns.

Skin cancer is extremely common; one in every five Americans will develop skin cancer. The biggest risk factor in developing skin cancer is exposure to ultraviolet (UV) radiation from the sun. Table 5-2 lists the most common skin cancers.

Table 5-3 lists some of the more common dermatologic diseases that may be seen on the exam. Table 5-4 lists descriptions of dermatologic lesions. A lesion is defined as an abnormal change caused by either injury or disease.

Table 5-1 Burn Classifications

Burn	Description
First degree	Superficial damage to epidermis only; superficial sunburn
Second degree	Damage to epidermis and dermis; blistered, pink skin
Third degree	Damage to epidermis, dermis, and subcutaneous tissue, also potential damage to muscle below; charred black-brown skin

Table 5-2 Skin Cancers

Carcinoma	Description
Actinic (solar) keratoses	Considered the earliest stage in the development of skin cancer (pre-squamous cell carcinoma); appear as small, scaly spots.
Basal cell	Most common and least harmful type of skin cancer; the tumor is derived from the basal cell layer of the epidermis. Lesions are pink, smooth, and raised with a depression in the center.
Squamous cell	The tumor is derived from the squamous cells of the epidermis. Lesions appear to be crusty sores that will not heal.
Melanoma	Most dangerous because of metastasis; sometimes fatal. Lesions are derived from melanocytes. Remember the ABCDEs of melanoma: Asymmetry, Border, Color, Diameter, and Evolving.

Table 5-3 Common Skin Diseases

Disease	Description
Acne vulgaris	Most common type of acne; caused by overproduction of sebum, often triggered by hormones in puberty.
Albinism	Inherited absence of pigment in the skin, hair, and irises due to a missing enzyme necessary for production of melanin.
Alopecia	Partial or complete loss of hair.
Decubitus ulcer	A pressure ulcer or bedsore from prolonged pressure, which may cause tissue death (decubitus = lying down).
Eczema	Dermatitis associated with itching and redness.
Furuncle	A large, tender area around a hair follicle caused by a staphylococcal infection; also known as a boil.
Hemangioma	A benign tumor in children made of newly formed blood vessels; they appear and enlarge through the first year of life. They regress approximately 10%/year; usually gone by age 10.
Herpes simplex	Viral infection caused by Herpes simplex virus I/II; causes a cold sore (fever blister).
Herpes zoster (shingles)	Viral infection caused by the *Varicella zoster* virus (same virus that causes chickenpox); occurs in people who have had chickenpox and is a reactivation of the dormant virus. It causes painful skin eruptions that follow the underlying route of the inflamed nerve.
Hirsutism	Excessive facial and body hair in women.
Impetigo	Bacterial skin infection characterized by pustules that become crusted and rupture.
Kaposi's sarcoma	A malignant tumor of the skin seen in people of Mediterranean descent and the HIV population.
Lupus erythematosus	Autoimmune disorder characterized by a red, scaly rash on the face and upper trunk; it may also affect the joints, kidneys, and other organs (systemic lupus erythematosus).
Pediculosis	Lice infestation.
Psoriasis	A disorder of the skin with flare-ups of red plaques covered with thick, silvery scales mostly on the elbows, knees, and scalp.
Scleroderma	Autoimmune disease that causes connective tissue to harden; the skin becomes hard and tight.
Tinea	A fungal infection: • Tinea capitis (head) • Tinea pedis (foot): "athlete's foot" • Tinea corporis (body) • Tinea cruris (groin): "jock itch"
Urticaria	Hives; wheals caused by an allergic reaction.
Verrucae	Warts; caused by the human papilloma virus.
Vitiligo	An autoimmune disease characterized by a loss of melanin, resulting in white spots on the skin.

Table 5-4 Dermatologic Lesions

Lesion	Description
Abrasion	Scrape
Atrophy	Thinning of the skin, with wrinkling
Avulsion	A tearing away of the skin
Bulla	Large, fluid-filled blister in the epidermis
Cyst	A subcutaneous sac filled with fluid
Erosion	Skin breakdown in the epidermal layer
Eschar	Scab
Excoriation	Scratch
Fissure	Linear break in skin
Keloid	Abnormally raised and thickened scar; genetic predisposition
Macule	Flat lesion, <1 cm
Nevus	Benign mole
Nodule	Well-defined, raised lesion, >1 cm
Papule	Raised lesion, <1 cm
Patch	Flat lesion, >1 cm
Plaque	Raised lesion, >1 cm
Pustule	Small area filled with pus in the epidermis
Scale	Flaking stratum corneum
Telangiectasia	Prominent, superficial capillary
Ulcer	Skin breakdown through the epidermis
Vesicle	Small, fluid-filled blister in the epidermis
Wheal	Raised bump that itches, often caused by an allergic reaction (hive)

MUSCULOSKELETAL SYSTEM

Diseases of the musculoskeletal system can affect the body's muscles, joints, tendons, ligaments, and nerves. The musculoskeletal system can be further divided into the muscular system and the skeletal system.

Muscular System

Some of the common diseases and pathology of the muscular system are found in Table 5-5. Skeletal muscle dysfunction may involve pathology to any of the components of the motor unit. The motor unit includes the somatic nerve innervating the skeletal muscle, the neuromuscular junction in which the nerve and muscle communicate, and the muscle itself. For example, myasthenia gravis affects the neuromuscular junction whereas muscular dystrophy causes damage to the muscle fibers.

Skeletal System

The pathology of the skeletal system is diverse. Tables 5-6, 5-7, and 5-8, provide information about various diseases of the skeletal system that may be seen on the exam.

The spine has normal curvatures that develop in infancy as a result of lifting the head and walking. Each of the naturally occurring and normal soft curves serves to distribute mechanical stress incurred as the body is at rest and during movement. There are three main abnormal curvatures of the spine, which are listed in Table 5-6.

Table 5-5 Common Diseases of the Muscular System

Disease	Description
Atrophy	Weakness and wasting of the muscle; may be a symptom indicative of a pathologic disease
Fasciitis (also spelled as fascitis)	Inflammation of the fascia; typically seen in plantar fasciitis, a painful inflammatory condition of the foot caused by excessive wear to the plantar fascia that supports the arch
Fibromyalgia	A syndrome of unknown cause characterized by uncontrollable fatigue and widespread pain in the muscles, ligaments, and tendons
Muscular dystrophy	An inherited muscle disorder that causes muscular weakness without affecting the nervous system
Myasthenia gravis	A chronic autoimmune disease that affects the neuromuscular junction and produces serious weakness of voluntary muscles
Sprain	An injury to a ligament as a result of overstretching
Strain	An injury to a muscle as a result of overstretching
Tendonitis	Inflammation of the tendons caused by excessive use of the joint

Table 5-6 Abnormal Curvatures of the Spine

Curvature	Description
Kyphosis	Outward curvature of the thoracic spine; "humpback" or "dowager's hump"
Lordosis	Inward curvature of the lumbar spine; "swayback"
Scoliosis	Lateral, sideways curvature of the whole spine; "c"- or "s"-shaped curve of the spine

Table 5-7 Arthritis

Type of Arthritis	Description
Gout	Excess uric acid in the body causing pain and inflammation of the joints, typically in the big toe of middle-aged men.
Osteoarthritis	Arthritis associated with aging; "wear and tear" arthritis.
Rheumatoid arthritis	Autoimmune arthritis usually seen in young to middle-aged women; the synovial membranes of the joints are inflamed and thickened.
Septic arthritis	A serious bloodstream bacterial infection attacking the joints.

Arthritis is an inflammatory condition of one or more joints. There are many forms and causes of arthritis. Table 5-7 provides a list of the more comment forms.

Fractures are breaks in the bone. The various types are listed in Table 5-8.

Congenital disorders are abnormal conditions that exist at the time of birth. Various factors may contribute to these disorders including prenatal influences, genetic and chromosomal abnormalities, premature birth, or injuries during birth. Two more common congenital disorders are cleft palate and spina bifida. Cleft palate is a congenital deformity in which the maxillary bone fails to close, leaving an opening in the roof of the mouth; it may also involve the upper lip and hard or soft palate. Spina bifida is a congenital deformity in which there is a malformation of the vertebrae (the spine fails to close properly during the early stages of pregnancy) and the spinal cord may be exposed. It is the most common neural tube defect.

Table 5-8 Fractures

Fracture	Description
Closed (simple)	Broken bone but *no* open wound in the skin.
Colles'	A fracture of the wrist (the distal radius); occurs when falling with an outstretched arm.
Comminuted	Bone is crushed into small pieces.
Compound (open)	Broken bone *with* an open wound in the skin.
Compression	A spontaneous fracture in which the bone is pressed together (typically seen in osteoporosis of the spine).
Greenstick	Bone is bent or partially broken; occurs in children.
Impacted	Broken ends of the bone are forced into each other.
Oblique	Fracture occurs at an angle.
Pathologic	Bone breaks because of a disease process (e.g., cancer).
Spiral	Bone breaks in a twisting motion (sports injury).
Stress	Small break in a bone because of chronic, excessive overuse (e.g., running).
Transverse	Bone breaks straight across.

Two other common skeletal diseases are osteomyelitis and osteoporosis. Osteomyelitis is the inflammation of the bone marrow and adjacent bone. Osteoporosis is decreased bone density associated with aging, especially in women.

NERVOUS SYSTEM

A wide variety of diseases affect the nervous system. Table 5-9 describes some of the more common diseases and conditions seen on the exam.

Table 5-9 Common Diseases of the Nervous System

Disease	Description
Alzheimer's disease	Degenerative changes in the brain that lead to progressive memory loss, impaired cognition, and personality changes; etiology is unknown.
Amyotrophic lateral sclerosis (ALS, Lou Gehrig's disease)	Degenerative disease of the motor nerves that innervate the muscles; patients become progressively weaker until they are completely paralyzed.
Bell's palsy	Paralysis of the seventh cranial nerve (facial nerve) that causes drooping of one side of the face; may be temporary.
Cerebral palsy	Congenital condition characterized by poor muscle control, spasticity, speech defects, and other neurologic deficiencies.
Cerebrovascular accident (CVA)	Damage to the brain that occurs when blood flow is disrupted; also called a stroke.
Dementia	A slowly progressive decline in mental abilities including memory, thinking, judgment, and personality changes.
Encephalitis	Inflammation of the brain.
Epilepsy	A condition in which a person has recurrent seizures.

(continues)

Table 5-9 Common Diseases of the Nervous System (Continued)

Disease	Description
Guillain-Barré syndrome	Inflammation of the myelin sheath in the peripheral nerves that leads to muscle weakness and possible paralysis.
Hydrocephalus	Abnormally increased cerebrospinal fluid (CSF) within the ventricles of the brain.
Multiple sclerosis	Autoimmune disorder in which there is progressive inflammation and hardening of the myelin sheath of nerve fibers in the brain and spinal cord; may cause loss of balance, fatigue, paralysis, and speech disturbances.
Parkinson's disease	A chronic, degenerative central nervous system disease characterized by slowing of movement, tremors, pill-rolling, shuffling gait, and little or no facial expression; symptoms tend to worsen as the disease progresses.
Poliomyelitis	A viral disease (poliovirus) that causes paralysis; preventable by the vaccine; children in the United States are now routinely vaccinated against the disease.
Sciatica	Inflammation of the sciatic nerve causing pain in the lower back, buttock, and/or various parts of the leg and foot.
Transient ischemic attack (TIA)	Temporary interruption of the blood supply to the brain; TIA symptoms are the same as those of stroke, only temporary; "mini-stroke."

CARDIOVASCULAR SYSTEM

Disorders of the heart may affect one of four things: the muscle itself, the electrical conduction system (which causes it to beat), the valves (which help the blood to flow correctly), or the blood supply to the heart (giving it the oxygen it needs to function). Table 5-10 illustrates the more common diseases of the cardiovascular system. Disorders of the blood vessels are described in Table 5-11.

Table 5-10 Cardiovascular Diseases

Disease	Description
Angina pectoris	Episodes of severe chest pain because of inadequate blood flow to the myocardium.
Arrhythmia	A change in the rhythm of the heartbeat; many types exist, some are life threatening.
Congenital heart disease	A malformation in one or more structures of the heart or major blood vessels that occurs before birth; many types exist. Symptoms may appear at birth, during childhood, or sometimes not until adulthood.
Congestive heart failure	A syndrome in which the heart is unable to pump enough blood to meet the body's needs. Fluid builds up in the lungs (pulmonary edema) and/or the abdomen and lower legs.
Heart valve disease (prolapse and stenosis)	Valvular prolapse is the abnormal protrusion of the valve so that it cannot close properly. Valvular stenosis involves abnormal narrowing of the valve so that it cannot open properly. Both conditions affect blood flow through the heart.
Myocardial infarct	A blockage of one or more of the coronary arteries so that the myocardium does not get enough oxygen to pump blood throughout the body; also called a "heart attack."
Rheumatic heart disease	Inflammation and dysfunction of the heart valves that results from rheumatic fever. Rheumatic fever begins with a strep throat from an untreated streptococcal infection.

Table 5-11 Disorders of the Blood Vessels

Disease	Description
Aneurysm	A localized weak spot of balloon-like enlargement of an artery; abdominal aorta and brain aneurysms are most common.
Arteriosclerosis	Abnormal hardening of the walls of an artery.
Embolus	A foreign object that travels through the bloodstream, lodges in a blood vessel, and blocks it; emboli may be composed of blood, a quantity of air or gas, a bit of tissue, fat, or tumor.
Hypertension	Abnormally elevated blood pressure (above 140/90); untreated hypertension is a risk factor for stroke, atherosclerosis, heart failure, and kidney disease.
Thrombus	A blood clot attached to the interior wall of an artery or vein.

HEMATOPOIETIC SYSTEM

Diseases of the hematopoietic system affect blood cells. Table 5-12 discusses various diseases of the blood.

Anemia is one of the more common blood disorders; it occurs when the level of healthy red blood cells (RBCs) in the body becomes too low. This can lead to health problems because RBCs contain hemoglobin, which carries oxygen to the body's tissues. Anemia can cause a variety of symptoms, including fatigue, paleness, dizziness, irritability, numb/cold hands or feet, and arrythmias. Some of the various types of anemias are described in Table 5-13.

Table 5-12 Diseases of the Blood

Disease	Description
Anemia	A disorder characterized by low levels of red blood cells circulating in the blood; many causes and types of anemia exist, as seen in Table 5-13.
Hemophilia	A hereditary condition in which one of the clotting factors is missing so that a person bleeds uncontrollably.
Leukemia	A malignancy characterized by an increased number of abnormal white blood cells.
Multiple myeloma	A malignancy in which plasma cells (which produce antibodies) invade bone marrow.

Table 5-13 Types of Anemia

Anemia	Description
Anemia of chronic disease	A chronic infection or inflammation or malignancy causes an abnormally increased demand for new RBCs.
Aplastic anemia	Failure of blood cell production in the bone marrow causes the absence of all blood cells, including RBCs.
Hemolytic anemia	RBCs are destroyed more rapidly than the bone marrow can replace them.
Iron-deficiency anemia	Too little iron causes a decrease in the production of RBCs; may be caused by inadequate iron intake, chronic blood loss, pregnancy, or lactation.
Megaloblastic anemia	A deficiency of folic acid or vitamin B_{12} causes an abnormal production of RBCs that are bigger than normal and dysfunctional.
Pernicious anemia	An autoimmune disorder in which the RBCs are abnormally formed due to the inability to absorb vitamin B_{12}; vitamin B_{12} injections are needed.
Sickle cell anemia	A genetic anemia characterized by sickle-shaped RBCs that break down faster then normal red blood cells; most often seen in people of African descent.
Thalassemia	A genetic anemia characterized by absent or decreased production of normal hemoglobin.

LYMPHATIC AND IMMUNE SYSTEM

An autoimmune disorder is one in which the immune system reacts incorrectly and inappropriately to the body's own antigens. Abnormal antibodies are produced against the body's own tissues, which results in various symptoms. Many of the body systems are affected. Table 5-14 describes some of the more common autoimmune diseases. Other diseases of the lymphatic and immune system are found in Table 5-15.

The cause of autoimmune diseases is unknown, but it appears that in many cases there is an inherited predisposition to develop autoimmune disease. For reasons that are not understood, autoimmune diseases tend to affect women more during the childbearing years.

Table 5-14 Autoimmune Diseases

Autoimmune Disorder	System	Description
Alopecia areata	Integumentary	Autoimmune disorder in which there is disruption of normal hair formation; hair loss results.
Lupus erythematosus	Integumentary	Autoimmune disorder characterized by a red, scaly rash on the face and upper trunk; it may also affect the joints, kidneys, and other organs (systemic lupus erythematosus).
Scleroderma	Integumentary	Autoimmune disease that causes connective tissue to harden; the skin becomes hard and tight.
Vitiligo	Integumentary	Autoimmune disease characterized by a loss of melanin, resulting in white spots on the skin.
Myasthenia gravis	Muscular	Chronic autoimmune disease that affects the neuromuscular junction and produces serious weakness of voluntary muscles.
Rheumatoid arthritis	Skeletal	Autoimmune arthritis usually seen in young to middle-aged women; the synovial membranes of the joints are inflamed and thickened.
Multiple sclerosis	Nervous	Autoimmune disorder in which there is progressive inflammation and hardening of the myelin sheath of nerve fibers in the brain and spinal cord; may cause loss of balance, fatigue, paralysis, and speech disturbances.
Pernicious anemia	Hematopoietic	Autoimmune disorder in which the RBCs are abnormally formed due to the inability to absorb vitamin B_{12}; vitamin B_{12} injections are needed.
Graves' disease	Endocrine	Autoimmune *hyperthyroidism*; body inappropriately stimulates the thyroid gland; symptoms of hyperthyroidism along with goiter and exophthalmos may be seen.
Hashimoto's thyroiditis	Endocrine	Autoimmune *hypothyroidism*; body inappropriately attacks the thyroid gland; symptoms of hypothyroidism may be seen.
Type 1 diabetes mellitus	Endocrine	Insulin-dependent diabetes mellitus (IDDM); high blood sugar due to autoimmune destruction of insulin-producing beta cells of the pancreas; treatment is with exogenous insulin, usually via injections.

RESPIRATORY SYSTEM

Diseases of the respiratory system may affect the upper respiratory tract (nose, pharynx, epiglottis, larynx, and trachea) or the lower respiratory tract (bronchial tree and lungs). Respiratory diseases range from mild and self-limiting, such as the common cold, to more life-threatening, such as bacterial pneumonia or pulmonary edema. Common diseases are listed in Table 5-16.

Table 5-15 Diseases of the Lymphatic and Immune Systems

Disease	Description	
Acquired immune deficiency syndrome (AIDS)	The advanced stage of an HIV infection characterized by unusual opportunistic infections and tumors.	
Lymphoma	A general term applied to malignancies that develop in the lymphatic system; the two most common types are Hodgkin's lymphoma and non-Hodgkin's lymphoma.	
	Hodgkin's lymphoma: Cancer originating from white blood cells; characterized by the presence of Reed-Sternberg cells on microscopic examination.	*Non-Hodgkin's lymphoma:* A diverse group of cancers that include any lymphoma other than Hodgkin's lymphoma.
Mononucleosis	Infection caused by the Epstein-Barr virus; symptoms include constant fatigue, fever, sore throat, loss of appetite, and swollen lymph nodes.	

Table 5-16 Respiratory System Diseases

Disease	Description	
Asthma	A chronic allergic disorder characterized by episodes of severe breathing difficulty, coughing, and wheezing.	
Bronchitis	Inflammation of the bronchial walls characterized by coughing.	
Chronic obstructive pulmonary disease (COPD)	A general term used to describe diseases characterized by chronic airflow limitations, namely chronic bronchitis and emphysema. COPD is usually caused by smoking and is a common source of respiratory problems and death in the United States.	
	Chronic bronchitis: Breathing is difficult because of inflammation, irritation, and mucus in the bronchial airways; patients commonly are referred to as "blue bloaters" because of the bluish color of the skin and lips.	*Emphysema:* Breathing is difficult because of destruction of alveolar walls with enlargement of the remaining alveoli; patients tend to have a pink color to their face because of the effort to exhale, and may be called "pink puffers."
Croup	An acute respiratory syndrome with a barking cough because of obstruction of the larynx; seen primarily in infants and children.	
Cystic fibrosis	A genetic disorder in which the lungs and pancreas are clogged with large quantities of abnormally thick mucus.	
Pertussis	A bacterial infection of the upper respiratory tract with recurrent episodes of paroxysmal cough; also called whooping cough because of the sound of the cough; can be prevented by vaccination.	
Pharyngitis	Inflammation of the pharynx; also called sore throat.	
Pleurisy	Inflammation of the pleura that produces sharp chest pain with every breath; also called pleuritis.	
Pneumonia	A serious infection of the lungs in which the bronchials and alveoli fill with pus and fluid; the infection may be caused by bacteria, viruses, fungi, or parasites. Symptoms include cough, chest pain, fever, and difficulty in breathing.	

(continues)

Table 5-16 Respiratory System Diseases (Continued)

Disease	Description
Pneumothorax	Accumulation of air in the pleural space, which causes a pressure imbalance and may cause the lung to collapse.
Pulmonary edema	Fluid in the lungs due to either heart failure (with backup of fluid in the lungs) or direct injury to the lung itself; the main symptom is difficulty breathing.
Pulmonary embolism	The blockage of a pulmonary artery usually occurring when a venous thrombus from one of the deep veins of the legs becomes dislodged and travels to the lungs; may cause sudden death.
Tuberculosis (TB)	Infectious lung disease caused by *Mycobacterium tuberculosis*; spread by respiratory droplets.

DIGESTIVE SYSTEM

The digestive system is made up of the alimentary canal, which starts at the mouth and ends at the anus. It is made up of a series of muscles that coordinate the movement of food and other cells that produce enzymes and hormones to aid in the breakdown of food. Along the way are three other organs that are needed for digestion: the liver, gallbladder, and pancreas. Digestive diseases and disorders are diverse. Some of the more common ones are described in Table 5-17.

Table 5-17 Digestive Diseases and Disorders

Disease	Description
Adhesions	Scar tissue that binds two different parts of tissue/organs together; classically seen after abdominal surgery.
Anorexia	The loss of appetite for food; may be caused by disease (e.g., cancer) or psychosis (e.g., anorexia nervosa).
Appendicitis	Inflammation of the appendix; a medical emergency; classic symptoms are right lower quadrant pain (McBurney's point tenderness), fever, and vomiting.
Botulism	Food poisoning characterized by paralysis and possible death; caused by the bacteria *Clostridium botulinum*.
Cholelithiasis	Gallstones in the gallbladder or bile ducts; symptoms range from asymptomatic to intense pain in the upper abdominal region and between the shoulder blades with possible nausea and vomiting.
Cirrhosis	End stage liver disease in which scar tissue replaces normal liver; symptoms include jaundice, portal hyertension, and failure of liver function.
Diverticulitis	Inflamed, abnormal pouches in the wall of the colon.
Gastroesophageal reflux disease (GERD)	Abnormal reflux of stomach acid and juices into the esophagus.
Giardia	Infectious diarrhea caused by *Giardia lamblia* found in contaminated water.
Hemorrhoids	Painful, inflamed, dilated veins in the rectum and anus.
Hepatitis	Inflammation of the liver; can be either acute or chronic depending on the type (A, B, C, D, or E).

(continues)

Table 5-17 Digestive Diseases and Disorders (Continued)

Disease	Description	
Inflammatory bowel disease	Refers to two chronic diseases that cause inflammation of the intestines: Crohn's disease and ulcerative colitis.	
	Crohn's disease: Can attack any part of the digestive tract, most commonly the last part of the small and some parts of the large intestine; Crohn's disease causes inflammation that extends much deeper into the layers of the intestinal wall than ulcerative colitis.	*Ulcerative colitis:* Only the mucosa lining reddens and swells and develops ulcers; most often in the rectal area, which can cause frequent diarrhea, and mucus and blood in the stool.
Intussusception	One section of the intestine telescopes into another section, causing blockage and potential gangrene.	
Irritable bowel syndrome	Refers to a group of symptoms in which the colon doesn't function correctly, causing cramping, bloating, gas, diarrhea, and/or constipation.	
Jaundice	A yellow discoloration of the skin and eyes caused by greater-than-normal amounts of bilirubin in the blood.	
Peptic ulcer disease	Lesions of the mucosa, most often in the duodenum or the stomach; many are associated with infection of *Helicobacter pylori* bacteria.	
Pyloric stenosis	Hypertrophy of the pylorus muscle, which causes obstruction of the stomach outlet and projectile vomiting; most often seen in infants.	
Thrush	An infection caused by the candida fungus, also known as yeast; it can occur in the mouth of breastfed infants, in the diaper area, or as vaginal yeast infections in women.	
Volvulus	A loop of bowel abnormally twisted on itself.	

URINARY SYSTEM

The urinary system produces, stores, and eliminates urine. Disease may affect the kidneys, ureters, bladder, or urethra. Common diseases are listed in Table 5-18.

Table 5-18 Urinary System Diseases

Disease	Description
Enuresis	Involuntary discharge of urine.
Glomerulonephritis	Acute or chronic inflammation of the kidney glomeruli; symptoms include edema, hematuria, and proteinuria.
Hydronephrosis	Distention and dilation of the kidney with urine, caused by backward pressure on the kidney when the flow of urine is obstructed.
Incontinence	The inability to control excretory functions.
Polycystic kidney disease	A genetic disorder in which the kidneys are enlarged with multiple cysts; may lead to kidney failure.
Pyelonephritis	An infection of the renal pelvis and kidney, usually from bacteria that have spread from the bladder.
Renal calculi	Kidney stones; pain is a main symptom.
Renal failure	Loss of kidney function, from either an acute situation or chronic problems.
Uremia	A toxic condition caused by excessive amounts of urea and waste products in the blood.

REPRODUCTIVE SYSTEM

Some of the common diseases and pathology of the male and female reproductive systems are described in Tables 5-19 and 5-20, respectively. There may be questions on the exam about sexually transmitted diseases (STDs). STDs are diseases that are passed from one person to another during sex (vaginal, anal, and oral sex). There are at least 25 different sexually transmitted diseases that can affect both men and women with a range of different symptoms. Some of the more common ones are described in Table 5-21.

Table 5-19 Male Reproductive Disorders

Disease	Description
Benign prostatic hypertrophy (BPH)	Enlargement of the prostate that is not malignant.
Cryptorchidism	During fetal development, the testes fail to descend into the scrotum.
Hypospadias, epispadias	Congenital abnormality of the placement of the urethral opening; in hypospadias, the urethral opening is on the under surface of the penis. In epispadias, the urethral opening is on the upper surface of the penis.
Impotence	Erectile dysfunction in which there is inability to achieve or maintain penile erection.
Phimosis	Tightness of the foreskin so that it cannot be fully retracted from the head of the penis.
Priaprism	Abnormal, painful erection lasting more than 4 hours and not caused by sexual excitement.
Prostate cancer	Symptoms range from nothing to difficulty urinating and erectile dysfunction; may be diagnosed with the PSA (prostate-specific antigen) blood test.
Testicular cancer	Usually discovered by testicular examination.

Table 5-20 Female Reproductive Disorders

Disease	Description
Abruptio placentae	An abnormal condition in which the placenta separates from the uterine wall before the birth of the fetus.
Amenorrhea	The absence of menstrual periods for three or more months.
Carcinomas	Five main types: cervical, ovarian, uterine, vaginal, and vulvar; as a group, they are referred to as gynecologic cancer. (A sixth type—fallopian tube cancer—is very rare.) Each gynecologic cancer is unique, with different signs and symptoms; a woman's risk of getting gynecologic cancer increases with age.
Eclampsia/preeclampsia	Toxemia of pregnancy characterized by hypertension, edema, and proteinuria.
Ectopic pregnancy	Pregnancy outside of the uterus, most often in the fallopian tubes.
Endometriosis	A condition in which patches of endometrial tissue attach to other organs in the pelvic cavity; a leading cause of infertility.
Erythroblastosis fetalis	Also called hemolytic disease of the newborn; a pregnant mom and her baby have different blood types and she produces antibodies that attack the developing baby's red blood cells.
Fibroid	Benign tumors in the walls of the uterus; also called leiomyoma.

(continues)

Table 5-20 Female Reproductive Disorders (Continued)

Disease	Description
Pelvic inflammatory disease (PID)	Inflammation of the female reproductive organs as a result of untreated sexually transmitted disease; causes infertility.
Placenta previa	Abnormal implantation of the placenta in the lower uterus; may cause sudden, painless bleeding during the third trimester.
Premenstrual syndrome (PMS)	A group of symptoms experienced by some women prior to menstruation; symptoms include bloating, edema, headaches, mood swings, and breast discomfort.
Toxic shock syndrome	Caused by the bacteria *Staphylococcus aureus* and has been associated with the use of tampons.
Yeast vaginitis	Caused by the fungus (yeast) *Candida albicans* when the immune response is weakened, especially in the vagina, causing a yeast infection, often characterized by vaginal itching and a cheese-like discharge or in the mouth, causing oral thrush, often seen in babies characterized by white deposits in the mucosal membranes.

Table 5-21 Sexually Transmitted Diseases

Disease	Description
AIDS	The advanced stage of an HIV infection characterized by unusual opportunistic infections and tumors; no cure.
Chlamydia	Most common STD; caused by the bacteria *Chlamydia trachomatis*. It may be undetected and, unless treated with antibiotics, can cause sterility in females and urethritis in males.
Gonorrhea	Caused by the bacteria *Neisseria gonorrhoeae*; characterized by painful urination and abnormal discharge from the penis or vagina.
Herpes (genital)	Caused by the herpes simplex virus; symptoms include itching, burning, and sores; antiviral drugs may ease symptoms but there is no cure.
HIV	Caused by the human immunodeficiency virus; patients are susceptible to many illnesses and opportunistic infections; one of the biggest health concerns globally and in the United States.
Syphilis	Caused by the bacteria *Treponema pallidum*; may progress through three stages: primary causes a chancre; secondary causes a rash; tertiary causes gummas (granulomas) and a chronic inflammatory state in the body.
Warts (genital)	Caused by human papilloma virus; the virus increases the risk for cervical cancer.

ENDOCRINE SYSTEM

Diseases of the endocrine system are dependent on the gland involved. Table 5-22 lists the diseases of the pituitary gland, Table 5-23 the pineal gland, Table 5-24 the thyroid gland, Table 5-25 the parathyroid gland, and Table 5-26 the adrenal cortex.

Thyroid Gland

Thyroid disease occurs when the thyroid gland doesn't supply the proper amount of hormones needed by the body. If the thyroid is overactive, it releases too much thyroid hormone into the bloodstream, resulting in hyperthyroidism. If the thyroid is underactive, it produces too little thyroid hormone, resulting in hypothyroidism.

General Knowledge

Table 5-22 Diseases of the Pituitary Gland

Disease	Description
Acromegaly	Excessive secretion of growth hormone (GH) *after* puberty; causes enlargement of the face, hands, and feet
Gigantism	Excessive secretion of growth hormone (GH) *before* puberty; causes abnormal overgrowth of the body
Diabetes insipidus	Insufficient production of antidiuretic hormone (ADH); causes abnormal increase in urine output, fluid intake, and thirst

Table 5-23 Disease of the Pineal Gland

Disease	Description
Seasonal affective disorder (SAD)	Excessive production of melatonin during dark, winter months; causes depression

Table 5-24 Diseases of the Thyroid Gland

Disease	Description
Cretinism	A congenital form of hypothyroidism; if not treated immediately, can cause mental and physical retardation.
Goiter	Enlarged and swollen thyroid gland; may be the result of either hyperthyroidism or hypothyroidism.
Graves' disease	Autoimmune *hyperthyroidism*; the body inappropriately stimulates the thyroid gland. Symptoms of hyperthyroidism along with goiter and exophthalmos may be seen. The most common form of hyperthyroidism.
Hashimoto's thyroiditis	Autoimmune *hypothyroidism*; the body inappropriately attacks the thyroid gland. Symptoms of hypothyroidism may be seen.
Hyperthyroidism	Overactive thyroid; symptoms include trouble sleeping, nervousness, trouble getting pregnant, frequent bowel movements, irritability, increased metabolic rate (weight loss without dieting), sweating, changes in vision, light menstrual flow, tachycardia, and hand tremors.
Hypothyroidism	Underactive thyroid; symptoms include fatigue, depression, sensitivity to cold, and decreased metabolic rate (weight gain).
Myxedema	Severe, prolonged hypothyroidism; causes edema and puffiness of the hands and face.

Table 5-25 Disease of the Parathyroid Gland

Disease	Description
Hyperparathyroidism	Increased parathyroid hormone (PTH) causes very high calcium levels in the blood; symptoms are diverse and include loss of energy, changes in personality, osteoporosis, pain in the bones, and kidney stones.
Hypoparathyroidism	Decreased parathyroid hormone (PTH) causes very low calcium levels in the blood; symptoms include painful muscle cramps which may lead to tetany and tremors or convulsions (increased nervous excitability).

102

Table 5-26 Diseases of the Adrenal Cortex

Disease	Description
Addison's disease	Adrenal cortex *does not produce enough* cortisol; symptoms include muscle atrophy, tissue weakness, and increased skin pigmentation.
Cushing's syndrome	Adrenal cortex *produces too much* cortisol (or patient overdoses on glucocorticoid hormone medication used to treat asthma or rheumatoid arthritis); symptoms include "moon" round face, fat pad on the back of the neck ("buffalo hump"), excessive weight gain, thin skin, and high blood sugar.

Table 5-27 Types of Diabetes

Disease	Description
Diabetes mellitus type 1	Insulin-dependent diabetes mellitus (IDDM); high blood sugar due to autoimmune destruction of insulin-producing beta cells of the pancreas; treatment is with exogenous insulin, usually via injections.
Diabetes mellitus type 2	Non-insulin-dependent diabetes mellitus (NIDDM); high blood sugar due to the body developing resistance to insulin, so it cannot properly use what it produces; typically seen in the obese population; treatment is initially with diet and exercise.

Table 5-28 Diabetic Emergencies

Diabetic Emergency	Description
Diabetic ketoacidosis (can lead to diabetic coma)	Caused by extremely high blood sugar; treatment is prompt administration of insulin.
Insulin shock	Caused by extremely low blood sugar; treatment is prompt administration of juice/sugar.

Pancreas

Diabetes mellitus is a very common endocrine disorder, one in which the pancreas does not function correctly. Table 5-27 describes the two types of diabetes. Common early signs of diabetes are polydipsia (excessive thirst), polyuria (frequent urination), polyphagia (excessive hunger), sudden weight loss, and fatigue. However, these early symptoms of diabetes may go unrecognized, and serious problems may arise such as heart disease and stroke, diabetic nephropathy (renal disease), retinopathy (disease of the retinal vessels), blurred vision (macular degeneration and eventual blindness), peripheral neuropathy (numbness and/or tingling in the hands and feet), slow healing of minor scratches and wounds (impaired immune system function), and dry or itchy skin (peripheral neuropathy also affects circulation and proper sweat gland function). These complications of diabetes are related to chronic levels of high blood sugar.

Diabetic emergencies are due to either too much or too little blood sugar. Diabetic emergencies include diabetic ketoacidosis and insulin shock which are described in Table 5-28.

SPECIAL SENSES: THE EYES AND EARS

Table 5-29 lists some of the more common eye diseases, and Table 5-30 lists the most common ear disorders. Both the eye and ear are complex and sensitive structures. Thus, diseases of these special sense organs tend to be complicated and diverse.

Table 5-29 Common Eye Diseases

Disease	Description
Astigmatism	Impaired vision because of uneven curvatures of the cornea; corrected with glasses.
Cataract	Loss of transparency of the lens; corrected with surgery.
Conjunctivitis	Infection or allergy causing inflammation of the conjunctiva; "pink eye."
Diabetic retinopathy	Poorly controlled diabetes leads to hemorrhage and damage of the retinal vessels.
Exophthalmia	Abnormal protrusion of the eyes, typically seen with thyroid disease.
Glaucoma	Increased intraocular pressure causes damage to the optic nerve and potential blindness; treatments include medication (eye drops and pills), laser procedures, and incisional surgery.
Macular degeneration	Loss of central vision because of abnormal growth of blood vessels or other materials in the macula; potential blindness is slowed by laser surgery.
Strabismus	Eyes point in different directions because the eye muscles are unable to focus; "lazy eye" or "cross-eyed."

Table 5-30 Common Ear Disorders

Disease	Description
Deafness	Complete or partial loss of hearing.
Ménière's disease	Dizziness, loss of balance, deafness; unknown cause; treatment is for relief of the symptoms.
Otitis media	Inflammation and infection of the middle ear; common in toddlers and treated with antibiotics.
Otosclerosis	Stiffening of the bones in the middle ear, which results in hearing loss; surgery may improve condition.
Tinnitus	A ringing sound in one or both ears.
Vertigo	Sensation of dizziness, loss of balance, and spinning; may be seen with nausea and/or vomiting.

QUESTIONS

5-1. A pregnant woman in the third trimester presents with swelling of the legs and headaches. Her blood pressure is elevated and urinalysis showed 4+ protein. These findings are most consistent with which of the following conditions?

    A. Miscarriage
    B. Abruptio placentae
    C. Endometriosis
    D. Preeclampsia
    E. Ectopic pregnancy

5-2. The pediatrician tells the parents that their child has a greenstick fracture. In layman's terms, what is a greenstick fracture?

    A. A break that can be seen with a bone scan but not an ordinary x-ray
    B. A break in which the bone is crushed
    C. A break that results in the broken edges of the bone piercing and/or tearing the skin
    D. Any break in the bone
    E. A partial break that results in one side of the broken bone bending

5-3. Osteoporosis

    A. is the thickening of bone due to excessive calcitonin production.

    B. may be prevented by swimming regularly.

    C. affects women, men, and children equally.

    D. is treated primarily through administration of testosterone.

    E. is a condition in which bone resorption exceeds bone deposition.

5-4. A young boy was bitten by a wild dog and contracted rabies. He subsequently suffered from fever, headache, photophobia, and seizures. An MRI showed inflammation of the brain. He is suffering from

    A. encephalitis.

    B. cerebral palsy.

    C. poliomyelitis.

    D. cerebral palsy.

    E. Bell's palsy.

5-5. Which of the following conditions is characterized by a shuffling gait, tremors, pill-rolling, and muscular rigidity?

    A. Parkinson's disease

    B. Cerebral palsy

    C. Hydrocephalus

    D. Epilepsy

    E. Alzheimer's disease

5-6. Which of the following conditions is a neural tube defect?

    A. Osteomyelitis

    B. Poliomyelitis

    C. Spina bifida

    D. Cleft palate

    E. Cerebral palsy

5-7. Which of the following dermatologic conditions is caused by a bacterial infection?

    A. Eczema

    B. Herpes zoster

    C. Pediculosis

    D. Impetigo

    E. Tinea pedis

5-8. Pelvic inflammatory disease is managed aggressively because long-term effects can include

    A. Preterm labor

    B. Renal failure

    C. Infertility

    D. Transmission to the fetus

    E. Toxic shock syndrome

5-9. A 21-year-old female is infected with HPV (human papilloma virus) following unprotected sexual intercourse. She is now at higher risk of developing which of the following cancers?

    A. Breast

    B. Ovarian

    C. Endometrial

    D. Vulvar

    E. Cervical

5-10. A 54-year-old male was recently diagnosed with osteoarthritis. Which of the following symptoms is he most likely experiencing?

    A. Redness of the joints
    B. Hypermobility of joints
    C. Contractures
    D. Joint pain
    E. Headaches

5-11. Which disease is characterized by thick, silvery, scaly, erythematous plaques surrounded by normal skin?

    A. Acne vulgaris
    B. Lupus erythematosus
    C. Psoriasis
    D. Pityriasis rosea
    E. Vitiligo

5-12. A 50-year-old male recently underwent a liver transplant and is taking immunosuppressive drugs. He now has pain and vesicular eruptions on the trunk that follow one nerve line. He reports that he had chickenpox as a child. Which of the following is the most likely diagnosis?

    A. Erysipelas
    B. Poliomyelitis
    C. Warts
    D. Herpes zoster
    E. Psoriasis

5-13. An 11-year-old male is newly diagnosed with type 1 diabetes mellitus. Before treatment he most likely experienced

    A. recurrent infections, fatigue, and paresthesias.
    B. polydipsia, polyuria, polyphagia, and weight loss.
    C. abdominal pain; sweet, fruity breath; and Kussmaul breathing.
    D. weakness, vomiting, hypotension, and mental confusion.
    E. numbness and blurred vision.

5-14. Congenital hypothyroidism that is not managed is a serious concern because of the risk for

    A. tetanus.
    B. respiratory distress.
    C. seizures.
    D. mental retardation.
    E. heart disease.

5-15. Graves' disease is an autoimmune disease in which there is excess _____ hormone secretion.

    A. growth
    B. antidiuretic
    C. parathyroid
    D. cortisol
    E. thyroid

5-16. An autoimmune disease that blocks the acetylcholine receptors of the sarcolemma, causing extreme muscle weakness, is

    A. infectious mononucleosis.
    B. myasthenia gravis.
    C. muscular dystrophy.

D. tetanus.

E. multiple sclerosis.

5-17. Which of the following viruses causes infectious mononucleosis?

    A. Human papilloma virus

    B. Human immunodeficiency virus

    C. Influenza virus

    D. Herpes simplex virus

    E. Epstein-Barr virus

5-18. Which of the following STDs is viral?

    A. Gonorrhea

    B. Chlamydia

    C. Syphilis

    D. Genital herpes

5-19. Which of the following disorders is associated with upper gastrointestinal bleeding?

    A. Diverticulosis

    B. Demorrhoids

    C. Esophageal varices

    D. Colon cancer

    E. Crohn's disease

5-20. All of the following could result in a mechanical bowel obstruction EXCEPT

    A. volvulus.

    B. intussusception.

    C. adhesions.

    D. cirrhosis.

    E. impacted feces.

5-21. The cardinal sign of pyloric stenosis is

    A. constipation.

    B. watery diarrhea.

    C. projectile vomiting.

    D. heartburn.

    E. bloody stools.

5-22. Infection with *Helicobacter pylori* is associated with which of the following?

    A. Appendicitis

    B. Crohn's disease

    C. Hemorrhoids

    D. Peptic ulcer disease

    E. Cirrhosis

5-23. A patient presents with McBurney's point tenderness, a high leukocyte count, fever, and vomiting. What does this patient most likely have?

    A. Peptic ulcer disease

    B. Sickle cell anemia

    C. Chlamydia

    D. Appendicitis

    E. Rheumatic heart disease

5-24. A 28-year-old female presents with severe chest pain and shortness of breath. She is diagnosed with pulmonary embolism, which most likely originated from the

    A. left ventricle.
    B. systemic arteries.
    C. deep veins of the leg.
    D. superficial veins of the arm.
    E. brain.

5-25. The most common cause of pulmonary edema is

    A. right heart failure.
    B. left heart failure.
    C. asthma.
    D. lung cancer.
    E. pneumonia.

5-26. A 53-year-old male with a 20-year history of smoking is diagnosed with emphysema. He is having difficulty breathing because of

    A. excessive mucus production.
    B. destruction of alveolar septa.
    C. infection and inflammation.
    D. airway edema.
    E. all of the above.

5-27. A 30-year-old male prison inmate contracted tuberculosis during an outbreak. He may transmit the disease to others through

    A. skin contact.
    B. fecal-oral transmission.
    C. respiratory droplets.
    D. blood transfusions.
    E. sexual activity.

5-28. A 25-year-old female is diagnosed with urinary tract obstruction. She has not urinated for 36 hours. A renal ultrasound shows

    A. glomerulonephritis.
    B. hydronephrosis.
    C. pyelonephritis.
    D. cystitis.
    E. polycystic kidney disease.

5-29. A 60-year-old male is diagnosed with chronic renal failure. Which of the following lab values would be most consistent with this diagnosis?

    A. Elevated plasma creatinine level
    B. Decreased plasma potassium level
    C. Metabolic alkalosis
    D. Increased uric acid
    E. Increased ferritin

5-30. Hearing loss caused by stiffening of the bones of the middle ear is called

    A. strabismus.
    B. tinnitus.
    C. otitis media.
    D. Ménière's disease.
    E. otosclerosis.

ANSWERS

5-1. The correct answer is D. Preeclampsia is also known as "toxemia of pregnancy" and is characterized by hypertension, edema, and proteinuria. Typically, the condition progresses rapidly and requires immediate medical attention. Apart from abortion, caesarean section, or induction of labor, and therefore delivery of the placenta, there is no known cure. Eclampsia is the final and most severe phase of preeclampsia.

5-2. The correct answer is E. A greenstick fracture is a partial break that results in one side of the broken bone bending. Because a child's bone is more pliable, an incomplete or greenstick fracture is more likely to occur.

5-3. The correct answer is E. Osteoporosis is decreased bone density associated with aging. With aging, particularly after menopause, bone resorption gradually begins to exceed bone formation, resulting in a slow loss of bone mass. If loss of bone mass continues long enough, osteoporosis results. Osteoporosis tends to affect women more than men. Treatment includes calcium supplements, weight-bearing exercise, and menopausal hormone replacement therapy.

5-4. The correct answer is A. Encephalitis is inflammation of the brain. Rabies is one potential cause of encephalitis. Symptoms of encephalitis include fever, headache, photophobia, and seizures.

5-5. The correct answer is A. Parkinson's disease is a chronic, degenerative central nervous system disease characterized by slowing of movement, tremors, pill-rolling, shuffling gait, and little or no facial expression. Symptoms of Parkinson's disease tend to worsen as the disease progresses.

5-6. The correct answer is C. Neural tube defects are birth defects of the brain and spinal cord. Spina bifida is the most common neural tube defect. It is a congenital deformity in which there is a malformation of the vertebrae (the spine fails to close properly during the early stages of pregnancy) and the spinal cord may be exposed. Anencephaly is another, more severe neural tube defect in which the brain fails to develop.

5-7. The correct answer is D. Impetigo is a bacterial skin infection characterized by pustules that become crusted and rupture. Impetigo is generally caused by one of two bacteria: *Staphylococcus aureus* or *Streptococcus pyogenes*. Tinea is a fungal infection; pediculosis is a lice infestation; herpes zoster is a viral infection; and eczema is an inflammation of the dermis (caused by genetic and environmental influences).

5-8. The correct answer is C. Pelvic inflammatory disease is inflammation of the female reproductive organs (fallopian tubes, uterus, ovaries) as a result of untreated sexually transmitted disease, especially chlamydia and gonorrhea. PID can lead to serious consequences including infertility and ectopic pregnancy.

5-9. The correct answer is E. Exposure to the human papilloma virus (HPV) increases the risk for cervical cancer as well as genital warts.

5-10. The correct answer is D. Osteoarthritis is arthritis associated with aging and is commonly referred to as "wear and tear" arthritis. One of the main symptoms of osteoarthritis is joint pain.

5-11. The correct answer is C. Psoriasis is a disorder of the skin with flare-ups of red plaques covered with thick, silvery scales on the elbows, knees, and scalp. The plaques are surrounded by normal skin.

5-12. The correct answer is D. His diagnosis is most likely herpes zoster, commonly known as shingles. It is a viral infection caused by the *varicella zoster* virus, the same virus that causes chickenpox.

Herpes zoster occurs in people who have had chickenpox and is a reactivation of the dormant virus. The virus causes painful skin eruptions that follow the underlying route of the inflamed nerve.

5-13. The correct answer is B. Early symptoms of diabetes are polydipsia (excessive thirst), polyuria (frequent urination), polyphagia (excessive hunger), and weight loss. These symptoms are the result of the body's cells not being able to use the glucose that is available in the body because of the lack of insulin. All of the other choices describe later symptoms seen with untreated or poorly controlled diabetes resulting in diabetic emergencies.

5-14. The correct answer is D. Cretinism is the result of congenital hypothyroidism that is not treated. It is a serious concern because of the risk for mental and physical retardation.

5-15. The correct answer is E. Graves' disease is an autoimmune hyperthyroidism in which the body inappropriately stimulates the thyroid gland.

5-16. The correct answer is B. Myasthenia gravis is a chronic autoimmune disease that affects the neuromuscular junction, specifically the acetylcholine receptors of the sarcolemma, and produces serious weakness of voluntary muscles.

5-17. The correct answer is E. Epstein-Barr virus causes infectious mononucleosis. Symptoms include constant fatigue, fever, sore throat, loss of appetite, and swollen lymph nodes.

5-18. The correct answer is D. Genital herpes is the only sexually transmitted disease that is viral. Herpes simplex virus type 2 (HSV2) causes most cases of genital herpes. Gonorrhea, chlamydia, and syphilis are all caused by bacteria.

5-19. The correct answer is C. Esophageal varices are extremely dilated veins in the esophagus that are associated with bleeding; hence, they are a cause of upper gastrointestinal bleeding. All of the other choices are associated with lower gastrointestinal bleeding.

5-20. The correct answer is D. Volvulus, intussusception, adhesions, and impacted feces could all cause mechanical bowel obstruction. The only one that has nothing to do with obstruction of the bowel is cirrhosis (end-stage liver disease).

5-21. The correct answer is C. The cardinal sign of pyloric stenosis is projectile vomiting. Pyloric stenosis is most often seen in infants when there is hypertrophy of the pylorus muscle, which causes obstruction of the stomach.

5-22. The correct answer is D. As many as 80% of cases of peptic ulcer disease are associated with infection by the bacterium *Helicobacter pylori*.

5-23. The correct answer is D. This condition is appendicitis; classic symptoms are right lower quadrant pain (McBurney's point tenderness), fever, vomiting, and a high leukocyte count.

5-24. The correct answer is C. This patient has a pulmonary embolism and needs immediate medical attention. Most pulmonary embolisms occur when a venous thrombus from one of the deep veins of the legs becomes dislodged and travels to the lungs.

5-25. The correct answer is B. Left heart failure is the most common cause of pulmonary edema. Another name for this condition is congestive heart failure.

5-26. The correct answer is B. Breathing is difficult in emphysema because of destruction of alveolar walls with enlargement of the remaining alveoli. Patients tend to have a pink color in their faces because of the effort to exhale, and may be called "pink puffers."

5-27. The correct answer is C. Tuberculosis is an infectious lung disease spread by respiratory droplets and caused by *Mycobacterium tuberculosis*.

5-28. The correct answer is B. Hydronephrosis is distention and dilation of the kidney with urine caused by backward pressure on the kidney when the flow of urine is obstructed.

5-29. The correct answer is A. Chronic renal disease is identified by a blood test for creatinine. Higher levels of creatinine indicate a decrease in glomerular filtration rate (GFR), the rate at which the kidneys filter blood. Therefore, the kidneys are not able to excrete waste products sufficiently.

5-30. The correct answer is E. Otosclerosis is a common loss of hearing caused by stiffening of the bones of the middle ear.

Psychology

The exam will contain questions about the basic principles of psychology, developmental stages of the life cycle, and defense mechanisms. The highlights of those areas are presented in this chapter.

BASIC PRINCIPLES

The following sections outline some of the important figures in psychology and behavioral theories that you may be asked about.

Sigmund Freud: Id, Ego, and Superego

Sigmund Freud was an Austrian physician who lived from 1856 to 1939. Even though many of his theories are no longer accepted, he provided the foundation for the modern study of psychology and psychoanalysis. He introduced the concept of the id, ego, and superego in personality structure. Figure 6-1 illustrates how the three concepts interrelate.

Id: According to Freud, the id represents whatever feels good at the time (such as comfort, food, sleep, and sexual, aggressive drives). The id is an important part of our personality because as newborns, it allows us to get our basic needs met. Freud believed that the id is based on our pleasure principle. Freud claims that we are born with our id.

Ego: Within the next 3 years after birth, as the child interacts more and more with the world, the ego is developed. The ego is based on reality. It understands that other people have needs and desires and that sometimes our desires have to wait. The major function of the ego is to maintain a relationship with the outside world and to be flexible with life's frustrations.

Superego: By the age of 5, the superego likely develops; it represents moral values and conscience. The superego controls the id.

Abraham Maslow: Hierarchy of Human Needs

Maslow's theory contends that humans are motivated by their needs. There is a progression of needs, with basic survival (food, oxygen, water) being the first need that has to be met. In general, a person cannot progress from one level to the next without meeting the needs in the lower levels.

Maslow's pyramid (see Figure 6-2) relates to health care in terms of communication with patients. For example, a patient who is struggling to feed his or her family will not be concerned about lowering his or her blood pressure.

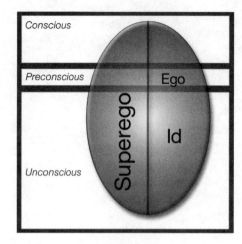

Figure 6-1 How Id, Ego, and Superego Relate

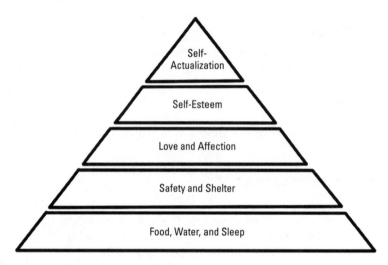

Figure 6-2 Maslow's Hierarchy of Needs

Ivan Pavlov: Conditioned Reflex

Pavlov was able to condition his dogs to salivate when he rang a bell. Thus, Pavlov discovered that environmental events (such as a bell sound) that previously had no relation to a given reflex could, through experience, trigger a learned reflex (salivation). This kind of learned response is called a conditioned reflex, and the process whereby dogs or humans learn to connect a stimulus to a reflex is called conditioning. Another example occurs when one learns to be afraid of snakes. A young child would be fascinated by a snake and is only taught fear after his or her parents warn about getting too close.

Elisabeth Kübler-Ross: Five Stages of Grief

Elisabeth Kübler-Ross was a Swiss-born psychiatrist who was appalled by the medical treatment of terminally ill patients. She proposed that there are five stages of death and grief. These stages are now accepted as an emotional cycle seen in most people who have been affected by bad news—not just death. Figure 6-3 illustrates the concept. Note that not all patients go through all five stages or experience them in the order given. The five stages of grief are:

Denial: The patient refuses to believe that he or she is dying.

Anger: The patient becomes angry (perhaps with the doctor or hospital).

Bargaining: The patient may try to strike a bargain with God in order to get better.

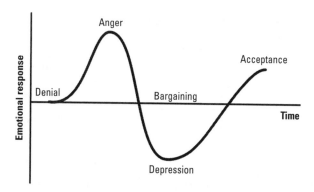

Figure 6-3 Roller Coaster of the 5 Stages of Grief

Depression: The patient finally realizes the inevitable.

Acceptance: The patient is calm and accepting of his or her fate.

DEVELOPMENTAL STAGES OF THE LIFE CYCLE

The developmental stages of the life cycle is a fascinating area of psychology. Although Erik Erikson based his developmental stages on Freud's original work, he expanded his theory to include outside cultural, societal, and genetic influences.

Erik Erikson: Developmental Stages

Erikson extended Freud's theory on personality. He organized life into eight stages that extend from birth to death. (Many developmental theories only cover childhood.) Adulthood covers a span of many years, so Erikson further divided the stages of adulthood into the experiences of young adults, middle-aged adults, and older adults. Erikson noted that personality traits come in opposites; for example, we may think of ourselves as extraverted or introverted, courageous or cautious, or aggressive or passive. Many of these are inborn temperament traits, but other characteristics, such as feeling either competent or inferior, appear to be learned, based on life experiences and upbringing.

Although he was influenced by Freud, Erikson, who lived from 1902 to 1994, believed the course of development is determined by the interaction between genetics and psychological, societal, and cultural influences. Table 6-1 illustrates the developmental stages.

Psychology of the Life Cycle: Stages of Development

The psychology of the life cycle is a branch of psychology that tries to relate the place where an individual is in the course of his or her life with the kinds of issues that the person is facing. It is based on Erikson's work. Table 6-2 describes the stages of development:

DEFENSE MECHANISMS

Many people react to adversity with defensive behavior. Many times people do not realize they are responding to events in this way. This unconscious behavior helps to decrease an individual's anxiety as well as maintain their sense of safety and self-esteem. Sigmund Freud was the first person to develop the concept of defense mechanisms. Today, they are classified as illustrated in Table 6-3.

Empathy

Empathy in a medical setting is appreciation of the patient's emotions and expression of that awareness to the patient. By displaying empathy, a medical assistant can best understand a patient's emotional and physical needs.

There may be a question on the exam about the difference between empathy and sympathy. Unlike empathy, sympathy is seen as the inclination to think or feel like the patient. It is a subtle, but distinct difference.

Table 6-1 Erikson's Eight Developmental Stages

Ages	Basic Conflict	Important Event	Summary
Birth–1 year	Trust vs. mistrust	Feeding	The newborn establishes a basic trust with his or her primary caregiver (or develops a sense of mistrust).
2–3 years (toddler)	Autonomy vs. shame and doubt	Toilet training	The toddler develops motor skills, including sphincter control. The child learns independence but may develop shame if not handled well.
3–6 years (preschool)	Initiative vs. guilt	Preschool	The young child begins to take risks to become more responsible. There is a fear of punishment and a sense of guilt.
6–12 years (school age)	Industry vs. inferiority	School	The child acquires new skills to become competent; otherwise, he or she risks inferiority.
12–18 years (adolescence)	Identity vs. role confusion	Peer relationships	The adolescent develops a sense of identity in all aspects of life or risks role confusion.
19–40 years (young adulthood)	Intimacy vs. isolation	Intimate relationships	The young adult must develop intimate relationships or suffer in isolation.
40–66 years (middle age)	Productivity vs. stagnation	Work/parenting	The middle-aged adult finds satisfaction in work and parenting or suffers stagnation.
66–death (maturity)	Ego integrity vs. despair	Reflection on one's life	The mature adult reflects on feeling fulfilled in life or is forced into despair.

Table 6-2 Stages of Development

Prenatal Development Pregnancy and prenatal development Intrauterine environment Birth Alterations and risk factors
0–2 years Motor development Intellectual development Affectionate and social development Acquisition of language
2–7 years Motor development Intellectual development Affectionate and social development Linguistic development
7–12 years Continued development of motor and coordination skills Intellectual development Affectionate development Social development

(continues)

Table 6-2 Stages of Development (Continued)

Adolescence
Rapid growth resulting in physical sexual maturity
Relationships with peers
Environmental influences: family, academics, and emotional support
Self-esteem issues
Planning for the future
Young adulthood
Survey of a situation and prior considerations, consequences
Cognitive processes: memory, attention, perception, problem solving
Affectionate behavior
Planning for the future
Adult age
Work
Parenting
Cognitive processes: memory, attention, perception, problem solving
Affectionate behavior
Relationships with social surroundings
Planning for the future
Potential for mid-life crisis
Old age
Physical degeneration
Concept of old age as a differential process
Psychosomatic aspects defining the stage
Relationships with social surroundings
Potential for depression and suicide

Table 6-3 Defense Mechanisms

Classification	Definition
Acting out	Performing an action(s) that is usually destructive to oneself or others. *The teenager started shoplifting so that her parents would pay attention to her.*
Altruism	Unselfish assistance of someone else. *Volunteering to help with the visually impaired.*
Compensation	Overemphasizing certain behaviors to compensate for real or imagined weaknesses. *Buying a child expensive gifts because of the parents' guilt of not spending enough time with them.*
Denial	Disbelief about reality. *A patient continues to run marathons with a diagnosed stress fracture.*
Displacement	Transferring negative feelings to someone or something unrelated to the situation. *You are rude to the medical assistant because your insurance won't cover the visit.*
Humor	Happiness is evoked to reduce anxiety. *Making light of a serious situation to reduce tension.*
Isolation	Isolation of affect, meaning that you can "think" the feeling but don't really feel it. *Someone states, "I am kind of mad at her, sort of."*
Projection	Placing blame on someone else (the actions or negative feelings are actually committed by the person him- or herself). *Stating the professor hates you, when you really hate the professor.*

(continues)

Table 6-3 Defense Mechanisms (Continued)

Classification	Definition
Rationalization	An irrational behavior or feeling is made to appear reasonable; justifying your thoughts or actions. *Nothing went right today. I deserve to go shopping.*
Regression	Returning to child-like, immature behavior because of stress, physical illness, or hospitalization. *An older child wets his bed after being hospitalized.*
Repression	Experience of true temporary amnesia in order to deal with a difficult situation. *A child witnesses a crime but cannot remember what she saw after she was threatened by the criminal.*
Sublimation	Redirecting unacceptable thoughts or behaviors into acceptable, socially productive thoughts or behaviors. *Attending Gamblers Anonymous meetings to avoid gambling.*
Suppression	Being vaguely aware of a thought or feeling but trying to hide it. *You try to be nice to someone whom you find annoying.*

QUESTIONS

6-1. Which of the following is NOT one of the five stages of grief and loss according to Elisabeth Kübler-Ross?

  A. Denial
  B. Bargaining
  C. Pleasure
  D. Anger
  E. Acceptance

6-2. Which one of the following defense mechanisms would a person be displaying by blaming her health problems on her troubled relationship rather than admitting to depression as the cause?

  A. Regression
  B. Altruism
  C. Denial
  D. Humor
  E. Splitting

6-3. In young adulthood (ages 19–40), when there is a reappraisal of one's life, which one of Erikson's theories applies?

  A. Intimacy vs. isolation
  B. Autonomy vs. shame and doubt
  C. Identity vs. role confusion
  D. Industry vs. inferiority
  E. Ego integrity vs. despair

6-4. A terminally ill patient states, "I am not really sick; I am just having a bad day." This patient is most likely in which stage of dying, according to Elisabeth Kübler-Ross?

  A. Denial
  B. Bargaining
  C. Acceptance
  D. Depression
  E. Anger

6-5. Which of the following statements about the elderly is FALSE?

   A. Suicide is rare among the elderly.
   B. Alzheimer's disease is more common in the elderly than in young people.
   C. The elderly experience thin and sagging skin.
   D. Presbyopia is common among the elderly.
   E. Elderly men have difficulty achieving and maintaining erections.

6-6. Which is the most common psychiatric disorder in the elderly?

   A. Personality disorder
   B. Alzheimer's disease
   C. Anxiety
   D. Depression
   E. Schizophrenia

6-7. Which of the following does Maslow say is the most basic human need that needs to be met before any others?

   A. Sex
   B. Food and water
   C. Money
   D. Respect
   E. Love

6-8. Who provided the foundation for the modern study of psychology?

   A. Maslow
   B. Jung
   C. Marks
   D. Freud
   E. Erikson

6-9. Which of the following is NOT a part of Freud's structure of personality?

   A. Id
   B. Ego
   C. Bravado
   D. Superego
   E. None of the above

6-10. According to Freud, which of the following is a function of the ego?

   A. Reality
   B. Morality
   C. Pleasure
   D. Aggression
   E. Sexuality

6-11. A previously toilet-trained child is hospitalized and then begins wetting the bed again. This is an example of which defense mechanism?

   A. Denial
   B. Displacement
   C. Projection
   D. Regression
   E. Intellectualization

6-12. Maslow's Hierarchy of Human Needs is based on the concept that

    A. self-respect is the most important need.
    B. there is a progression of human needs.
    C. security is the least important need.
    D. affection must come from those around us.
    E. human needs vary among people.

6-13. People use unconscious behaviors to protect themselves from guilt or shame. These are called

    A. therapeutic techniques
    B. human needs
    C. communication needs
    D. defense mechanisms
    E. special indicators

6-14. A mother gives her child expensive gifts to make up for not spending enough time with him. Which defense mechanism does this example describe?

    A. Compensation
    B. Denial
    C. Displacement
    D. Regression
    E. Sublimation

ANSWERS

6-1. The correct answer is C. Elisabeth Kübler-Ross was a Swiss-born psychiatrist who was appalled by the medical treatment of terminally ill patients. She proposed the five stages of death and grief: denial, anger, bargaining, depression, and acceptance.

6-2. The correct answer is C. Defense mechanisms are psychological behaviors that protect a person from guilt and shame. Denial is a common defense mechanism whereby a person refuses to accept unpleasant circumstances or unwanted information. In this case, the patient is in denial because she is blaming her health problems on her troubled relationship rather than admitting to depression as the cause.

6-3. The correct answer is A. Erikson developed eight psychosocial stages that humans encounter throughout their life: trust vs. mistrust, autonomy vs. shame and doubt, initiative vs. guilt, industry vs. inferiority, identity vs. role confusion, intimacy vs. isolation, productivity vs. stagnation, and ego integrity vs. despair. According to Erikson, young adulthood is the stage of intimacy vs. isolation. Responsibilities of early adulthood include development of an intimate relationship with another person. If the individual does not develop the ability to nurture an intimate relationship, he or she suffers emotional isolation.

6-4. The correct answer is A. Elisabeth Kübler-Ross would say that this person is in denial. It is frequently the first stage that a terminally ill person experiences. The patient refuses to believe that he or she is dying.

6-5. The correct answer is A. In the elderly, strength and physical health gradually decline. Older Americans are disproportionately likely to die by suicide. Although they comprise only 12% of the U.S. population, people age 66 or older accounted for 16% of suicide deaths in 2004. Elderly white men, in particular, are the most likely to commit suicide.

6-6. The correct answer is D. Depression is the most common psychiatric disorder in the elderly. Depression, one of the conditions most commonly associated with suicide in older adults, is a widely under-recognized and under-treated medical illness. The risk of depression in the elderly increases when the ability to function becomes limited.

6-7. The correct answer is B. Abraham Maslow's Hierarchy of Human Needs theory contends that humans are motivated by their needs. There is a progression of needs with basic survival (food, oxygen, water) being the first need to be met.

6-8. The correct answer is D. Even though many of his theories are no longer accepted, Sigmund Freud provided the foundation for the modern study of psychology and psychoanalysis.

6-9. The correct answer is C. Freud introduced the concepts of the id, ego, and superego in the personality structure.

6-10. The correct answer is A. According to Freud, the ego is based on the reality principle. The ego understands that other people have needs and desires and that sometimes our desires have to wait. The major function of the ego is to maintain a relationship with the outside world and to be flexible to life's frustrations.

6-11. The correct answer is D. This defense mechanism is called regression. The child regresses back to wetting the bed in order to escape the emotional unpleasantness of being in the hospital.

6-12. The correct answer is B. Maslow's hierarchy of human needs is based on the premise that human needs progress from physiologic (most essential) all the way up to self-actualization (most advanced).

6-13. The correct answer is D. Defense mechanisms are unconscious behaviors that people use to protect themselves from guilt or shame.

6-14. The correct answer is A. The defense mechanism in this example is compensation. The mother is compensating for her weakness—not spending enough time with her child.

Professionalism

The exam will have questions testing your knowledge of professional attitude, job readiness, and working as a team. All three areas are important in your success as a medical assistant.

DISPLAYING A PROFESSIONAL ATTITUDE

Throughout your educational program, your coursework focused on the areas identified by the American Association of Medical Assistants as important in the profession. The specific duties of a medical assistant will vary from office to office. Additionally, state law plays a role in determining what a medical assistant may do.

Before we discuss professional attitude, let's look at the general role of a medical assistant. The Commission on Accreditation of Allied Health Education Programs (CAAHEP) provides us with this description of the profession in its 2008 Standards and Guidelines:

> Description of the Profession: Medical assistants are multi-skilled health professionals specifically educated to work in ambulatory settings performing administrative and clinical duties. The practice of medical assisting directly influences the public's health and well-being, and requires a mastery of a complex body of knowledge and specialized skills requiring both formal education and practical experience that serve as standards for entry into this profession.

The CAAHEP works closely with the American Association of Medical Assistants (AAMA) to accredit educational programs in medical assisting. It is the AAMA who determines the educational curriculum through the Medical Assisting Education Review Board (MAERB) of the AAMA Endowment. The AAMA Certifying Board prepares the content outline for the medical assisting exam. Confused about the various organizations? The questions on the exam will probably focus more on your understanding of what a medical assistant does than the organizations that will be providing the certification. What is important about this alphabet soup is to remember that once you have passed the certification exam, it is important to for you to join your professional organization—the American Association of Medical Assistants. The website for more information is http://www.aama-ntl.org. Dues are reasonable, and national membership also entitles you to state and local membership without additional charge. Becoming active in your local AAMA chapter is an important part of staying current. As a health professional, you should participate in your professional organization. Acting like a professional is the first step in developing a professional attitude.

As a Certified Medical Assistant (CMA-AAMA), you are required to continue your education if you wish to remain certified. You also will be required to earn continuing education units (CEUs) over a 5-year period, or you will have to retake the certification exam. The AAMA website has specific details about the types of CEUs that are necessary. Continuing education is a sign of a competent professional.

Throughout your education and training as a medical assistant, you will use your critical thinking skills. In the work world, all is not simple and you will need to accept responsibility for your actions. It is always easy to blame someone else for the problem, but as a professional, it is important that you use your critical thinking skills along with a systematic approach to solving problems to be successful.

Most experts list five steps to problem solving:

1. *Identify the specific problem.* For example, patients may be complaining that they are waiting too long to see the physician. The wait isn't just in the lobby of the practice, but also in the exam room. The medical assistant is receiving a lot of complaints. She knows the problem is patient frustration with the waiting time, but her apologies to the patients are just temporary fixes.

2. *Gather information.* In the case of the patient wait time problem, are patients waiting because the physicians are running late from the hospital? Are there too many patients booked for the number of exam rooms available? Is one of the back office medical assistants slow to complete her intake and get the patient in the room? How long are the patients actually waiting? These and many other behaviors may be the cause of the consistent complaining.

3. *Evaluate the evidence.* By gathering as much information as possible, you will be able to focus on what is actually causing the problem.

4. *Identify solutions and the implications of those solutions.* If you determine that there is one cause for the problem, fix the problem if possible. If the patient waiting problem is because the physicians are trying to return too many phone calls in between patients, work on ways to limit the calls the physicians handle between patients. If the problem is due to a slow staff member, work with that staff member to improve their skills.

5. *Implement the best solution.* After you've implemented your solution for a period of time, reevaluate the solution if the problem persists.

The exam will probably have some general questions about being a certified medical assistant. It may have very short situations where you have to pick the most logical solution. Use the problem solving skills to think through those situational questions.

JOB READINESS AND SEEKING EMPLOYMENT

The exam may have questions about how to prepare a résumé and cover letter as well as methods for searching for a job. There also may be questions about interviewing skills. Let's talk about résumés and cover letters first.

Résumés provide employers with a snapshot of your education and experience. They also provide evidence of your written communication skills, so it is important that they be prepared with care. The résumé should be typed, concise, and professional in appearance. Use a good white bond paper for the printed version. Do not use colored paper or borders. Be sure to check your résumé for grammar and spelling errors. Your résumé should be saved in an electronic file in case the prospective employer wants it emailed first. If you do not have a professional-sounding email address, create one for your job search. If you are uncertain of how to prepare your résumé, get help from your school counselor or visit one of the many free websites that offer suggestions.

Your cover letter also is an important tool in presenting yourself to an employer. It is meant to be an introduction to your résumé. It should be only one page long. The first paragraph should tell the reader the position you are applying for or the general area of work that interests you. It should also include how you learned about the job opening. The second paragraph should give background information that helps the reader see how you can help fulfill the job requirements posted. It should not repeat what is on the résumé. Instead, use this one paragraph to relate how your background applies to the job. The last paragraph should close by making a specific request for an interview. You may say that you will follow up with a phone call to arrange a mutually convenient time for an interview. Finally, thank the potential employer for their time and consideration.

Searching for a job is never easy. Table 7-1 lists a variety of ways to begin your job search.

Table 7-1 Job Search Resources

- Use the career counselors at your school.
- Search the classified ads in the local newspaper or the local newspaper's website.
- Use job seeker websites where you can post your résumé.
- Check with the local employment office of your state.
- Sign up with employment agencies, but only if they are not charging a fee for their service.
- Network. Join your local chapter of the AAMA. Talk to other medical assistants.

Everyone is nervous when they interview. Being prepared before you go to the interview will help you present yourself as a professional. To prepare for and participate in interviews, try the following:

1. Practice interviewing with your friends or family member. Or sit in front of a mirror and watch your body language.
2. Learn about the practice or clinic. Find out how what type of medical practice it is. How many physicians are employed at the practice?
3. Be on time. Your first impression is very important. Make certain you know where the interview is and arrive a few minutes early. Allow for traffic jams and parking problems.
4. Dress appropriately. Wear clean, pressed, conservative business clothes in conservative colors. Do not wear the latest fashions. Keep your jewelry to a minimum. Make sure your hair and nails are clean. Do not carry a big purse.
5. Know the interviewer's title and the pronunciation of their name. Do not sit down until the interviewer does.
6. Smile. Offer a firm handshake. Sit up tall. Try to avoid any nervous habits like biting your fingernails, twisting your hair, or chewing gum.
7. Maintain eye contact. Try to speak with confidence.
8. Anticipate question types (see Table 7-2).

Table 7-2 Possible Interview Questions

- Tell me about your background and experience.
- Why do you think you are qualified for this job?
- What is your greatest strength? Your greatest weakness?
- Describe how you see teamwork.
- Will you be able to work overtime?
- Can you work various shifts?
- What would your medical assisting instructors say about you?
- Give me an example of your ability to work under pressure.
- Where do you see yourself in 5 years?
- What are your major accomplishments in the workplace?
- Why did you choose medical assisting as a career?
- What questions do you have about the job? The practice?

9. Relate your experience to the job. If you don't have any experience, illustrate how your school experience, volunteer work, or other leadership activities prepare you for the job. Express a willingness to learn.
10. When the interview ends, be sure to thank the interviewer for their time.
11. Send a thank-you letter within 2 days of the interview.

Employers may ask illegal questions. Questions that refer to race, age, sexual orientation, marital status, religion, or number of children are considered illegal. That does not mean employers will not ask inappropriate questions. You will have to decide whether you want to answer them, or simply indicate that you would prefer not to answer the question. If the interviewer persists in asking inappropriate questions, you may want to reconsider working for that practice.

WORKING AS A TEAM MEMBER TO ACHIEVE GOALS

As a medical assistant, you will be part of a work group. The group may be only two people, but the likelihood is that you will be working in an office with several employees. The first thing that everyone in the group must remember is that patients come first and everyone should be promoting safe and competent patient care. It is sometimes easy to forget that without patients, a medical assistant would not have a job. As a member of a group, you have a responsibility to be a part of the team effort. If there is conflict, it is important for you to examine your behavior to see if you are contributing to the problem. Group dynamics is the attempt to understand how people interact with, influence, and are influenced by others within groups. The exam will probably contain some questions that ask you to select the best choice for resolving a problem within a group. You will need to select the one best answer. The following are some basic rules you should remember as a team member:

- Good patient care is always the primary focus.
- Treat your fellow employees with respect.
- Be considerate of your fellow employees' responsibilities and duties.
- Take the extra step and help out whenever you can if a fellow employee is overburdened.
- Avoid interpersonal conflict if possible. If the conflict continues, be the first to reach out to get the problem resolved.

QUESTIONS

7-1. Before scheduling an interview for hiring, the individual responsible for hiring will review each candidate's

    A. dress and demeanor.
    B. accent and mannerisms.
    C. weaknesses, as disclosed by the candidate.
    D. application form.

7-2. The first impression the patient has of the medical office is the waiting room and reception area. The medical assistant should check the following when opening the office

    A. stock of medical supplies.
    B. recent incident reports.
    C. clinical procedures.
    D. neatness, cleanliness, and temperature setting.

7-3. When an individual is first interviewed for a position in a medical office, the office manager will discuss a number of issues with the candidate. One topic that is often not discussed until a second, follow-up interview is

    A. the applicant's education and experience.
    B. any unexplained gaps in the applicant's history.

    C. details of salary and benefits.

    D. the reasons for terminations from prior employment.

    E. the applicant's strengths and weaknesses.

7-4. You are having problems with a co-worker. The first step in problem solving for interpersonal relationships is to

    A. review you past behavior.

    B. implement a solution strategy.

    C. identify the problem.

    D. clarify your desired outcome.

    E. outline a plan for improvements.

7-5. Which of the following steps happens BEFORE the job interview?

    A. Inquire about salary and benefits.

    B. Complete federal tax withholding forms.

    C. Research the position and network.

    D. Tour the facility.

    E. Send a follow-up letter.

7-6. As a medical assistant working the front desk of the medical office, you notice that patients are consistently having to wait past their appointment times to see the physician. You ask the physician, and he tells you that he can never see the 9:00 AM scheduled patient on time because he stops by the hospital first thing each morning to see patients there and gets to the office at 9:30 AM. This discussion with the physician is which step in the five steps of problem solving?

    A. Identify the specific problem.

    B. Gather information.

    C. Evaluate the evidence.

    D. Identify solutions.

    E. Implement the solution.

7-7. A medical assistant assigned to the front desk of the medical office will need to have which of the following skills?

    A. Computer skills

    B. Proper handling of the daily mail

    C. Records management

    D. Operation of office equipment

    E. All of the above

7-8. Which of the following groups oversees the certification program for medical assistants?

    A. American Medical Association (AMA)

    B. American Association of Medical Assistants (AAMA)

    C. Occupational Safety and Health Administration (OSHA)

    D. None of the above

7-9. Experts generally concur that there are five steps in problem solving, presented here in scrambled order

    A. Evaluate the evidence.

    B. Implement the solution.

    C. Identify solutions.

    D. Gather information.

    E. Identify the specific problem.

7-10. The individual responsible for hiring new personnel in a large medical practice will be the

    A. physician.
    B. human resources director.
    C. director of laboratory services.
    D. office manager.

ANSWERS

7-1. The correct answer is D. Prior to bringing in candidates for interview, all application forms received will be reviewed and the candidates best qualified for the position will be scheduled for an interview.

7-2. The correct answer is D. At the start of the day, the medical assistant should make sure that the waiting room and reception areas are clean and orderly, and that the thermostat is set at a comfortable setting.

7-3. The correct answer is C. The first interview is part of the screening process to determine the applicant's ability to perform the responsibilities of the position. Frequently, salary and benefits will be discussed in a second interview after references have been contacted.

7-4. The correct answer is C. In dealing with problems with interpersonal relationships, the first step is always to identify the problem. Once the problem has been identified, dealing with the issues and implementing a solution will follow.

7-5. The correct answer is C. Once you have been selected for an interview, research the medical office as a potential employer for issues such as working conditions and treatment of employees. You should network with others in the field who have knowledge of this employer.

7-6. The correct answer is B. You identified the problem when you noticed that patients were in the waiting room past their appointment times. Your discussion with the physician was part of step two of the problem solving process, to gather information.

7-7. The correct answer is E. The medical assistant must be a multi-skilled health professional to be effective in the medical office. All of your education and training will be used to perform the job properly.

7-8. The correct answer is B. The American Association of Medical Assistants (AAMA) oversees the certification program for medical assistants

7-9. The correct answer is B. The proper order of the five steps in problem solving is: identify the specific problem, gather information, evaluate the evidence, identify solutions, and implement the solution.

7-10. The correct answer is B. In a larger medical office, the position of human resources director will be responsible for the recruiting and hiring of new personnel. In smaller offices, this responsibility will fall to the office manager or administrator, or even the physician.

Communications

The exam may contain a variety of questions about communications. In this chapter we will cover a variety of communication skills and techniques. Before you take the exam, it will be important for you to review some basic grammar and punctuation from your English textbooks.

THE COMMUNICATION PROCESS

The ability to communicate effectively with patients, physicians, and co-workers is an important part of the skill set of a medical assistant. Often the medical assistant is the first contact a patient has with the medical office; good communication will provide the proper medical attention to the patient and allows the patient to be comfortable with the process of care.

There are four basic components to the communication process: the sender, the receiver, the message, and feedback. As you (the sender) provide information (the message) to the patient (the receiver), you will always need to make sure that the message has been received and understood by the patient (feedback). Figure 8-1 illustrates how the communication process works. It is important to remember that the process is circular, sometimes you are the receiver and the patient is the sender. Also, the communication process is not limited to just patient and medical assistant, but it is important in all communications.

Many experts suggest that there are five "Cs" in communication. They are listed in Table 8-1.

COMMUNICATING WITH PATIENTS WITH SPECIAL NEEDS

A critical part of the communications process is recognizing and responding to each patient's limitations. A patient with a visual impairment cannot use the written information provided by the medical office and cannot respond to nonverbal actions of the medical assistant. The medical assistant will need to take extra care in explaining instructions to the visually impaired patient. The patient may be directed to a chair in the waiting room or the examination room by taking them by the arm, but only after obtaining their permission for physical contact.

The degree of hearing loss will determine how the medical assistant should respond to a patient with a hearing impairment. Speak slowly and clearly and always face the patient. Nonverbal communication and the use of written documents will aid in the communication process.

Dealing with the elderly brings its own set of special concerns. A decline in mental acuity sometimes comes with aging; however, each elderly patient will be different and the medical assistant will need to treat each one based on his or her determination of the patient's ability to understand and retain information. Feedback during the communication process with the elderly is critically important.

Figure 8-1 Four Basic Components of the Communication Process

Table 8-1 The Five "Cs" in Communication

Completeness	Assuring that the message provides all of the information required
Clarity	Assuring that the message is not vague or misleading
Conciseness	Keeping the message short and directly on point
Courtesy	Delivering the message with professionalism and respect to the receiver
Cohesiveness	Making sure the message is organized logically

When dealing with a patient who is a minor, make sure that the child is informed in simple terms of the medical care to be provided and allow the child to see and touch the medical equipment to be used. Also keep the parents involved in the process.

When dealing with a patient with a serious or terminal illness, maintain your professionalism and treat the patient and his or her family with respect and dignity. Recognize the extreme stress being experienced by both the patient and his or her family and respond to them with empathy.

Patients with a mental handicap will be especially challenging. Remain calm if the patient becomes agitated and do not raise your voice. Speak slowly and clearly and ask for feedback from the patient to assess whether your message has been received and understood.

Occasionally, the medical assistant will need to work with an illiterate patient. The medical assistant will need to carefully explain all written documentation and forms that need to be completed. If the patient comes to the medical office with a literate friend or family member, include the person in the conversation and instructions provided.

When dealing with a patient from a foreign country, you need to be aware of both language and cultural differences. When English is not the patient's primary language, speak slowly and clearly and make sure they understand what you are saying. Cultural differences should be respected so long as they do not impede effective medical care.

Many patients will exhibit anxiety in the medical office, with causes ranging from a fear of injections to concerns that their medical condition may be terminal. They may appear tense, irritable, or agitated, or have sweaty palms or elevated rates of breathing. The medical assistant should provide a professional and calming influence to the patient to control their anxiety.

Effectively communicating with an angry patient will always be difficult. Do not allow the patient's anger to affect your handling of the situation. Stay calm and request the patient to fully describe the cause of their anger. Do not argue with the patient, but state clearly what you can and cannot do to affect the situation. When possible, use an available office space to avoid bothering other patients, so long as you do not feel physically threatened by the patient. An angry patient needs to be dealt with calmly, focusing on the solution to the problem rather than the anger.

VERBAL AND NONVERBAL COMMUNICATION

Nonverbal communication is body language. The medical assistant's body language when dealing with patients is an important part of the communication process. Smiling, leaning forward to speak and listen, maintaining eye contact, and using welcoming hand gestures conveys to the patient that you are attentive and caring. Sitting back with arms folded and refusing to make eye contact will convey the opposite. You will encourage the communication process by actively listening, asking appropriate questions of the patient, providing feedback, and using positive body language. If you serve a culturally diverse population, you need to learn which standard U.S. gestures or symbols mean something different in the patient's native country .

The use of open-ended questions will aid in communication. Whereas a closed-ended question requires only a yes or no answer from the patient, an open-ended question will allow the patient to become involved in the communication process, providing as much information as they wish and discussing in depth their medical issues. Barriers to effective communication include the medical assistant being judgmental of the patient, offering inappropriate advice to the patient, and defending the medical practice when it may not be helpful to do so.

Always be attentive to the needs of the patient. A patient who is anxious or distraught over a medical condition or procedure will need to be comforted by the calmness and professionalism of the medical assistant. Provide full information to the patient to reduce the fear of the unknown.

Therapeutic communication is the ability to effectively communicate with each patient as an individual coming from a different background and circumstances, with individual needs. When discussing a patient's medical condition, it is very important to maintain professionalism. Never get emotional in the presence of the patient; stay calm and actively listen to the patient. You should show empathy to the patient. Empathy is listening carefully to the patient and expressing concern. Showing sympathy or pity to the patient is not appropriate. Never be judgmental of the patient and do not allow the patient to become defensive when you disagree with what the patient is saying.

PROFESSIONAL COMMUNICATION AND BEHAVIOR

The medical assistant will need to be able to communicate effectively with other professionals as well as patients. These will include physicians, co-workers, and outside agencies such as referral physicians, testing laboratories, and pharmacies. Physicians and co-workers in the medical practice expect and deserve to be treated with tact, diplomacy, and courtesy. The medical assistant needs to demonstrate responsibility and integrity. When a disagreement occurs with a co-worker, the medical assistant should first objectively review his or her actions to determine if he or she could be part of the problem. Meet with the co-worker in a private setting, away from other employees, and attempt to resolve the problem, taking responsibility when appropriate. When dealing with outside agencies on the phone, be friendly and open, and state your requests clearly and concisely. When difficulties are encountered, work on the solution, rather than establishing blame for the problem.

PATIENT INTERVIEWING TECHNIQUES

In the modern medical office, the patient may well spend more time with the medical assistant than with the physician. To make the physician's time with the patient as worthwhile as possible, the medical assistant needs to provide the physician with a detailed medical history and current symptoms of the patient. Interviewing techniques will include the use of exploratory, open-ended, and direct questions to get full information from the patient. The medical assistant will use observation of the patient, active listening techniques, and the appropriate use of feedback to assist in the process. The medical assistant must always be aware of the need for a private setting for the interview to protect the confidentiality of patient information. When dealing with individuals other than the patient, such as parents of minors, family members, and friends, patient confidentiality must always be protected.

RECEIVING, ORGANIZING, PRIORITIZING, AND TRANSMITTING INFORMATION

Information will come into the medical office from a number of sources: mail, fax, email, telephone, and delivered in person from the patient. Regardless of the mode of receipt, all information received needs to be handled properly. The medical assistant is responsible for organizing the information received and assuring that it is made available to the proper person. Depending on the information received, it may be necessary to bring it to the physician's attention quickly. For example, abnormal lab results should be brought to the physician's attention as soon as possible. Most offices have a procedure for getting abnormal lab results to the physician in between seeing other patients. Some offices have the medical assistant or nurse screen lab or other test results and call the patient to schedule an appointment. In contrast, something as simple as an invoice for office supplies will be given to the accountant or bookkeeper of the medical office. The medical assistant must be able to sort out all the forms of information that come into the office.

An important part of the process of handling information is prioritization. Each piece of information received comes with its own sense of importance and urgency that must be determined by the medical assistant.

TELEPHONE TECHNIQUES

Medical offices receive a large number of phone calls during a business day. Managing these calls is an important part of the business of the practice. Each phone call should be answered promptly, using a pleasant voice to make the caller feel welcome. Never eat or chew gum while on the telephone. Calls need to be screened so that they can be transferred to the appropriate person in the office. When transferring a call, give the caller the name and position of the person the call is being transferred to; for example, "I'm going to transfer your call to Bob in bookkeeping. I'm sure he can assist you with your issue on billing."

The medical assistant needs to be constantly aware of maintaining patient confidentiality when discussing patient issues on the phone. However, sufficient information needs to be gathered to properly respond to the caller.

Many offices have multiple telephone lines coming into a central location. The medical assistant needs to be competent with the system to be able to handle a number of calls concurrently. An appropriate greeting when the phone is answered would be: "This is Mary with Dr. Smith's office. How may I help you?" Each medical office will have procedures for the use of the phone to assist in training new employees. When taking a message, make sure that you understand the message by reading it back to the caller for clarification. Each phone call should be ended with a "thank you."

The medical assistant needs to be trained to be ready to handle nonroutine calls such as medical emergencies, calls from family members, and angry callers. The critical skill is to remain calm and know the proper steps to deal with these nonroutine calls. Handling an angry patient on the telephone is similar to handling the problem in the office.

FUNDAMENTAL WRITING SKILLS

Documents that are prepared in the medical office, including memoranda for internal use and business letters to outside agencies and patients, reflect on the professionalism of the practice. When creating the document, consider the key points that need to be covered in the correspondence and identify the action that is requested from the person receiving the correspondence.

The medical assistant needs to be comfortable with the basic language rules of sentence structure, grammar, and punctuation. Common errors are subjects and verbs not agreeing, run-on sentences, double negatives, improper use of commas and apostrophes, improper capitalization, and common word mistakes such as incorrectly using accept vs. except or affect vs. effect. Once the document has been prepared in draft form, you will need to review and edit the document. Although modern computer software has aids such as spell-check, a dictionary and thesaurus should be available to assist in document preparation. When you are not confident in your skills in document preparation, have a co-worker review and edit the document prior to having it finalized for signature. Remember that your written words reflect on the practice. If the practice communicates with patients, vendors, and others by email, it is important to remember that professional language still needs to be maintained at all times.

QUESTIONS

8-1. When conducting a patient history, which of the following types of listening behaviors will be most effective?

    A. Passive
    B. Active
    C. Closed
    D. Selective
    E. Evaluative

8-2. You should use which of the following to have effective communication with a patient?

    A. Detailed medical terminology
    B. Defensive body language
    C. Condescending remarks and negative body language to get the patient's attention
    D. Conversation at the patient's social and education level
    E. A loud voice to get the patient's attention

8-3. A patient in the medical office suffers from loss of memory. A technique useful in communicating with this patient is to

    A. speak loudly and slowly.
    B. use medical terminology.
    C. provide empathy about the patient's condition.
    D. direct the patient to perform one task at a time.
    E. ask the patient closed-ended questions.

8-4. Which of the following is important for communication with a hearing-impaired patient?

    A. Speak slowly and distinctly, and ask for feedback.
    B. Talk very loudly and shout if necessary to be heard.
    C. Never try to call the patient on the telephone.
    D. Communicate only in writing.

8-5. In which of the following ways should a medical assistant communicate with a difficult patient?

    A. Maintain a diplomatic attitude.
    B. Display an air of authority.
    C. Require any complaints to be put in writing.
    D. State that you know the office is right and the patient is wrong.

8-6. A medical assistant is on the phone with a patient when another call comes into the switchboard. The MOST appropriate action would be to

    A. request the second caller to "Please hold" and complete the first call.
    B. put the first caller on hold and answer the second call.
    C. only answer the second call after finishing the first call.
    D. put both callers on hold and ask for help.

8-7. A 4-year-old child is in the office for allergy testing. The BEST way to prepare the child for this procedure is to

    A. ignore the child and speak to the parents.
    B. use role-playing to demonstrate the procedure to the child.
    C. have the parents read an illustrated brochure about the procedure to the child.
    D. show the child a video of the procedure.

8-8. An elderly male patient comes into the office after the recent loss of his wife. His personal grooming has been neglected and he moves slowly and is noncommittal in responses. He tells the medical assistant he often wonders if life is still worth living. Which of the following would be the most sensitive response to the patient?

    A. "Your feelings are very normal after the loss of a spouse."
    B. "I hear you. I've felt that way sometimes."
    C. "Please discuss this with the physician."
    D. "You need to get your act together."

8-9. The medical assistant may repeat back a patient's statements as a way to encourage open communication. Which technique is this?

    A. Active listening
    B. Focusing
    C. Encoding
    D. Reflecting
    E. Decoding

8-10. The medical assistant is asked to compose a business letter. To make the letter more interesting to the reader, the medical assistant should increase the variety of the wording and use synonyms. Which of the following reference books would she consult?

    A. Dictionary
    B. Thesaurus
    C. Style manual
    D. Encyclopedia

8-11. The medical assistant will restate, reflect, or seek clarification of the patient's statements to encourage effective communication. This is referred to as which of the following?

    A. Communicating
    B. Messaging
    C. Judging
    D. Acknowledging
    E. None of the above

8-12. The physician has been involved in handling an emergency and appointments are running behind schedule. An appropriate statement to each patient in the waiting room would be to say

    A. "Please be patient. We'll get to you as soon as we can."
    B. "Read one of our magazines. This will take some time."
    C. "Dr. Brown has had to handle an emergency and will be about a half hour behind schedule. We are sorry for the inconvenience."
    D. "Why don't you go home and call us to reschedule?"

8-13. Effective methods of assisting visually impaired or blind patients include

    A. allowing the sighted caregiver to work with the patient.
    B. scheduling appointments at times convenient for transportation.
    C. informing the patient verbally in advance of all actions.
    D. assisting the patient in walking to the examination room.
    E. All of the above

8-14. A new patient comes into the office who obviously does not speak English. The most effective means of communication would be to

- **A.** speak slowly and loudly.
- **B.** ask closed-ended questions.
- **C.** maintain continuous eye contact.
- **D.** put messages to the patient in writing.
- **E.** encourage nonverbal communication.

8-15. A nonverbal method of displaying openness to communication would be

- **A.** sitting back with arms folded.
- **B.** frowning.
- **C.** looking down and avoiding eye contact.
- **D.** leaning forward, with eyes focused on the communicator.
- **E.** sighing.

8-16. Three of the elements required for communication are

- **A.** clarification, sender, feedback.
- **B.** message, feedback, body language.
- **C.** message, sender, receiver.
- **D.** sender, receiver, body language.

8-17. Which of the following is the best way to teach a patient how to perform a procedure for themselves, such as changing a dressing?

- **A.** Internet website
- **B.** Brochure
- **C.** Demonstration
- **D.** Verbal description
- **E.** Videotape

8-18. The relationship between an employee and employers, co-workers, and patients is influenced by a number of personal traits. Which of the following is the most important?

- **A.** Effectiveness in communication
- **B.** Genuineness
- **C.** Empathy with others' problems
- **D.** Respect

8-19. Which of the following statements shows proper grammar?

- **A.** This was an incorrect diagnoses.
- **B.** The meetings was scheduled for 2 PM
- **C.** Review of systems were negative.
- **D.** Every doctor and nurse are coming to the meeting.
- **E.** There was no recurrence of the tumor.

8-20. Questions that can be answered with yes or no are called

- **A.** open-ended questions.
- **B.** closed-ended questions.
- **C.** direct statements.
- **D.** indirect statements.

ANSWERS

8-1. The correct answer is B. Active listening provides the greatest opportunity to obtain a full and complete review of the patient's medical history.

8-2. The correct answer is D. To hold an effective conversation with a patient, speak in a normal tone of voice and avoid excessive technical terminology. Speak to the patient at their social and education level.

8-3. The correct answer is D. When dealing with a patient with loss of memory, provide directions one step at a time and request feedback from the patient to ensure the communication has been effective. When the first step has been completed, provide directions for the next step.

8-4. The correct answer is A. With a hearing-impaired patient, speak slowly and distinctly. Use the technique of asking questions of the patient to ensure he or she is receiving your message.

8-5. The correct answer is A. When the medical assistant has a confrontation with a difficult patient, maintaining a diplomatic attitude will keep the problem from getting worse and will provide an atmosphere in which the problem may be solved.

8-6. The correct answer is A. Calls should always be answered in the order they are received. Place the second caller on hold and finish the first call.

8-7. The correct answer is B. Showing the child exactly what will happen during the procedure is the most effective means of reducing the child's anxiety.

8-8. The correct answer is A. The best way to provide comfort to an individual grieving the loss of a loved one is to let them know that their feelings of loss are a normal part of dealing with the loss.

8-9. The correct answer is D. When interviewing a patient, an effective technique to encourage the patient to fully explain their issues is to repeat their statements back to them. This technique is called reflecting.

8-10. The correct answer is B. The thesaurus will provide synonyms of words, allowing the writer to use a wider variety of words.

8-11. The correct answer is D. Using restatement, reflecting, and seeking clarification are examples of the technique of acknowledging, used to encourage effective communication with the patient.

8-12. The correct answer is C. Patients appreciate as much information as is available and to be provided with an estimate of how long the delay will last. The medical assistant should keep patients as fully informed as possible without betraying patient confidentiality.

8-13. The correct answer is E. All of the above techniques will be effective in helping visually impaired or blind patients receive medical service as easily as possible.

8-14. The correct answer is E. When dealing with a patient who does not speak English, use non-verbal communication techniques such as gestures. Use a full body chart to try to determine the nature of the person's medical complaint.

8-15. The correct answer is D. To show that you are open to communication, lean forward and maintain eye contact.

8-16. The correct answer is C. For communication, there needs to be a person sending (sender), a person getting the communication (receiver), and something that is sent (message).

8-17. The correct answer is C. The most effective way of teaching a patient to perform a procedure for themselves is through a demonstration. The medical assistant can perform the procedure on themselves and then allow the patient to perform the procedure, providing feedback on proper technique.

8-18. The correct answer is A. Effectiveness in communication is the most important trait in establishing and maintaining relationships with employers, co-workers, and patients.

8-19. The correct answer is E. A common grammatical error is the mixing of singular and plural. In choice A, "this" is singular and "diagnoses" is plural; in choice B "meetings" is plural and "was" is singular; in choice C, "review" is singular and "systems" is plural; and in choice D the rule is that when the subjects are preceded by each or every the verb is singular.

8-20. The correct answer is B. Questions that begin with "Are you," "Do you," and "Is this" ask for a yes or no response, or at most a short response. These are referred to as closed-end questions. Open-ended questions ask for descriptions or explanations.

Legal and Ethical Issues

The exam will contain a variety of questions about the legal environment and the various legal requirements that medical assistants must follow. There are seven main areas that may be covered; this chapter breaks them down into separate sections. Reviewing your course materials on law and ethics is a good idea. The following information also will aid in your preparation.

LICENSES

Each state has a medical practice act that governs the professional conduct of physicians. Medical practice acts often cover other health care providers as well, such as physician assistants. The practice act usually covers four areas:

- Defining the practice of medicine for the state
- Providing the requirements and methods to obtain and maintain a medical license
- Establishing medical boards to review all licensing procedures
- Defining grounds for suspension or revocation of a physician license

The laws defining unprofessional conduct vary from state to state. The policies regarding revocation and suspension of medical licenses also vary. In general, however, the following behavior could result in either suspension or revocation of a license to practice medicine:

- Failure to recognize or act on common systems
- Writing excessive amounts of prescriptions without a legitimate medical reason
- Physical abuse of a patient
- Poor record keeping
- Inability to practice due to an addiction or physical or mental illness
- Performing beyond the scope of a license
- Failure to meet and maintain continuing education requirements

LEGISLATION

On the exam, there could be questions on eight different areas of legislation.

- *The Patient Self-Determination Act of 1990* was passed to encourage the use of advance directives. The act requires that hospitals and health care providers provide written information to patients on this subject. There are several documents that work together to provide for the advance directives of a patient. A *living will* documents the patient's wishes for end-of-life care.

A *durable power of attorney* allows the patient to name another individual to make decisions, including health care decisions, when the patient cannot. A health care proxy accomplishes the same goal, but deals specifically with health care decisions.

- *The Uniform Anatomical Gift Act of 1968* provides the authority to allow individuals to donate their organs or other body parts after death. Any individual at least 18 years of age and of sound mind may elect to make these donations. Following this legislation, the *National Organ Transplant Act of 1984* recognized the shortage of organs for transplant and provided funding to establish the Organ Procurement and Transplantation Network to encourage individuals to establish plans for organ donation after death.

- *Public health statutes* are in place in all states and cover a variety of occurrences that must be reported to the proper authorities. Vital statistics, such as births and deaths, must be reported. Communicable diseases that could spread rapidly throughout the local population must be reported in the public interest. Most states will require reporting of diphtheria, cholera, typhoid fever, and other diseases that could spread rapidly. Most states now also require reporting of cases of sexually transmitted diseases (STDs), such as HIV, gonorrhea, and syphilis. Legislation is in place in all states that requires that injuries resulting from assault, rape, and domestic violence be reported to the proper authorities. Mandatory reporting is generally covered by state laws; however, there are several pieces of federal legislation dealing with specific circumstances:
  - The *Child Abuse Prevention and Treatment Act of 1974* requires the reporting of all cases of suspected child abuse.
  - The *Amendments to the Older Americans Act of 1987* strengthened the original legislation passed in 1965 by defining the abuse, neglect, or exploitation of the elderly.
  - The *Unborn Victims of Violence Act of 2004* establishes federal penalties for anyone causing injury to or the death of a fetus.

- The *Occupational Safety and Health Act of 1970* created the Occupational Safety and Health Administration (OSHA) and gave that agency powers to create, administer, and enforce standards of employee safety and welfare in the workplace. OSHA conducts scheduled inspections of workplaces and also responds to mandatory reports from employers on deaths or serious injuries in the workplace. OSHA also conducts a workplace investigation when an employee files a formal complaint of unsafe or unsanitary working conditions. Employers have the responsibility of following all required safety procedures and requiring employees to use protective equipment for their specific occupation. Many states will have *right-to-know* laws that require employees to have access to important safety issues.

- The *Food and Drug Administration* is the federal agency that regulates the quality and standardization of drugs and must approve any new drugs prior to their being available to the public. The *Drug Enforcement Agency (DEA)* is involved in the regulation of drug use under provisions of the *Controlled Substances Act of 1970*. Any medical office that dispenses controlled drugs must register with the DEA, keep records on the inventory and dispensing of controlled drugs, secure the drug supply properly, and conduct a drug inventory every 2 years. There are five schedules of controlled substances, ranging from Schedule I drugs that have a high potential for abuse to Schedule V drugs that have a low potential for abuse.

- The *Clinical Laboratory Improvement Act (CLIA) of 1988* requires that controls be established by clinical laboratories dealing with the release of test results and reports. The requirement of the act is that test results and reports may only be released to authorized parties. Generally, this will limit the release of information to only the individual or the medical office ordering the tests.

- The *Americans with Disabilities Act of 1990* was written to mandate access improvements for disabled persons. All businesses and public facilities are required to make their buildings more accessible to the handicapped. Items such as steps and wheelchair ramps, elevators, counter heights, and handicapped restrooms are addressed. Employers are prohibited from discriminating against disabled persons and must provide accommodation for disabled employees.

- The *Health Insurance Portability and Accountability Act (HIPAA) of 1996* was the most sweeping legislation affecting health care providers in decades. The act established regulations to protect the health care rights of patients, including the privacy of medical records. The act also protects the continuity of health care insurance when employees change jobs and was designed to help to hold down rising health care costs resulting from fraud and abuse in the health care system. The HIPAA act has four sets of standards, each with sets of rules that were required to be implemented by covered entities within specified time frames. Table 9-1 provides a brief overview of HIPAA's four major standards. This subject will almost certainly be covered during the examination, and the student is encouraged to consult their medical law textbook for a review of the important details of this act.

HIPAA recognized the growing complexity of the medical profession and the need to bring standardization to the various software programs in use and the electronic transfer of information between parties in the health care field, such as between providers in the managed care setting and the billing programs used for insurance reimbursement. All health care providers, clearinghouses, and health care insurance companies are considered to be *covered entities* under the act. *Covered transactions* under the act include any electronic transmission of information between two covered entities.

Table 9-1 HIPAA Standards

Standard 1: Transactions and Code Sets	A transaction is defined as the movement of information between two covered entities, such as a medical office requesting payment for services from an insurance company. Code sets are the data formats used to transmit the information. HIPAA requires all covered entities to use a common set of codes for the electronic transmission of health care information.
Standard 2: Privacy Rule	This rule deals with the confidentiality of patient records. Covered entities must have written permission from the patient for each and every disclosure of patient health information (PHI). The medical office must take steps to verify that a request for PHI is based on a request from the patient. This may include asking the patient for proper identification and verifying that the patient has requested the release of PHI to their health insurance company.
Standard 3: Security Rule	Health care providers, as well as clearinghouses and health insurance companies, are required to establish policies and procedures to protect against the improper release of PHI contained in electronic form. The policies and procedures will include such issues as password control and firewall software.
Standard 4: National Identifier Standards	Under HIPAA provisions, a central national database has been established. Every covered entity now has a unique identifier, either numeric or alphanumeric, that identifies the entity. This is similar to the unique email address that you were required to establish for receiving and sending mail on your home computer.

DOCUMENTATION/REPORTING

The medical office is required to document and report a wide variety of information under federal and state law, as well as established business practice. When you are unsure of the requirements in a specific area, the county or state medical association will be able to provide you with detailed information. The following information on various laws follows the Content Outline of the AAMA.

The Drug Enforcement Administration (DEA) has established regulations dealing with the required record-keeping and reporting of dispensing controlled substances. If the medical office keeps controlled substances in the office, the office must record each and every use.

The Internal Revenue Service (IRS) has a wide variety of mandated forms in the employment and compensation areas. These include the W-4 form completed by employees to establish income tax withheld from pay, the W-2 form prepared annually by the employer showing employee compensation for the year, and the 941 form for quarterly filing with the IRS of all wages paid during the quarter.

Employers need to be aware of the requirements of a wide variety of employment laws. The Wagner Act of 1935 prohibits actions against an employee for union membership. The Civil Rights Act of 1964 prohibits discrimination in the workplace. The Age Discrimination in Employment Act of 1967 prohibits discrimination based on age. The Americans with Disabilities Act of 1990 mandates access for the disabled and prohibits discrimination against the disabled.

Laws have also been established dealing with employee compensation. The Social Security Act of 1935 established the system of payroll deductions and old age, survivors, and disability benefits that remains in place today. The Fair Labor Standards Act of 1938 set standards for overtime and minimum pay and prohibited child labor. The Employee Retirement Income Security Act of 1974 (ERISA) provides regulation of private pension plans.

Medical offices will purchase general liability insurance, protecting the practice from occurrences of personal injury. When an individual is injured in the medical office, such as from tripping and falling on your premises, the incident must be documented and reported to the insurance company providing the general liability policy.

The federal government and all states have enacted workers' compensation laws to protect the employee in cases of workplace accidents that affect the employee's ability to continue to work, on either a temporary or permanent basis. Workers' compensation will pay the costs of medical treatment and provide for the rehabilitation of the employee, and provide cash benefits in lieu of the normal paycheck from the employer. Workers' compensation comes with its own set of documentation and reporting requirements.

Medical records represent by far the greatest volume of documentation in the medical office. The medical record will contain personal and insurance data on the patient and the patient's health history. Each patient activity, such as phone calls from patients and arrivals for appointments, will be documented. Each item involved in patient care, including the physician's notes from every visit and vital signs and laboratory results, will be in the medical record. The medical office has the responsibility of maintaining the confidentiality of the patient's medical record and should never release information without the written permission of the patient. The information in the medical record belongs to the patient; however, the physical medical record belongs to the physician. If a patient requests his or her medical record, a photocopy of the requested documents will be provided. The original medical record is retained by the physician.

Employee personnel files are an additional area of required documentation. Each employee's personnel file will contain their completed job application and résumé, employment forms documenting the right to work in the United States, and payroll forms for income tax withholding. Written performance appraisals will always be included in the personnel file and may serve to protect the medical office in cases where discrimination is alleged. The medical office must respect the privacy of personnel files.

RELEASING MEDICAL INFORMATION

In general, as mentioned earlier, the release of medical information requires the written authorization of the patient. The confidentiality of medical records is protected by HIPAA. Drug and alcohol rehabilitation records have even more restrictive release requirements.

There are, however, exceptions to the prohibition of release of medical information without the consent of the patient. Communicable diseases must be reported to local health authorities for the public good. Incidents of sexually transmitted diseases (STDs), such as HIV, must also be reported. When the medical office receives a *subpoena duces tecum* from the court, requiring the release of medical records, the records must be provided.

The patient has the right to rescind authorization for release of medical records at any time. If a patient wishes to rescind the authorization to release his or her medical records, the request must be in writing.

THE PHYSICIAN–PATIENT RELATIONSHIP

The relationship between the physician and the patient falls under contractual law. A contract is an agreement between two parties, with one party making specific promises and the second party offering a consideration (some type of compensation). In the medical setting, the physician is offering to provide his or her services in the area of medical care in return for the payment of fees for services provided. Normally, contracts in the medical setting are implied, rather than written.

The *standard of care* refers to the professional duties of the physician. The physician is expected to carry out his or her professional duties at the level expected of the profession. The *"reasonable person"* rule holds an individual to a standard of action that could be expected of any reasonable person. Physicians are held to a higher standard, in that the medical care provided to a patient needs to be at a level that could reasonably be expected to be received from a trained professional.

When the patient feels that the physician has not provided the proper standard of medical service, he or she may bring a course of legal action against the physician. Suit may be brought against the physician for malfeasance, misfeasance, or nonfeasance.

- *Malfeasance* is the conduct of a wrong or unlawful act.
- *Misfeasance* is a legal act that is performed in an improper or illegal manner.
- *Nonfeasance* is the failure to act when the circumstances dictated that action should have taken place.

When a patient brings suit against a physician for the medical care received, the physician can use a number of methods to remove or limit the possible liability. These are termed *affirmative defenses*. A lawsuit will not be heard by the court if the action is not properly filed with the court during a specific period of time, referred to as the statute of limitations. The physician may claim that there was comparative/contributory negligence, where actions of the patient contributed to the impairment of the patient. For example, a patient sues the physician when knee surgery does not result in the freedom of movement expected by the patient. The physician may claim that the patient is wholly or partially responsible for the results due to the patient's failure to follow the rehabilitation regimen prescribed by the physician. The physician may also claim assumption of risk, meaning that the patient was informed of possible negative outcomes and made the informed decision to have the procedure.

Both the physician and the patient have certain rights and responsibilities under the implied contract for medical services. The patient has the right (sometimes limited by managed care plans) to select their physician and to change physicians when not pleased with the medical care they receive. The physician has the right to set up a medical practice within his or her license to practice medicine. The physician has the obligation to use skill and judgment in treating the patient and to stay up to date on improvements in medical care. Except for emergency room physicians, physicians have the right to choose the patients to receive medical care. The primary responsibility of the medical assistant is to protect patient confidentiality. Medical information must never be released without the written authorization of the patient or under limited legal exceptions (discussed in the previous section).

Third-party agreements are those where a separate, independent agency becomes involved in the contractual relationship between physician and patient. Most commonly, this will be the health care insurance company of the patient. The promise side of the contract remains the same, with the physician providing medical care. The consideration side of the contract is modified in that compensation is provided from a fee schedule agreed to between the physician and the insurance company.

Consent, in the medical setting, means that the patient has agreed to a certain course of action. When a patient sets an appointment for a physical examination, the patient has provided implied consent for the physician to take the appropriate steps required in the examination. *Informed consent* deals with more serious medical issues, such as surgeries, and sets a higher standard on physicians to ensure that the patient fully understands their consent. The patient has the right to receive a full explanation of his or her current condition, the proposed method of treatment, why the treatment is necessary, options and risks of treatment alternatives, and risk if a course of treatment is not followed. The patient then will be asked to sign an informed consent form.

As court dockets have become more and more crowded, courts have come to rely heavily on alternative dispute resolution (ADR). Under ADR, both parties will agree to mediation or arbitration to resolve civil disputes. In mediation, a neutral third party listens to both sides and helps resolve the dispute. However, a mediator does not have the authority to order a solution. In arbitration, both parties agree to abide by the arbitrator's decision. When a patient has agreed to and signed an arbitration agreement prior to surgery, the resolution of any dispute arising from the surgery will be handled by a neutral arbitrator rather than the court system.

Although a patient can end the physician–patient relationship at any time and for any reason, the physician is held accountable to higher standards when terminating the relationship with a patient. The physician may terminate the relationship if the patient will not pay for services provided, does not keep scheduled appointments, or will not follow the instructions of the physician, or when the patient states that he or she will be receiving future medical care from another physician. The medical office should have a written policy for terminations. The patient needs to be notified in writing, preferably by certified mail return receipt, and a copy of the letter must be placed in the patient's medical record. The patient must be provided with sufficient time to seek treatment from another physician.

The medical assistant exam will require that the student have a good working knowledge of medico-legal terms and doctrines. A number of these have been discussed above. Two Latin terms commonly used in the legal profession are *res ipsa loquitur* and *res judicata*. The first term means that the issue is so obvious that it speaks for itself without the need for expert witnesses. This is also called the doctrine of common knowledge; an example would be when a physician inadvertently leaves a sponge in the patient during surgery. *Res judicata* means that the issue has been decided. Under this principle, when a claim has been decided by the court, it cannot be retried. An additional important term is *respondeat superior*, which means that physicians are held liable for the actions of their employees.

MAINTAINING CONFIDENTIALITY

The medical assistant is an agent of the physician; under the terms of *respondeat superior*, mentioned in the previous section, the physician may be held responsible for the actions of the medical assistant. Patients have certain rights, and the right to the confidentiality of their medical records is one of the most important. Medical assistants need to be vigilant in dealing with the release of medical records to ensure that the privacy of the patient is always protected. Always obtain written authorization from the patient prior to the release of medical information and make sure you know who you are releasing information to.

A *tort* is an action, not involved in a breach of contract, that causes injury to another party. When the person knows, or should have known, the result of the action, then the action is an *intentional tort*. An *unintentional tort* is a mistake or when the action has consequences that could not have been predicted. For the medical assistant, *invasion of privacy* is an intentional tort and occurs when confidential medical information is inappropriately released. *Defamation of character* is also an intentional tort, and concerns the damages to an individual's reputation and character from false and malicious words. *Slander* is when defamatory words are spoken; *libel* is when the defamation is in writing.

PERFORMING WITHIN ETHICAL BOUNDARIES

All personnel in the medical office have the responsibility of adhering to professional and ethical standards. Guidelines for ethical standards in the medical profession are available in both the AAMA Code of Ethics and the AMA Principles of Medical Ethics. All medical assistants should become familiar with the AAMA Code of Ethics, even if they do not join the organization.

Core ethical principles deal with patient dignity; honest communications with patients; promoting the principles of the medical profession; constant improvement of knowledge, skills, and abilities; commitment to expose unacceptable behavior; and promoting individual health and well-being for the good of society. A critical component of ethical medical behavior concerns the rights of patients. The American Hospital Association has outlined these in its Patient Bill of Rights. These patient rights include the right to information concerning diagnosis and course of treatment, the right to make decisions on medical care, the right to have advance directives, and the right to privacy.

Recent scientific advances have brought about new ethical considerations. The new field of bioethics considers ethical issues dealing with subjects such as cloning, the appropriate uses of genetic testing, and the future impacts of genetic technology. The allocation of scarce health care resources, abortion, stem cell research, and in vitro fertilization are other current bioethical issues.

QUESTIONS

9-1. Law that is based on prior rulings from a court is

- **A.** common law.
- **B.** regulatory law.
- **C.** constitutional law.
- **D.** statutory law.

9-2. Which of the following actions requires that the physician file a report with the proper authorities?

- **A.** The medical office conducts an abortion on an adult woman.
- **B.** The physician conducts experiments in genetic research.
- **C.** The physician dispenses a narcotic drug.
- **D.** The physician treats a cancer patient.
- **E.** The physician has suspicions that an individual is guilty of elder abuse.

9-3. HIPAA provides standards for the interchange of electronic data to protect the privacy and confidentiality of electronically stored and transmitted health information. One of the goals of HIPAA is NOT

- **A.** to increase the reliability of shared data.
- **B.** to reduce fraud.
- **C.** to reduce the use of computer networks in health care.
- **D.** to accelerate processes and reduce paperwork.
- **E.** to improve tracking of health information.

9-4. Confidential medical record information is stored on the office computer. To maintain patient confidentiality, the medical assistant should NEVER

- **A.** share their personal computer password with co-workers.
- **B.** leave the computer unsecured during lunch break or at the end of the day.
- **C.** print out confidential information without monitoring the print function.
- **D.** All of the above.

9-5. An effective tool to ensure patient confidentiality would be to

- **A.** release confidential information over the telephone.
- **B.** allow an insurance adjustor access to the medical office file room.
- **C.** provide independent verification of a fax number before faxing confidential data.
- **D.** dump old medical records in the trash.

9-6. Which of the following actions may be performed using a patient's implied consent?

    A. An electrocardiogram
    B. Donation of organs after death
    C. A blood transfusion
    D. Release of medical records
    E. Gall bladder surgery

9-7. A patient has had open heart surgery and is in a coma. The patient's spouse brings suit against the physician, alleging that the patient was not informed of the possible complications from use of general anesthesia. The suit will be filed on the following basis

    A. malfeasance.
    B. misfeasance.
    C. nonfeasance.
    D. negligence.

9-8. An order of the court that requires the individual named to appear in court on a set date and time is a(n)

    A. summons.
    B. tort.
    C. subpoena.
    D. appeal.
    E. verdict.

9-9. Malfeasance is one form of

    A. nonfeasance.
    B. misfeasance.
    C. misinformation.
    D. malpractice.

9-10. Which of the following is NOT a felony under the law?

    A. Assault
    B. Rape
    C. Murder
    D. Embezzlement
    E. Tort

9-11. An expressed contract is

    A. implied.
    B. in writing.
    C. witnessed by an attorney.
    D. filed with the court.

9-12. In which of the following instances is consent not required?

    A. When the patient is not mentally competent
    B. When the patient is not conscious
    C. In an emergency situation
    D. When the patient is a minor

9-13. Which of the following may be found in an advance directive?

    A. Written distribution of assets
    B. Arrangements for cremation

    C. Medical power of attorney
    D. Diagnosis and treatment plan

9-14. The testimony provided by an individual in a sworn, pretrial setting is

    A. a statement of intention.
    B. a deposition.
    C. a verdict.
    D. an inquisition.
    E. None of the above.

9-15. The doctrine of *respondeat superior* applies to

    A. the responsibility of the physician for his or her actions as well as actions by staff members.
    B. the requirement of subordinates to respond to superiors.
    C. a court-ordered subpoena.
    D. a ruling received at arbitration.

9-16. The medical assistant sees an apparent conflict between ethics and patient confidentiality in a situation not covered under the law. The medical assistant should

    A. make the best decision possible and relate the decision to the patient.
    B. take the matter to court.
    C. discuss the issue with co-workers and come to a majority decision.
    D. refer the conflict to the physician for his or her decision.

9-17. The reasonable person rule compares an action with one that would be performed by a prudent and reasonable person under similar circumstances. Failure to act in this manner would constitute

    A. fraud.
    B. libel.
    C. abuse.
    D. negligence.
    E. None of the above.

9-18. By law, the physician MUST report

    A. births.
    B. deaths.
    C. communicable diseases.
    D. suspected abuse.
    E. All of the above.

9-19. Which of the following is NOT a part of the Patient Bill of Rights?

    A. The right to privacy notices
    B. A reasonable response from the physician when medical services are requested
    C. The right to negotiate fees for medical services received
    D. The right to refuse treatment under circumstances prescribed by law

9-20. A minor child comes into the medical office for immunizations required by the school. The medical assistant notices bruising on the patient and suspects child abuse. The appropriate first step for the medical assistant is to

    A. immediately call the police.
    B. tell the parents you suspect they are abusing the child.
    C. notify the physician privately of your concern.
    D. take no action.
    E. file a notification of child abuse with the proper authorities.

ANSWERS

9-1. The correct answer is A. The body of law that is derived from precedents of prior court rulings is common law.

9-2. The correct answer is E. The law requires that suspicion of elder abuse be reported to the proper authorities.

9-3. The correct answer is C. HIPAA does not have a goal of reducing the use of computer networks in health care.

9-4. The correct answer is D. Maintain the security of confidential information by protecting your password, always locking your computer when not at your workstation, and making sure print jobs are secured while printing.

9-5. The correct answer is C. When dealing with an individual allowed to receive confidential information, verify the fax number where the information is to be sent prior to faxing the information.

9-6. The correct answer is A. A noninvasive procedure, such as an electrocardiogram, may be performed using a patient's implied consent.

9-7. The correct answer is D. The suit will be filed on the basis of negligence. The physician must inform the patient of all risks, potential negative outcomes, and alternatives.

9-8. The correct answer is C. A subpoena is a written order from the court requiring appearance in court and providing penalties for failure to comply.

9-9. The correct answer is D. Malfeasance, nonfeasance, and misfeasance are all forms of malpractice. Any of these may subject a physician to legal action.

9-10. The correct answer is E. A tort is a civil wrong committed against either a person or property. It may not be prosecuted as a felony.

9-11. The correct answer is B. An expressed contract is always in writing.

9-12. The correct answer is C. In an emergency situation, consent is not required. The medical necessity of treatment in an emergency situation outweighs the protections of consent when the patient may not be able to provide consent and next of kin may not be immediately available. For the unconscious patient, not in an emergent/urgent situation, every effort to obtain consent from the appropriate family member for care is appropriate.

9-13. The correct answer is C. An advance directive may contain a power of attorney for authorization of medical procedures.

9-14. The correct answer is B. A deposition is sworn testimony provided in advance of trial.

9-15. The correct answer is A. *Respondeat superior* is the doctrine that the physician is responsible not only for his or her actions, but also for the actions of staff members.

9-16. The correct answer is D. In matters of ethics and patient confidentiality, the physician bears ultimate responsibility and should be fully briefed on the conflict and allowed to make the decision.

9-17. The correct answer is D. Failure to act in a manner that would be used by a prudent and reasonable person is negligence.

9-18. The correct answer is E. Physicians are required to report births, deaths, communicable diseases, and suspected abuse to the proper authorities.

9-19. The correct answer is C. The Patient Bill of Rights does not provide patients with the right to negotiate fees for medical services received.

9-20. The correct answer is C. Child abuse must be reported to the proper authorities; however, the physician should make the final decision on the suspected child abuse and order the notification.

Administrative Knowledge

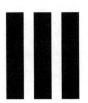

Administration and Technology

The exam will contain a variety of questions about the administration of the medical office. In this chapter we will cover data entry, computer concepts, records management, and appointment management. Chapter 11 covers many of the other administrative topics.

DATA ENTRY

Computer word processing programs are used to generate a number of written documents used in the medical office. Documents commonly used in the medical office include business letters, memoranda for circulation internal to the medical office, reports, and chart notes transcribed from physician dictation or written notes.

Keyboard Fundamentals and Functions

The keyboard of the computer system is composed of a standard typewriter keyboard with letters and numbers, but also has keys for specific computer operations. Arrows on the keyboard serve as cursor controls. The Backspace and Delete keys allow for easy corrections. The Enter key allows inputting of data into the system. There are 12 function keys, F1 through F12, that perform specific computer functions. Shift and Caps Lock keys allow for capitalization.

Formats for Written Communication

Letters

The standard business letter will be printed on letterhead purchased for the medical office, containing the name, address, and phone number of the business office. Generally, business letter stock measures 8.5 by 11 inches. The standard business letter will have 1-inch margins.

The personal preference of the physician may dictate that a rough draft of the letter be prepared and provided to the physician for editing. Computerized word processing programs allow for easy changes from the rough draft to the final document.

The basic components of the business letter are the date line, inside address, salutation, subject line, body of the letter, complimentary closing, signature block, identification line for the initials of the sender and preparer of the letter, and, finally, notations to show courtesy copies (cc) and enclosures.

Most letters from the medical office will contain the original signature of the physician. Other letters are signed by the Office Manager or other staff members in the office.

The date line is normally typed 2.5 inches below the top of the page, or 1/2 inch below the letterhead. The date should not be abbreviated (e.g., use September 3, 2010, not Sept. 3, 2010). The inside address identifies the addressee by name and address and will be identical to the address block on the envelope. Degrees are always abbreviated. The salutation line will be in the format "Dear Mrs. (or Mr. or Ms.) Thompson:" with a full colon, and starts at the left margin of the letter. A subject line is optional. If used, it will identify the nature of the correspondence and will be located two lines below the salutation and two lines above the start of the body of the letter. Two lines below the body of the letter is the complimentary closing, such as "Sincerely Yours," or "Yours Truly,". Four lines below the complimentary closing is the signature block, containing the writer's full name on the first line and title on the second line. If an identification line is used, it should consist of the three initials of the sender in capital letters, then a slash sign, followed by the two initials of the preparer of the letter in lowercase letters (e.g., JMS/tl). The final item(s) in the business letter are notations to identify any courtesy copies (cc:) or enclosures (Encl.) being sent with the letter. Courtesy copies, sometimes referred to as carbon copies, identify who is receiving a copy of the letter. Both the identification line and the enclosure notation should appear two lines below the signature block.

The letter style will reflect the personal preference of the physician. In the full block style, all lines will be flush with the left-hand margin. In the modified block style, the date line and the complimentary closing are moved to the center of the letter. In the semi-block style, all lines are flush with the left-hand margin except the first line in each paragraph of the body of the letter, which is indented five spaces. The simplified style is the same as full block, but eliminates both the salutation line and complimentary closing. The simplified style is not recommended for formal business correspondence. Figure 10-1 illustrates a sample letter in modified block style.

Cardiology Practice

October 18, 2009

Marie Anderson
1822 Delgado Lane
Naples, FL 34119

Dear Mrs. Anderson:

Thank you for your invitation to speak at the American Heart Association meeting on January 18, 2010. I am pleased to accept this invitation and have enclosed my C.V. for your review.

As you requested, I will be discussing the incidence of heart problems in student athletes. This is a timely issue given the recent incident at one of our local high schools.

If you would let me know the location and specific time, I will make arrangements to clear my schedule.

Again, thank you for this opportunity.

Sincerely,

Rafael Palmetto, MD

RP:sw
Enc.
cc. S. Webster (scheduler)

Figure 10-1 Sample Cover Letter

Memos

Memos are written communications within a business such as a medical practice. A memo is only for internal use and should not be used to communicate with patients, vendors, insurance companies, or any other organizations. Some small practices use the memo as a way to create policies and procedures for the practice. Some practices may even be using email in place of memos.

Reports

Reports vary in nature. Sometimes a physician may prepare a paper for presentation or create a report for the local medical association. The medical assistant may assist in the preparation of the presentation or report by gathering data or preparing a rough draft.

Envelopes

Envelopes are used to mail letters and other documents. Letters are normally sent using a No. 10 envelope. Reports and other documents may be sent by using different size envelopes. Students are encouraged to do a quick Internet search using the words "envelope size" to learn about all the different sizes of envelopes available. However, there are usually only one or two questions about envelope size, so don't spend a lot of time trying to memorize all the different sizes. Envelopes, regardless of size, will generally be preprinted with the return address of the medical office.

Chart Notes

Chart notes are sometimes called progress notes. Each practice selects the type of chart note format they will be using. Chart notes are discussed further in the Records Management section in this chapter.

PROOFREADING

There are usually at least one or two questions about proofreader marks and making corrections from rough draft. Figure 10-2 illustrates some of the more common proofreader marks.

You may be asked to proof rough drafts of reports, letters, or other documents. You will use some of the proofreader marks to make those corrections. Additionally, if the document is in Microsoft

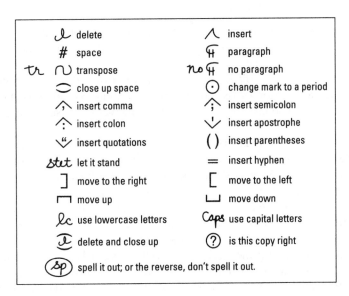

Figure 10-2 Proofreader Marks

Word, you can use its comment function. Also, a PDF document may be corrected using PDF software. However, due to the cost of PDF software to create sophisticated documents, many practices do not purchase the software.

OFFICE EQUIPMENT

In today's medical office, automated electronic equipment has replaced the pegboard and the typewriter. Offices will have electronic calculators, photocopy and facsimile (fax) machines, scanners, and telephone systems with modern capabilities of voice mail, call transferring, and transmitting credit card payments. All of these are tools that make management of the office more efficient; however, they require a new skill set from employees. Each piece of equipment will come with an instruction manual to assist the user in the proper operation of the equipment. Each will also come with a manufacturer's warranty, and more sophisticated equipment will have a service agreement and repair service negotiated with a local vendor. All documentation dealing with the equipment needs to be properly filed to be accessible when needed to train new employees on proper operation and in case of malfunction.

COMPUTER CONCEPTS

An understanding of computer systems and their use in the medical office is a critical skill for medical assistants. Large practices may use a server and workstation system that has the power to meet the needs of larger businesses. Smaller medical offices will use personal computers. These will include desktop computers and notebook (portable) computers. Individual personal computers will be networked (linked) to provide central storage of computer data and for sharing of information among system users.

Computer hardware consists of the physical components of the system. These include the central processing unit (CPU), monitor, keyboard, mouse, and printer. Computer operation is divided into four stages, each requiring distinct hardware: input, processing, storage, and output. Data is entered into the system in the input phase with a keyboard, a mouse or other pointing device, or a scanner. The central processing unit (CPU) handles the processing of the data. The hard drive is located inside the CPU and serves for storage of the data. Data may be stored in a variety of ways, including:

- *Floppy disk:* A square rigid disk that holds data. This type of storage has become outdated.
- *Hard drive:* This is a large capacity storage device housed in a rigid case. The hard drive may contain data, operating systems, programs, or files.
- *Jump, thumb, or flash drive:* A small device used to store data. These types of drives are portable and are installed in a USB port.
- *Optical disc:* A high capacity storage medium. Discs are read by a laser light, so most practices do not use this type of data storage.

Additionally, there may be a question on the exam about scanners or scanning capability. A scanner is a device that captures images from paper or other hard copy for editing and storage. Scanners are often used to prepare files for storage.

Finally, output is when data is displayed on the monitor or sent to the printer.

The exam may ask a question or two about basic computer commands such as Enter, Delete, and Tab. These questions are usually easy for students to answer because most students use computers routinely.

Computer applications or software provide the operating instructions that allow the computer to function. Software comes in two basic types: system software that controls the basic operations of the computer, such as Windows XP and Vista, and application software, such as Microsoft Word, Microsoft Excel, and Medical Manager, which performs specific tasks.

Computers are used for a number of important applications in the medical office. A word processing program is used for preparing letters and memoranda, and for producing doctors' notes. A database management program or medical management software is used for storage and management of patient records, including medical charts, billing records, and insurance information. A spreadsheet program, such as Microsoft Excel, is used for bookkeeping and accounting. Specialized programs for accounting and billing allow the medical office to track patient accounts, generate statements, and prepare accounting and tax records.

Appointment software has become much more sophisticated, allowing for storing of patient preferences on appointment times and listing available appointment times based on these preferences. The combination of programs for accounting and billing as well as appointments is often referred to as a practice management system or medical management software.

Computers in the medical office allow access to the unlimited reference possibilities of the Internet. Electronic mail (email) allows for near-immediate communication between two or more parties. All medical professionals should be cautious in using email to communicate personal medical information, however. Privacy concerns must be the first consideration for any type of communication, and email often lacks privacy.

The security of the computer system and the confidential data stored on the system is always an important consideration. When the computer or the computer network is connected to the Internet, anti-virus software is essential. All computer workstations need to be secured with password control to assure that unauthorized use is prohibited. Employees need to be cautioned to keep their passwords private and required to change them on a regular basis. More sophisticated computer systems will monitor activity on the system as a means to ensure appropriate use. The individual responsible for the computer network will back up the system on a regular basis to protect against loss of data in case of computer malfunction.

RECORDS MANAGEMENT

The exam will have several questions about different types of filing systems used in the medical office. They are outlined below.

- *Alphabetical filing:* Files are listed alphabetically by the last name of the patient, followed by the first name and middle name or initial. Records may be color coded, with each section of the alphabet given a different color, as an aid in locating improperly filed records. A common system of color coding is to break down the alphabet as follows and assign specific colors to each group of letters. Each practice may choose its own colors.

  Red   = A–D
  Lavender = E–H
  Yellow   = I–M
  Blue   = N–Q
  Green   = R–Z

- *Numeric filing:* In a smaller medical office, a simple numeric system of assigning consecutive numbers to new patients will be effective. For larger medical practices, a terminal last digit system is preferred. In the terminal digit system, a file number is assigned with numbers separated into groups of two or three. The numbers are read in groups, from right to left, and filed in that manner. Numeric filing provides greater confidentiality to patients than an alphabetic system. The numeric filing system, like alphabetical, is color coded. A quick review of your medical assisting textbooks, as well as your experience in your internship, will provide you with a review of the common color coding systems.
- *Subject filing:* Records are indexed according to subject and then filed either alphabetically or numerically. This system is generally used for files other than patient medical records. You will find most subject files in the business office, but everyone in the office probably has a small set of files by subject.
- *Tickler file:* A tickler file is used to alert the medical assistant of date-sensitive actions that need to be taken. These will be filed chronologically, beginning with the nearest action date. Items in the tickler file will include invoices and taxes that need to be paid and licenses that need to be renewed.
- *Electronic data processing:* The use of computers is expanding into the records management field, especially in large medical practices. The electronic medical record (EMR), in which all

information about the patient is entered and stored electronically, is beginning to make headway in the medical office. These types of systems will become the standard in the future.

Some offices maintain a cross-reference or master file list. This is particularly helpful in offices where several people have access to the same files.

Care must be taken when storing and protecting various records. Every office should have a plan in place in the event a disaster of any kind occurs. Because most physician offices are still paper based, rather than electronically based, all records should be protected as best as possible from damage occurring as a result of water, fire, and other disasters. Records may be copied onto CDs or optical disks for long term storage.

The transfer of medical records to another entity is a legal process that differs state by state. The medical record legally belongs to the physician. Medical records need to be in an area that can be properly secured to protect the records, either in file cabinets that can be locked or on open shelves in a room that can be separately locked for security. When a medical record is removed by the medical assistant, an out guide is placed in the spot vacated by the removed medical record, with the out guide dated and initialed by the medical assistant.

Maintaining accurate medical records is an essential part of the proper operation of a medical office. Up to date medical records allow the physician to provide the best medical care to patients by providing for continuity of care. The medical record for each patient will contain the patient registration form, medical history, results of physical examinations and laboratory tests, prescription information, diagnosis and treatment plans, progress notes, and other relevant documents such as informed consent forms, discharge summaries, and correspondence. The organization of the record will usually be done by using tabs to mark the various areas.

In a problem-oriented medical record (POMR), vital information such as allergies, medications, and major health problems are in a prominent location in the chart, usually in a one-page summary form that is on top of one side of the chart. Then the individual medical problems are identified by number. The chart is then built around the numbered problems. The progress notes for each medical problem are usually organized in the SOAP format:

S = subjective impression

O = objective clinical information

A = assessment or diagnosis

P = plan for treatment, further studies, or other medical management

The source-oriented medical record (SOMR) is the second way in which a medical record may be organized. In SOMR, information is organized by the source of the information. A tab may be created for each source (i.e., lab reports, radiology reports, surgeries, progress reports, physical examination, and other sources).

The medical information is collected and filed in chronological order. That means that the most recent information is at the top of the folder or tabbed section.

The steps to correct a medical record are listed in Table 10-1.

Retention schedules, detailing how long a medical record or other record must be maintained, are governed by both federal and state law. Each medical office should have a policy in place that lists all of the records maintained by the office and noting how long each record is kept.

Table 10-1 Steps in Correcting a Medical Record

To make a correction in the medical record
1. Draw a single line using a red ink pen through the error.
2. Make the correction.
3. Write "correction" above the area corrected.
4. Initial and date the correction.

SCHEDULING AND MONITORING APPOINTMENTS

The scheduling of patients in the medical office is one of the most important functions on the administrative side of the organization. Most people lead busy lives, and lengthy waits to see the physician are not appreciated. Appointment books may be maintained manually, but it is more common to use specialized computer software for appointments. With either the manual or computer system, a daily appointment schedule is generated and must be maintained as a legal document. The Health Insurance Portability and Accountability Act (HIPAA) requires the daily schedule to be posted where it may not be viewed by patients.

Medical offices use a number of different scheduling techniques to maintain an effective patient schedule, as illustrated in Table 10-2. The appointment interval, or length of each appointment, is based on physician preference and proven past practice. Physician preference is also used to block out certain times on the schedule for lunch breaks, catch-up, and short meetings with pharmaceutical representatives. Full days or weeks are blocked off for vacations and attendance at conferences.

Special scheduling situations are not uncommon in the medical office. A patient with a severe issue will need to be seen by the physician immediately. In some instances, the patient's condition is so severe that an ambulance will need to be called. Referrals from other physicians should be scheduled to be seen as soon as possible. When the physician orders medical tests, the revisit must be scheduled far enough ahead to allow for the tests to be completed and the results returned to the physician. The schedule must be established taking into consideration the limits of equipment in the office.

When a patient schedules a return appointment in person, he or she should be provided with an appointment card to serve as a reminder. One or two days in advance of the appointment, the patient should be given a courtesy call as a reminder. The medical assistant should determine from the patient whether it is acceptable to leave appointment information on a telephone answering machine.

The office should have a policy dealing with patients habitually late for appointments. "No-shows," patients who don't call to cancel an appointment that will not be kept, and cancellations the day of the appointment should be noted in the patient's records.

Table 10-2 Types of Schedules

Type of Scheduling	Description
Stream (time-specified)	This is the most common method of scheduling. Patients are scheduled at separate times, with time provided based on the nature of the visit. Visits from established patients may be scheduled for 15 minutes each, with longer times scheduled for new patients and complete physicals.
Wave	With this method of scheduling, a number of patients are scheduled for the same time, with patients seen by the physician in the order of arrival in the office. As an example, three routine visits from established patients are scheduled for 9:00 AM, using the assumption that each will take 10 minutes. If one patient is late, the other two on-time patients will be seen first and make efficient use of the physician's time.
Modified wave	This type of scheduling is used to meet extended time needs of certain patients. For example, three routine visits may be scheduled on the hour and one new patient visit or a complete physical scheduled on the half-hour. Physician offices apply modified wave in a variety of ways.
Double booking	Two or more patients are scheduled for the same time. This may be effective when one patient is scheduled for a diagnostic procedure, such as an electrocardiogram, or when a patient needs to be added to an already full schedule due to the nature of their illness or injury.
Open booking	Patients are directed to come into the office in a specified time range, such as 1–3 PM. Patients with injuries or severe illnesses may be seen by the physician ahead of patients on routine visits.
Clustering (categorization)	Based on the purpose of the visit, patients are scheduled in groups. An example would be a series of pre-employment medical examinations.

QUESTIONS

10-1. Which of the following situations should be considered an emergency appointment?

   A. A pre-employment physical so that the patient can start a new job
   B. A child who sprained an ankle at school
   C. An older man with breathing difficulties
   D. A patient who ran out of medication and needs a refill

10-2. The ability of the computer system to recognize printed letters and numbers is known as

   A. universal product code (UPC)
   B. optical character recognition (OCR)
   C. fax machine
   D. image scanner

10-3. The standard envelope size for general business correspondence is

   A. No. 7.
   B. No. 9.
   C. No. 10.
   D. No. 12.

10-4. The appointment book of a medical office is set up by crossing off all times that will not be used for patient visits. This is known as setting up a

   A. matrix.
   B. calendar.
   C. schedule.
   D. timeframe.

10-5. A computer system consists of a number of pieces of hardware required for the operation of the unit. Which of the following is NOT a unit of hardware?

   A. Keyboard
   B. Database
   C. Central processing unit (CPU)
   D. Printer
   E. Monitor

10-6. Medical offices will use a number of different types of reminders for patient appointment reminders, EXCEPT

   A. telephone reminder calls.
   B. appointment cards.
   C. facsimile (fax) machine messages.
   D. postcards.

10-7. The file that is inserted on the shelf when a medical record is in use is a(n)

   A. closed file.
   B. inactive file.
   C. file label.
   D. out guide.

10-8. The use of electronic mail (email) has one major disadvantage, which is that it

   A. adds to the time to get back to a patient.
   B. facilitates a rapid response.

    C. is not secure.

    D. may be used at a time convenient to the physician.

10-9. A patient is scheduled for an appointment and is a "no show." The missed appointment is documented in the patient's file to

    A. schedule another patient in that time slot.

    B. show all missed appointments in case the patient needs to be counseled on no shows.

    C. erase the patient from the appointment book.

    D. refuse further appointments for that patient.

    E. report the no show to the patient's insurance company.

10-10. "Double booking" in appointment scheduling refers to

    A. one patient being booked into two consecutive appointment slots due to the nature of the appointment.

    B. two patients being booked into the same appointment time.

    C. two physicians practicing in the same office, using the same appointment book.

    D. three patients being scheduled on the hour and three more on the half hour.

    E. six patients being scheduled at the top of each hour.

10-11. The salutation line of a business letter reads "Dear Mr. Smith". The punctuation mark that follows the salutation is a

    A. hyphen.

    B. period.

    C. semicolon.

    D. colon.

10-12. The medical assistant should do which of the following to protect against the loss of computerized data?

    A. Make a back-up copy.

    B. Format a disk.

    C. Use application software.

    D. Use spell check.

    E. Use electronic mail.

10-13. Which of the following names will come first in alphabetic filing?

    A. Smith, William Paul

    B. Smith, Paul William

    C. Smyth, William

    D. Smythe, Bill

10-14. When releasing medical records

    A. never release the original medical record, only a copy.

    B. it is appropriate to release a medical record based on a verbal request from the patient.

    C. when discussing the medical record with someone other than the patient, only release a limited the amount of medical information.

    D. send the patient the original record, when requested.

10-15. When the computer is turned on, the process of loading the operating system is called

    A. booting.

    B. back-up.

C. networking.
D. anti-virus.

10-16. The medical assistant should take which of the following steps when the physician is delayed in arriving at the office for appointments?

A. Offer patients in the waiting room the chance to reschedule to avoid delays.
B. Cancel all appointments for the day.
C. Reschedule all appointments for the day.
D. Offer to refer the patients to another physician.

10-17. All of the following pieces of information about the patient will need to be provided to the hospital when calling to schedule inpatient surgery, EXCEPT the

A. physician's name.
B. time and day requested for the procedure.
C. urgency of the procedure.
D. anesthesia required.
E. insurance co-payment required from the patient.

10-18. A tickler file is a(n)

A. appointment card for patients' future visits.
B. chronological file of time-sensitive items by date.
C. file of patients that were "no shows."
D. temporary file for documents before filing them in patient medical records.

10-19. A filing system using a combination of numbers and letters is

A. alphabetic filing.
B. numeric filing.
C. subject filing.
D. alphanumeric filing.

10-20. Medical records are organized and sequenced based on all of the following factors EXCEPT

A. where the practice is located.
B. the type of medical practice.
C. the preference of the physician.
D. the frequency of access to records.

ANSWERS

10-1. The correct answer is C. Breathing difficulties in a senior citizen can be a sign of a serious condition and should be seen by the physician on an expedited basis.

10-2. The correct answer is B. Optical character recognition (OCR) is a process in which a printed document is scanned and the computer recognizes the letters and numbers. An example of OCR is a bank scanning checks and recognizing the preprinted account number.

10-3. The correct answer is C. No. 10 is the standard size envelope used for business correspondence.

10-4. The correct answer is A. Setting up a matrix for the appointment book involves crossing out all of the times that are not to be made available for patient appointments. These will include lunch breaks, days off, and vacations for the physician.

10-5. The correct answer is B. A database is a software application program, not a piece of hardware.

10-6. The correct answer is C. A fax machine is not an appropriate way to remind patients of appointments. Fax machines are generally located at the patient's place of work and may be seen by co-workers, violating confidentiality.

10-7. The correct answer is D. The out guide, updated with the initials and date of the medical assistant, is placed on the shelf in place of the file removed for active use.

10-8. The correct answer is C. The one major disadvantage of email is that it is only as secure as the internal controls over computer systems established on the systems of both sender and receiver.

10-9. The correct answer is B. Chronic no shows will need to be counseled on the need to keep appointments or, at a minimum, to call the medical office when an appointment cannot be kept.

10-10. The correct answer is B. Double booking is the process of booking two patients into the same appointment time.

10-11. The correct answer is D. A full colon is the appropriate punctuation mark following "Dear Mr. Smith" on the salutation.

10-12. The correct answer is A. When using a personal computer not networked to a larger system, the medical assistant should make a back-up copy of records to protect against loss of data. In a larger, networked system, back-ups are the responsibility of the network manager.

10-13. The correct answer is B. In the alphabetic filing system, medical records are filed alphabetically using the spelling of the last name of the patient. When the last names are the same on two or more records, the order of filing is then determined by the first name.

10-14. The correct answer is A. The original medical record should never be released to the patient. Upon the proper request from the patient, the record may be copied and delivered to the patient.

10-15. The correct answer is A. Booting is the process of the computer loading the operating system when the computer is turned on.

10-16. The correct answer is A. When the physician is delayed, the most effective step is to offer the patients currently in the waiting room the opportunity to reschedule to avoid lengthy delays. Patients who have appointments but have not yet arrived should be reached by phone and also offered the opportunity to reschedule.

10-17. The correct answer is E. Each of the above is important information to provide to the hospital, except information on the patient's insurance. The hospital will ask the patient for insurance information on intake.

10-18. The correct answer is B. A tickler file is used to remind the medical assistant of items that must be handled by a specific date, such as completing a license renewal form or paying an invoice.

10-19. The correct answer is D. Alphanumeric filing uses a combination of numbers and letters to determine the proper order of filing.

10-20. The correct answer is A. The location of the practice will have no bearing on the organization and sequence of medical records.

Administrative Functions and Management

The exam will contain a variety of administrative questions. In this chapter, we cover screening and processing of mail, resource information and community services, maintaining the office environment, and office policies and procedures.

SCREENING AND PROCESSING MAIL

The medical assistant will need to understand the types of mail used by the U.S. Postal Service and use the type most appropriate for the item to be mailed. Table 11-1 lists the types of mail used in the United States.

Medical offices that process a reasonable amount of outgoing mail will want to consider using a postage meter, which prints the appropriate amount of postage on the envelope to be mailed, eliminating the need for keeping books of stamps or having to go to the post office. The postage meter is loaded with a check written to the local post office for a dollar amount of available postage. As mail is processed and postage stamped on envelopes, the available balance is reduced and will need to be replenished as necessary.

The medical office will receive a wide variety and volume of incoming mail each business day. A medical assistant will be given the responsibility of handling the mail and needs to perform the task on a daily basis. Payment checks will be received from patients and from insurance companies. These should be immediately stamped on the back with a restrictive endorsement and forwarded to bookkeeping. Invoices and monthly statements will be received for items purchased by the medical office and should also be forwarded to bookkeeping. Business correspondence will need to be reviewed as to the appropriate recipient in the office. Mail that needs to be reviewed by the physician should be stacked for review with the most important documents on top and the least important on the bottom.

Mail should be reviewed to make sure that any indicated enclosures have been received. If not, the sender should be notified. Packages should be inspected to determine that all contents noted have been received and are not damaged. Any mail that is addressed to the physician and marked "personal" or "confidential" should not be opened by the medical assistant, but given directly to the physician.

For outgoing mail, the medical assistant needs to ensure that correspondence has been properly signed and that any enclosures indicated on the letter are included for mailing. When window envelopes are used, make sure that the address of the recipient shows through the window. Prior to taking the day's mail to the post office, the medical assistant will use the postage meter to stamp the envelopes with the proper postage. Mailing labels may be used for mailing bulk items such as patient newsletters.

Some large medical offices have begun to use OCR (optical character recognition) in the sorting of mail and to process checks and credit cards. OCR uses a computer to recognize printed or written text characters. The delivery of mail is much faster when OCR machines are in use.

Table 11-1 U.S. Mail Classifications

Mail Classifications	Definitions
First class mail	Used to mail general business correspondence weighing less than 13 ounces. First class mail provides second day service to major metropolitan areas and 3-day service elsewhere in the United States.
Priority mail	Used for mail within the United States for parcels over 13 ounces but less than 70 pounds. Priority mail provides the same delivery schedule as for first class mail.
Express mail	Used when the delivery schedule for first class or priority mail is not fast enough. For an additional fee, the postal service will guarantee overnight delivery. For overnight delivery, the medical office may also use private-sector business services such as Federal Express and the United Parcel Service (UPS).
Certified mail	Mail sent by first class or priority mail may be certified for an additional fee. Certified mail guarantees that the item mailed is delivered by requiring that the recipient sign for delivery. The receipt signed by the recipient is held at the receiving post office. For an additional fee, the sender may receive a return receipt as proof of delivery.
Registered mail	First class or priority mail that contains an item of value may be sent by registered mail. The item mailed is controlled at each step in the process and is insured for the value of the item being mailed.

RESOURCE INFORMATION AND COMMUNITY SERVICES

Being able to provide patients the contact information of resources available in the community is an important service. The medical assistant should have a comprehensive listing of services that may have a bearing on a patient's health and well-being. These will include financial aid available from local charities; alcohol, substance abuse, and addiction recovery services; counseling services; and legal services. To be able to appropriately respond to the needs of patients, the medical assistant should know the appropriate agencies to contact immediately when there is imminent danger to the patient. Such agencies include child protective services and emergency medical services. The medical assistant should maintain contact information for the local medical society and national medical organizations. Finally, written reports sometimes will need to be filed with the local public health department; the medical assistant should have the appropriate forms and addresses for filing those reports.

The Internet is a good source for information about local community resources. When using the Internet to research health issues, it is important to verify that the site is a reliable site. Sites whose addresses end in .gov, .edu, and .org are almost always good sources of information.

MAINTAINING THE OFFICE ENVIRONMENT

The exam will contain questions about the management of the office environment. The reception area is the patient's first contact with the medical office and should both put the patient at ease and create an atmosphere of professionalism. The furniture should be functional and comfortable and the area needs to be clean and uncluttered. Furniture should be arranged so that patients have easy access to the receptionist and the area is free of dangerous obstacles, such as throw rugs or children's toys left on the floor. If reading material is provided for the patients' use, make sure that newspapers and magazines are maintained in an orderly fashion and retired when they become outdated or have excessive wear from use. The temperature and lighting should be at a setting that is comfortable. Provide a coat rack and an umbrella stand for use by patients when weather dictates.

The medical assistant serving as receptionist should be seated behind a counter and will have a clear view of the reception area. During the work day, the medical assistant must make sure to keep the work area free of clutter. All medical assisting staff need to maintain high standards for personal hygiene and professional appearance and dress. The medical assistant should always behave in a professional manner and demonstrate a friendly, caring, and respectful attitude towards the patients.

Every medical office is responsible for assuring compliance with a variety of federal, state, and local requirements in establishing and running the office environment. The Occupational Safety and

Health Administration (OSHA) of the U.S. Department of Labor has established standards for basic workplace safety, including infection control, and has penalties for noncompliance. Table 11-2 outlines the basic standards.

The Americans with Disabilities Act of 1990 (ADA) mandates equal access and employment rights for the disabled. Guidelines also have been established by the Centers for Disease Control and Prevention (CDC) for the handling of epidemics such as the flu. On the local level, medical offices need to comply with fire safety regulations and access rules.

Table 11-2 OSHA Standards

OSHA Standard	Definitions
Bloodborne Pathogens	Intended to reduce exposure to bloodborne pathogens, this standard targets HIV and the hepatitis B and C viruses. Basic rules require a written exposure control plan that is updated annually, use of safer needles and sharps, use of personal protective equipment, universal precautions, no-cost hepatitis B vaccines for staff, follow-up after exposure, proper containment of waste, proper identification of waste containers, and employee training.
Hazard Communication	This standard requires that employees are made aware of any hazardous chemicals in the office. It also requires the maintenance of the material safety data sheets (MSDS) by the designated safety officer.
Clearly Marked Exit Routes	This standard includes the requirements for providing safe and accessible building exits in case of fire or other emergency.
Electrical Outlets and Wiring	This standard addresses electrical safety requirements for hazardous locations. If you use flammable gases, you may need special wiring and equipment installation.

EQUIPMENT AND SUPPLY INVENTORY

Many medical assistants are responsible for maintaining an inventory of all capital equipment, including all of the clinical and laboratory equipment, as well as the office equipment and furniture in the reception and administrative areas. The capital equipment inventory will include all of the assets of the medical office with a value over a certain minimum level, which is determined by the accountant retained to do year-end accounting and tax work. The minimum level will generally be in the range of $500 to $1000. Purchases with a lower value will be treated as consumable supplies. The inventory will include a description of the asset, serial number, vendor, date purchased or leased, and cost. The inventory should be updated on an annual basis and is used in the preparation of the year-end financial statements.

Many assets will come with an operating manual and may include a warranty and possibly an extended warranty purchased by the medical office. For specialized equipment, the medical office may have purchased a service contract to cover the maintenance requirements of the equipment. This information should be maintained in a separate file for each individual piece of equipment and should be readily accessible.

Many pieces of equipment may be leased rather than purchased. The lease will be for a fixed period of time and will generally include a service contract for needed maintenance and repairs of the equipment. For example, many businesses will lease, rather than purchase, the office photocopier due to the unique service needs of that piece of equipment.

Supplies in the medical office will include all of the items that are used (consumed) on a regular basis. Medical offices may set up a standing order with a vendor for restocking of frequently used supplies based on usage. Medical assistants are often responsible for the ordering and maintenance of supply items. A medical assistant should review the weekly use of supply items and determine from the selected vendor how long it will take to get delivery of an order. From this information, the medical assistant can determine the level of the supply item that should be set to assure that the practice does not run out of the item. As an example, let's say the medical office uses an average of 10 items of a specific supply each business day. The selected vendor has informed you that the normal delivery time is 1 week, which is 5 business days. To protect against delays in receiving shipments from the vendor, you set a safety stock level of 25 items, equal to a one-half week supply. From this information, you would set the re-order point for this item at 75 items—a 1-week supply of 50 to cover the 1-week lead time for delivery and the safety stock of 25. Whenever the supply inventory drops to 75 items, you would place an order for delivery. The amount to be ordered at one time will be based on a number of considerations. The vendor may offer a discount for a larger order; however, cash flow and the ability to store a larger number of supply items must be taken into account.

If possible, the medical office should have a separate entrance for deliveries, so that supplies do not need to be brought into the office through the reception area. The contents of each delivery must be compared to the packing slip received with the shipment. Any discrepancies or back-ordered items need to be noted. The packing slip should be initialed and dated and provided to bookkeeping as part of the documentation to pay the vendor invoice.

LIABILITY COVERAGE

The medical practice will need to obtain insurance policies to cover a variety of exposures that could lead to substantial financial loss to the practice. Appropriate insurance coverage will include property insurance to protect against fire losses and other damage to the building and equipment owned by the practice. A general liability policy will protect against exposures such as a slip and fall in the office and the inadvertent release of confidential medical information. Coverage for workers' compensation will be mandated by the state the practice is domiciled in to cover the costs of an employee injured on the job. Individual physicians will be covered by professional liability insurance, designed to protect the physician in case of malpractice claims. Medical offices may maintain group health insurance coverage for employees, paid for by the practice, by the employee, or through joint contribution.

TIME MANAGEMENT

The ability of the medical assistant to manage his or her time effectively is a critical skill in a busy medical office. A "to-do" list, with the items properly prioritized to assure that the most important issues are addressed first and completed on a timely basis, is a key tool in time management. At the end of the business day, cross out the items on the to-do list that have been completed, transfer the incomplete items to a new list for the next day, and add any new items that must be addressed the next day, again prioritized in order of importance. Make sure you have a desk calendar or small pocket calendar to keep track of appointments and a listing of important phone numbers.

OFFICE POLICIES AND PROCEDURES

Many medical offices will prepare written information to provide to the patient, describing the practice and services provided, listing the qualifications of the physicians, and introducing the staff members. Office hours, procedures for scheduling appointments, and insurance and payment policy will be covered. A key issue to be discussed will be the medical practice's statement on confidentiality. The format in which to provide this information to patients will range from a simple, one-page document to a professionally prepared brochure including pictures of physicians and staff. Additional information may be provided to patients relating to specific procedures. These may include booklets describing the procedure, anatomical models, and videotapes.

Another common document in the medical office is the personnel manual. The manual is designed to provide the employee with information on their rights and responsibilities. The manual will commonly start with a statement of the medical office's mission, vision, and philosophy. Included will be sections dealing with pay frequency and overtime policy, holidays and vacation time, benefits paid for by the employer and optional group benefits that may be purchased by the employee, and the dress code of the practice. Also included will be policies dealing with illegal drug use and disciplinary actions. The personnel manual will be readily available to all employees; some practices will require new employees to sign a statement attesting that they have read and understand important policies contained in the manual.

Most medical offices will also have a policies and procedures manual. This manual will provide detailed directions for the approved process of accomplishing a specific task. Each task will be handled separately and will normally be maintained in a loose-leaf notebook so that task procedures may be easily updated as technology and techniques improve. For example, there will be separate procedures for the handling of incoming mail and for the proper process to follow in creating a medical record for a new patient. The policies and procedures manual is a valuable tool in the orientation of a new employee and an easy refresher for the seasoned employee.

QUESTIONS

11-1. The medical office has been cited for storing boxes of medical supplies in front of an emergency exit. The agency or person citing this infraction is

    A. the enforcement agency for the Americans with Disabilities Act (ADA).
    B. a Medicare inspector.
    C. the local fire inspection agency.
    D. An inspector for the Centers for Disease Control and Prevention (CDC).

11-2. The medical office will maintain referral information for the convenience of patients. This will include referral information for

    A. drug and alcohol abuse counselors.
    B. agencies providing financial aid to the needy.
    C. legal services.
    D. All of the above.

11-3. Certified mail is special handling for which classification of mail?

    A. Express mail
    B. First-class mail
    C. Second-class mail
    D. Third-class mail
    E. Bulk mail

11-4. The most appropriate first step when processing the daily mail is to

    A. discard advertisements.
    B. place all mail on the physician's desk.
    C. date stamp each item.
    D. distribute mail to staff members.
    E. prepare bank deposit of insurance payments.

11-5. Which type of insurance pays benefits when an accident or serious illness results in loss of pay?

    A. Medicare
    B. Disability insurance
    C. Major medical insurance
    D. Medicaid
    E. Workers' compensation

11-6. Business correspondence and postcards are mailed by

    A. first-class mail.
    B. second-class mail.
    C. third-class mail.
    D. bulk mailing.
    E. expedited mail.

11-7. When the medical office needs to have a mailed document received the next business day, which type of mailing is used?

    A. First-class mail
    B. Certified mail
    C. Registered mail
    D. Express mail
    E. Bulk mailing

11-8. A multi-physician medical practice uses two boxes of syringes daily, with each box containing 25 syringes. How many boxes of syringes will need to be ordered each month?

    A. 40
    B. 30
    C. 20
    D. 10
    E. 5

11-9. The most appropriate FIRST step before using new equipment is to

    A. sign and date the warranty card.
    B. contact the manufacturer.
    C. read the product accessory literature.
    D. ask a co-worker about proper operation.
    E. review the user manual.

11-10. The annual premium for the physician's malpractice insurance needs to be paid by May 12, 2011. A note to make this payment would be found in which of the following filing systems?

    A. Alphabetic
    B. Numeric
    C. Alphanumeric
    D. Tickler
    E. Subject

11-11. Which of the following documents guarantees that a service provider will maintain the equipment at no additional cost for a specific period of time?

    A. Service contract
    B. Preventive maintenance schedule
    C. Purchase order
    D. Warranty
    E. Packing slip

11-12. Express mail

    A. includes insurance in the charge for service.
    B. guarantees next day delivery.
    C. is eligible for mailings up to 70 pounds.
    D. All of the above.

11-13. Which of the following would NOT be appropriate for use in a medical office's reception area?

    A. End tables with lamps
    B. An aquarium
    C. Live plants
    D. Magazines and newspapers
    E. Throw rugs

11-14. Water is accidentally left on the floor of the restroom. A patient is asked to provide a urine sample and slips and falls on the wet floor. If the patient brings a lawsuit against the medical office, the insurance policy that will provide protection is

    A. general liability.
    B. professional liability.
    C. malpractice insurance.
    D. workers' compensation.
    E. disability insurance.

11-15. The quote "Our medical staff, working together as a team, will provide the best possible medical care to each of our patients" would be an example of which of the following?

    A. A clinical procedure
    B. An administrative procedure
    C. A statement of risk management
    D. An office procedure
    E. A mission statement

11-16. Which of the following would NOT be included in a medical office's personnel manual?

    A. Policy for handling incoming mail
    B. Holidays and vacations
    C. Illegal drug policy
    D. Employee benefits
    E. Disciplinary action

11-17. Which of the following is the correct two-letter abbreviation for Michigan?

    A. MN
    B. MI
    C. MA
    D. MG
    E. MH

11-18. The medical assistant mistakenly opens a letter to the physician marked "Personal." The appropriate action to be taken is to

    A. discard the letter.
    B. page the physician to inform him or her of the mistake.
    C. take the letter to the physician's office immediately.
    D. write "opened in error" on the envelope and initial.
    E. reseal the letter in an office envelope.

11-19. The process of ranking tasks for the day based on their importance is

    A. prioritizing.
    B. projecting.
    C. prescribing.
    D. procrastinating.
    E. presuming.

11-20. Items such as deeds and wills are valuable documents, but do not have a significant monetary value. The best way to mail this type of document would be by using

    A. express mail.
    B. first-class mail.
    C. registered mail.
    D. priority mail.
    E. certified mail.

ANSWERS

11-1. The correct answer is C. The local fire agency will inspect commercial properties for compliance with fire codes.

11-2. The correct answer is D. The medical office will be able to provide patients with information on local agencies providing drug and alcohol abuse counseling, financial aid, and legal services.

11-3. The correct answer is B. Certified mail is special handling, at an additional charge, of first class mail.

11-4. The correct answer is C. The first step in processing the daily mail is to date stamp each item received.

11-5. The correct answer is B. Disability insurance, commonly offered to employees as an employee-paid group benefit, will provide, after a mandatory waiting period, monthly cash benefits to compensate the employee for the loss of a paycheck.

11-6. The correct answer is A. Business correspondence and postcards, up to 13 ounces, are considered to be first-class mail.

11-7. The correct answer is D. Express mail from the post office guarantees delivery the next business day.

11-8. The correct answer is A. Two boxes daily for 5 business days each week is 10 boxes. Ten boxes per week for each of 4 weeks will total a monthly order of 40 boxes.

11-9. The correct answer is E. When a new piece of equipment is delivered to the medical office, the first step will always be a thorough review of the user (operator's) manual.

11-10. The correct answer is D. A tickler file is used to record actions that need to be taken on a future date.

11-11. The correct answer is A. A service contract, which is purchased for a specific piece of equipment, will provide the medical office with a guarantee that the equipment will be properly maintained for a specific period of time.

11-12. The correct answer is D. Express mail may be used for any mailing of up to 70 pounds, includes insurance in the fee, and guarantees next day delivery.

11-13. The correct answer is E. Any items that may be dangerous to patients should not be placed in areas used by the patients. Throw rugs may be a slip and fall hazard and are examples of items that should not be used.

11-14. The correct answer is A. A general liability insurance policy will provide insurance coverage in the case of slips and falls in the medical office.

11-15. The correct answer is E. The mission statement of a medical office will establish the standards for providing superior medical care to the patients. The mission statement will commonly be part of a patient information booklet.

11-16. The correct answer is A. Operating policies and procedures, such as the policy for handling incoming mail, would be located in the policy and procedures manual of the medical office.

11-17. The correct answer is B. The correct two-letter abbreviation for Michigan is MI. Care must be taken to use the correct two-letter abbreviation for states when mailing.

11-18. The correct answer is D. Unless specifically authorized by the physician, correspondence addressed to the physician and marked "personal" or "confidential" should not be opened as part of the daily activity of processing incoming mail. If such a letter is opened by mistake, write "opened in error" on the envelope and deliver it to the physician with the rest of the day's mail.

11-19. The correct answer is A. Prioritizing is the process of arranging the tasks or functions that need to be accomplished in the order of their importance.

11-20. The correct answer is E. Certified mail is the preferred method of mailing important documents that do not have a significant monetary value. Certified mail provides a proof of mailing, and a receipt of delivery can be requested.

Finance

Medical assistants are expected to have an understanding of basic bookkeeping functions, as well as some accounting, banking, and payroll procedures. This chapter outlines the material that may be covered on the exam. This topic will continue in Chapter 13, which covers third-party billing, and Chapter 14, which reviews basic coding information.

BOOKKEEPING PRINCIPLES

Bookkeeping is the process of recording items into the accounting system. In the medical office, this will include charges for services provided to patients, payments received from patients and their insurance companies, and adjustments made to patient accounts. On the expense side, bookkeeping will include checks issued for the purchase of office and medical supplies and the payroll process to compensate employees for their service to the medical practice.

Bookkeeping and accounting processes have improved dramatically over the years with the expanded use of computers in the medical office. Specialized software, designed solely for the medical profession, has reduced bookkeeping and accounting time and provides control over errors. Some medical offices, however, continue to use a manual system or a combination of automated and manual systems. An understanding of these manual systems continues to be important.

The single-entry bookkeeping system is the oldest form of bookkeeping, requiring only a single entry for each item being recorded. Although it is easy to use, it is highly prone to errors because there is no built-in check and balance, as is found with the double-entry system. In the double-entry system, both a debit and a credit of equal size must be recorded for every item entered into the system. This follows the basic accounting equation that assets equal liabilities plus equity. Assets, such as cash, accounts receivable, furniture and equipment, and supplies inventory, are debits and are shown on the left side of the balance sheet. Liabilities (such as the balance of unpaid vendor invoices and any bank loans outstanding) and equity are credits and are on the right side. Revenues are credits and expenses are debits. In a simple example, a patient receives a medical service and pays cash. Posting of this transaction would be a debit to cash (increasing the asset balance for cash). The corresponding credit will be to medical services revenues (increasing the revenue balance in the account). At any time, but at least on a monthly basis, a trial balance is prepared to assure that the accounting records are in balance. The trial balance will highlight any errors made and facilitate their correction.

Still used in some medical offices is the pegboard system (or "one-write" system). This manual system consists of a board with a series of pegs along the left-hand side. Fitted onto the pegs are a series of bookkeeping sheets. These sheets will include the day sheet, ledger cards, patient charge slips, and receipt forms. With the proper alignment of the forms, a single entry will post the necessary information to each of the forms. Even in smaller medical offices, however, the pegboard system is being phased out in favor of a computer-based system.

Whether manual or computer-based, individual bookkeeping entries will flow into the accounting records of the medical office. The total of the individual patient account balances will equal the control account of accounts receivable in the general ledger. At the end of the business year, a final trial balance will be prepared. From that trial balance will flow the income statement for the medical office, summarizing the revenues and expenses to determine the profit or loss for the year. A balance sheet will also be prepared at the end of the year, detailing the assets, liabilities, and equity of the medical office.

On a daily basis, the medical assistant may have responsibility for balancing the day sheet, which is the record of daily charges and payments received. Table 12-1 lists the basic steps for balancing the day sheet. The day sheet does not include payments received on account (ROAs). The ROAs are those payments received in the mail or electronically for previous services rendered.

Table 12-1 Steps to Balancing the Day Sheet

1. Review the appointment schedule to determine the cancellations and no-shows for the day.
2. Collect all encounter forms for every patient seen that day.
3. Run your first trial balance for the day. This is also called a daily edit report.
4. Verify that information from all encounter forms has been entered into the trial balance.
5. Count the day's cash, total checks, and credit card payments for patients seen that day. Verify that the total amounts of cash, credit card charges, and checks match with the trial balance.
6. If the day does not balance, review each posting made. Typical errors include posting a cash payment as a credit card payment or a $205 payment as $200.
7. You must balance the day before you close the day. In most electronic practice management systems if you do not balance the day, the system will not allow you to open for the next day's business. Additionally, electronic claims forms may not automatically be sent if the day does not balance.

CHARGES, PAYMENTS, AND ADJUSTMENTS

In the days prior to widespread health insurance, the physician would establish a fair and reasonable charge for a medical service and bill the patient that amount. The patient would pay the bill and the account balance for that patient would be at zero. Today, medical offices agree to accept payments from insurance companies that provide health insurance coverage to patients. Each insurance company will have its own fee schedule that the physician agrees to accept.

As part of the agreement between the physician and the insurance company, the physician agrees to accept the approved amount for a specific medical service in lieu of the standard fee schedule of the physician. For example, the medical office has established a fee of $100 for a specific medical procedure. The patient is covered by insurance and requests that the medical office bill the insurance company. The specific medical procedure is approved for payment by the insurance company at $70. The patient has an office visit co-payment requirement of $25; the insurance company pays $45 to the medical office (approved charge of $70 less co-payment of $25). The medical office has posted $100 as revenue and an account receivable for the procedure. After applying the $45 payment from the insurance company and the $25 co-payment received from the patient, the account has a $30 balance that needs to be addressed. The proper practice is to post a $30 credit to the patient account; the debit to offset the credit is $30 to reduce office revenues. Under the terms of the agreement with the insurance company, the medical office is prohibited from "balance billing," which is billing the patient for the uncollected balance.

PETTY CASH FUND

A medical office will maintain a small cash fund to pay for miscellaneous business expenses, such as postage due on mail delivered or minor business purchases at a vendor where the office does not have an account. Cash will be withdrawn from the fund and a petty cash slip completed with the date, amount, and subject of expense. When the petty cash fund is in need of replenishment, a check will be written to cash for the total of the petty cash slips and taken to the bank. The accounting entry will be debits to appropriate expense accounts and a credit to cash, each balancing to the amount of the replenishment check. The petty cash fund will always be replenished to the original balance at the end of the medical office's business year.

BILLING PROCEDURES

Billing procedures differ slightly in every medical practice. As mentioned in Chapter 13, all bills sent to insurance companies and Medicare and Medicaid must be itemized on the CMS-1500 form. Also, most billing today is done electronically. Depending on your practice, you may send electronic versions of the CMS-1500 on a daily, weekly, or monthly basis. If there are questions regarding billing cycles on the exam, it is best to select the most frequent cycle as the correct item.

AGING PROCEDURES

The best practice for the medical office is to ask patients to arrange for payment of medical services at the time the services are provided. However, many patients have health insurance that requires that you bill the insurance company first, collecting only the co-pay at time of service.

The first step in the collection process is the preparation of an aging analysis. This analysis will provide you with needed information on how long balances due to the medical office have been outstanding. Most electronic patient management systems will provide the medical assistant with a list not only of 30-, 60-, and 90-day overdue balances, but also balances by insurance company. This allows the medical assistant to follow up with an insurance company for multiple claims.

COLLECTION PROCEDURES

All outstanding accounts that are owed by the patient should be billed at least on a monthly basis. However, once the account is overdue 30 days, legitimate collection activities may begin. A combination of telephone calls to the patient and written correspondence to the patient should be used. All contacts should be handled professionally and must not be abusive or threatening. A firmer tone may be used in follow-up contacts when initial contacts have been unsuccessful. After a series of unsuccessful attempts at collection, the account is termed uncollectible and should be immediately turned over to a collection agency under contract to the medical office. Alternative means of collection include small claims court or action through the attorney of the medical office. When notified that a patient with an outstanding balance has filed for bankruptcy, the medical office must suspend all collection activities and file a claim with the bankruptcy court.

CONSUMER PROTECTION ACTS

The exam may contain questions about the following three federal laws regarding collection:

- The Equal Credit Opportunity Act, which prohibits discrimination in providing credit
- The federal Truth in Lending Act, which regulates interest charges and installment payments of more than four payments
- The Fair Debt Collection Practices Act, which prohibits certain activities in the collection of debts, such as harassment, frequent phone calls, and phone calls to the patient's place of employment

ACCOUNTS PAYABLE

The purchase of goods or services will generate accounts payable. Medical and office supplies are ordered from vendors where credit accounts have been established. When a delivery is received, the items received should be verified against the packing slip received with the shipment. When the invoice is received from the vendor, packing slips are reconciled to the invoices for accuracy. Most vendors will expect payment to be received within 30 days and may impose delinquent charges on payments not received in that time. The medical office should have procedures in place that will provide for timely payments and avoid late charges.

BANKING

A commercial checking account with a bank is an important part of the financial management of a medical practice. During each business day, patients have paid in person for medical services with cash or a personal check, and additional checks are received as the daily mail is processed. Once each of the items has been appropriately entered into the accounting system, a bank deposit is prepared using a preprinted deposit slip for the checking account. The individual responsible for preparing the bank deposit needs to double check the balance of cash to be deposited and ensure that each check has been properly endorsed. The most common form of endorsement is the restrictive endorsement. The medical office will have a stamp prepared with the words "For Deposit Only," followed by the name of the medical office and the number of the bank account. Other forms of endorsement are the blank endorsement, which is only the signature of the owner of the account; a limited endorsement with the words "Pay to the Order of," used to transfer the proceeds of the check to a third party; and a qualified endorsement used to protect from future liability. All payments received should be deposited on a daily basis.

Occasionally, the bank will refuse to honor a check because the issuer of the check does not have sufficient funds in his or her account to cover the amount of the check. This is an NSF, or non-sufficient funds, check. The medical office should redeposit the check immediately to see if the owner of the checking account has added funds to the account to be able to cover the amount of the check. If returned by the bank a second time, the medical office will follow standard collection processes to be paid the funds due from the patient.

Each month, the bank will supply the medical office with a statement on the checking account. This statement must be analyzed and banking activity posted to the accounting system in a process called reconciliation. Remember that there will be a delay of several days from the date of the bank statement to the time the statement is reconciled. In those days, the medical office has most likely issued checks that have not cleared the bank and are not on the bank statement, and may have one of more deposits that are not listed, also referred to as deposits in transit. The steps required for reconciliation of the bank statement are shown in Table 12-2.

Table 12-2 Steps for Reconciling the Bank Statement

1. *Identify deposits not posted by the bank.* Put a check mark on all deposits from the accounting records that are shown on the bank statement. Deposits that do not have a check mark are unposted deposits and need to be added to the bank statement balance.

2. *Identify checks that have not cleared the bank.* Put a check mark on all checks issued that have cleared the bank. Checks that do not have a check mark are outstanding and need to be deducted from the bank statement balance.

3. *Identify service fees and interest earned on the checking account.* Service fees, shown as a debit on the bank statement, need to be posted to the accounting records of the medical practice as a business expense. Interest earned, shown as a credit on the bank statement, needs to be posted to the accounting records as revenue. Make sure that all debits and credits on the bank statement have been accounted for.

4. Verify that the bank statement balance, adjusted for unposted deposits and outstanding checks, equals the balance in the accounting records, adjusted for any debits or credits on the bank statement.

PAYROLL

The largest area of expense for the medical office is compensating employees for the services they provide. Payroll is also the area most heavily regulated by the federal government and state law. When an employee is first hired, the medical office must determine that the new person meets the definition of an employee, rather than an independent contractor. The decision also must be made as to whether the new employee is exempt or non-exempt for required payment of overtime pay. The new employee will complete Form W-4, Employee's Withholding Allowance Certificate. This form directs the medical office on the calculation of tax withholding. At the end of the year, all employees are provided with a Form W-2, Wage and Tax Statement. This form identifies earnings and taxes withheld for the year. Employers must complete and file a Transmittal of Wage and Tax Statements (Form W-3) annually with Social Security, accompanied by copies of the W-2 forms for all employees. The employer is also responsible for filing Form 941, Employer's Quarterly Federal Tax Return each quarter. Last, employers must file a Form 940 known as the Employers Annual Federal Unemployment Tax Return.

Employees will commonly be paid on either a weekly or bi-weekly basis. The Fair Labor Standards Act (FLSA) requires that the employee be compensated at time-and-a-half for hours worked in excess of 40 hours per week. Gross pay is determined by multiplying the employee's rate of pay by the standard work week, commonly 40 hours, and multiplying overtime hours by the employee's rate of pay times 1.5 for overtime. For example, a medical assistant is hired at the rate of $12 per hour for a 40-hour workweek. Gross base pay is $480 weekly. In a given week, the medical assistant worked an additional 10 hours to cover for a sick employee. Overtime pay would be $180 ($12 per hour × 10 hours × 1.5 for overtime). Gross pay for the week would be $660.

There are required deductions from gross pay to determine the paycheck received by the employee. The Form W-4 completed by the employee to identify dependents will determine the tax withholding schedule used for federal and state income taxes. The employer will use the Employer's Tax Guide for federal withholding tables and withholding tables provided by the state government. The Federal Insurance Contributions Act (FICA) governs withholding for Old Age, Survivors, and Disability Insurance (OASDI) for Social Security at the rate of 6.2% and Medicare at 1.45%. These two deductions, totaling 7.65%, are required to be matched by the employer. Voluntary deductions from payroll for employees may include the employee's contribution to health care insurance, participation in a deferred compensation plan, or contributions to a credit union account. The Federal Unemployment Tax Act (FUTA) governs payments to support unemployment compensation. FUTA is based on payroll, but is paid only by the employer, not the employee.

QUESTIONS

12-1. The medical office maintains a record of each check issued that shows the date, the check number, the amount, and the payee. This is called a(n)

    A. aging report.
    B. ledger.
    C. journal.
    D. check register.
    E. accounts payable detail.

12-2. Susan is employed as a medical assistant and earns $15 per hour. The medical office pays employees each week. She works 42 hours during the current week. Her payroll deductions each week total $102.10. Her net pay for the week is

    A. $747.10.
    B. $702.10.
    C. $645.00.
    D. $522.90.
    E. $542.90.

12-3. When a check is endorsed "For Deposit Only," this is referred to as a

    A. simple endorsement.
    B. restrictive endorsement.
    C. qualified endorsement.
    D. special endorsement.
    E. blank endorsement.

12-4. Which of the following will list, by individual patient names, funds owed to the practice for services provided?

    A. Day sheet
    B. Accounts payable ledger
    C. Receipt
    D. Charge slip
    E. Accounts receivable ledger

12-5. The process of determining which patient accounts are past due is

    A. compiling a fee profile.
    B. aging analysis.
    C. posting managed care discounts.
    D. coordination of benefits.
    E. posting debits.

12-6. The delinquent account of a patient has been turned over to a collection agency. The patient calls the office and wants to make payment arrangements. The medical assistant should

    A. ask the patient how much he can pay today.
    B. set up a payment schedule with the patient.
    C. tell the patient that the total amount due must be paid immediately.
    D. direct the patient to the collection agency to discuss payments.
    E. warn the patient of pending legal action to collect the money owed.

12-7. The individual record of the amounts owed for medical services, payments made, and account balance for each patient is found in the

    A. financial journal.
    B. general ledger.
    C. patient's ledger.
    D. daily journal (day sheet).
    E. trial balance.

12-8. Accounts receivable are

    A. the record of expenses to be paid by the practice.
    B. the record of money owed to the practice.
    C. the record of health insurance companies.
    D. the record of payroll transactions.
    E. the record of disbursements.

12-9. The petty cash fund of the medical office is replenished when

    A. a check is written and arrangements made for it to be cashed.
    B. the medical assistant adds cash to the fund and requests reimbursement.
    C. cash is added from daily collections when funds are low.
    D. the physician contributes cash to the fund.
    E. the petty cash fund is closed.

12-10. The patient's ledger is actually a(n)

    A. accounts payable ledger.
    B. accounts receivable ledger.
    C. day sheet.
    D. income account.
    E. general ledger.

12-11. The trial balance of accounts receivable is prepared

    A. daily.
    B. weekly.
    C. monthly.
    D. annually.

12-12. Payments for professional services by cash, check, or credit card are called

    A. receipts.
    B. receivables.
    C. adjustments.
    D. payables.
    E. disbursements.

12-13. The medical assistant can find information regarding the filing of reports and taxes from the employee's earnings and employer's tax contributions in the

    A. IRS Employer's Tax Guide.
    B. medical office handbook.
    C. IRS Income Tax Guide.
    D. *Physician's Desk Reference.*

12-14. The medical assistant applies a discount to an unpaid balance on a patient account. This action is referred to as a(n)

    A. charge for service.
    B. account payable.
    C. adjustment.
    D. receivable.
    E. withholding.

12-15. The following ledger entry reduces the balance owed by a patient, but is NOT caused by either a charge for service or a payment.

    A. Debit
    B. Credit
    C. Adjustment
    D. Payable
    E. Receivable

12-16. A patient is charged $100 for treatment by the physician. The patient pays $60 and the medical office posts an adjustment to reduce the balance due by $15. What is the balance due on this account?

    A. $100
    B. $85
    C. $40
    D. $15
    E. $25

12-17. Employers are obligated by law to match which of the following?

    A. Local income tax withheld
    B. State income tax withheld
    C. Federal income tax withheld
    D. FICA
    E. FUTA

12-18. Of the following statements, the one MOST appropriate for use in a collection letter is

    A. "We will be happy to assist you in making payment arrangements."
    B. "We must receive payment within 10 business days or. . . ."
    C. "Did you lose our last billing?"
    D. "We are disappointed that you have not made payment on this account."
    E. "We cannot pay our employees without receiving your payment."

12-19. An emancipated minor sees the physician for a scheduled appointment. The charge for service should be

    A. billed to the parents.
    B. written off as uncollectible.
    C. forwarded to the insurance company of the parents.
    D. billed to the patient.
    E. filed with Medicaid.

12-20. When reconciling the bank statement for the medical practice, which of the following actions will cause an error?

    A. Deducting bank service charges from the checkbook balance
    B. Deducting outstanding automated teller machine (ATM) withdrawals from the bank statement
    C. Deducting outstanding checks from the bank statement
    D. Deducting NSF checks from the checkbook balance
    E. Deducting monthly interest paid by the bank from the checkbook balance

ANSWERS

12-1. The correct answer is D. The check register for a medical office lists all checks written, showing the check number, date written, payee, and amount.

12-2. The correct answer is E. Regular pay at $15 per hour for a 40-hour workweek is $600.00. Two hours at $15 per hour at time and a half for overtime is $45.00. Total gross pay would be $645.00. Deductions will include mandatory deductions for federal and, if applicable, state tax, Social Security, and Medicare. Additional deductions may include employee contribution to a health plan and retirement coverage. The $645.00 less $102.10 in deductions yields net pay of $542.90.

12-3. The correct answer is B. "For Deposit Only" is a restrictive endorsement. This should be stamped immediately on checks received at the medical office and will include the name and account number of the practice to assure that checks are deposited into the proper account.

12-4. The correct answer is E. Funds owed to the practice are accounts receivable and will be accounted for, by individual, in the accounts receivable ledger.

12-5. The correct answer is B. The aging analysis determines the past due status of patient accounts.

12-6. The correct answer is D. Once the medical office has turned over an account to a collection agency, all further contact should be between the individual and the collection agency. The appropriate action is to refer the patient to the collection agency.

12-7. The correct answer is C. The patient's ledger will contain all financial activity dealing with the individual, including charges for medical services, payments made, and current balance.

12-8. The correct answer is B. Accounts receivable are the net difference between charges for medical services and payments made on individual accounts. This is the money owed to the practice that has yet to be collected.

12-9. The correct answer is A. The petty cash fund of the medical office is replenished by writing a check payable to "Cash." An employee of the medical office will hand carry the check to the bank and receive cash to replenish the fund.

12-10. The correct answer is B. The term "patient's ledger" is the same as "accounts receivable ledger."

12-11. The correct answer is C. The trial balance of accounts receivable is prepared on a monthly basis to assure that any variances are reconciled on a timely basis. The daily trial balance is done to reflect only daily activity.

12-12. The correct answer is A. The term "receipts" is used for payments made on accounts for professional services provided by the medical office. Payment methods will include cash, check, or credit card.

12-13. The correct answer is A. The IRS Employer's Tax Guide will provide detailed information on the proper completion and filing of reports and taxes.

12-14. The correct answer is C. A discount to the unpaid balance on a patient account may result from a reduction in allowable charges from an insurance company. An adjustment is posted to the patient account, resulting in a smaller balance due from the patient for the unpaid balance.

12-15. The correct answer is C. An adjustment made to the patient account is an action that is not caused by either a charge for service or a payment received on the account.

12-16. The correct answer is E. The initial charge of $100 is reduced by the payment received of $60 and further reduced by the adjustment of $15, for a balance due on the account of $25.

12-17. The correct answer is D. FICA (Social Security) is a 6.2% deduction from the paycheck of the employee, up to a maximum established annually, and matched by the employer.

12-18. The correct answer is A. Collection letters need to be both unemotional and not confrontational. The letter should state the medical office will be willing to accept payments over a reasonable period of time and will work with the patient on a repayment schedule.

12-19. The correct answer is D. For purposes of medical billing, an emancipated minor is one responsible for the payment of his or her own charges. The charge for service should be billed to the patient.

12-20. The correct answer is E. Interest paid by the bank and posted to the bank statement of the medical practice must be *added to* the checkbook balance to accurately reconcile the account.

Third-Party Billing

A medical assistant is expected to have a good understanding of the third-party billing system. Many medical assistants also serve as the biller for the practice. The exam will contain a variety of questions about the types of third-party payment, and how to process claims, apply managed care principles, and handle fee schedules.

TYPES OF HEALTH INSURANCE

Health insurance is a contract between the patient and/or employer and the insurance company or other third-party payer. The contract states that the insurance company will pay a portion of the covered individual's medical expenses for sicknesses and injuries, and often for preventive care. The portion of the costs to be paid by the insurance company varies with every contract. The patient (and/or the employer) agrees to pay the insurance a premium each month for this service.

There are three general types of insurance plans: government-sponsored plans, group health plans, and individual health policies. In addition, both group health plans and government-sponsored plans can be either traditional insurance or managed care. Individual coverage is almost always traditional insurance.

Government-Sponsored Plans

The federal government sponsors a variety of plans. Additionally, at least one plan, Medicaid, has both federal and state government participation. On the exam, you will be expected to know the differences among the various government-sponsored plans.

Medicare

Medicare is a federal health insurance program financed through a Medicare payroll withholding tax. Both employers and employees contribute an equal percentage of the employee's pay. Medical bills are paid from trust funds created by the withholding tax for those eligible for Medicare.

Medicare is considered an entitlement program for people over 65, whatever their income. Disabled people and dialysis patients may also be eligible.

Medicare has four parts. Part A covers hospital services and inpatient stays in a skilled nursing facility. The nursing home care must be inpatient care. Custodial or long-term care in a nursing home is not covered by Medicare. Hospice care services and some home health care services are covered. As with all insurance plans, there are limits to what Medicare will cover. There is no premium for Part A if a recipient or their spouse paid Medicare taxes while working.

Medicare Part B covers doctors' services, outpatient care, some other medical services Part A does not cover, and some preventive services. A monthly premium must be paid. The costs to the patient will be different if they are a member of a Medicare Advantage Program (Part C of Medicare) or if the patient has other insurance like a Medigap policy or employer coverage.

Part C coverage from Medicare is called the Medicare Advantage Plan. This program is the managed-care portion of Medicare. Recipients may elect to join a Part C provider instead of Part B and sometimes Part D. The plans in the Medicare Advantage Plans are managed-care plans. Depending on the plan selected, recipients may receive better benefits from a Medicare Advantage Plan.

The newest part of Medicare is Part D, which is the prescription drug benefit. Some Part D plans work in conjunction with Part C.

Medicaid

Medicaid is an assistance program, technically not an insurance plan, serving a select group of low-income people. Funding for Medicaid comes from federal, state, and local tax funds. Medicaid will pay providers for the covered individuals. Patients usually pay none of the costs for covered medical expenses. A small co-payment is sometimes required, but no premium payment is required. Medicaid rules and payments differ from state to state.

State Children's Health Insurance Program

The State Children's Health Insurance Program (SCHIP) covers uninsured children under the age of 19 whose parents earn less than a certain amount annually. Families who earn too much to qualify for Medicaid may be able to qualify for SCHIP. For little or no cost, SCHIP pays for doctor visits, hospitalizations, immunizations, and emergency room visits.

Coverage for Military Members and Their Families

TRICARE is the federally funded program providing comprehensive health benefits for dependents of active duty military personnel and dependents of military personnel who died while on active duty, as well as retired military personnel and their dependents. It was originally known as CHAMPUS, but in 1993, changed its name to TRICARE. There are three choices for military families in TRICARE, as illustrated in Table 13-1.

TRICARE is different from CHAMPVA, the Civilian Health and Medical Program of the Veterans Administration, which is administered by the Department of Veterans Affairs. To be eligible for CHAMPVA, you cannot be eligible for TRICARE and you must be in one of the categories listed in Table 13-2.

Workers' Compensation Health Insurance

If a person is injured at work, workers' compensation covers health care costs for an injury or illness. Funding for workers' compensation comes from premiums paid by the employer into both a state fund and federal fund (Federal Unemployment Tax Act [FUTA] and State Unemployment Tax Act [SUTA]). Whenever a patient comes in with an injury, it is important for the medical assistant to find out if the patient was injured on the job. Not all workers may understand that they must report the injury or illness to their employer.

Table 13-1 TRICARE Coverage

Plan Type	Coverage
TRICARE Standard	This is similar to an indemnity plan and is often referred to as the old CHAMPUS plan. Patients have more choice in providers, but they pay a higher out of pocket cost.
TRICARE Extra	This is similar to a PPO in that patients must obtain their care from an approved list of providers.
TRICARE Prime	This plan is similar to an HMO in that patients are assigned a primary case manager and all care is coordinated through the case manager. It is the least expensive of the options.

Table 13-2 Eligibility for CHAMPVA

You are eligible for CHAMPVA if you are:

- The spouse or child of a veteran who has been rated permanently and totally disabled for a service-connected disability by a VA regional office.
- The surviving spouse or child of a veteran who died from a VA rated service-connected disability.
- The surviving spouse or child of a veteran who at the time of death was rated permanently and totally disabled from a service-connected disability.
- The surviving spouse or child of a military member who died in the line of duty, not due to misconduct. Most of the time, these survivors are eligible for TRICARE, so they are not eligible for CHAMPVA.

Table 13-3 Documentation Management for Workers' Compensation

- The physician must file a first report of injury with the employer, the employer's identified workers' compensation insurance carrier, and the state workers' compensation board.
- The employer, the insurance carrier, and the state are only entitled to information about treatment for the work-related injury or illness. It is important not to release any other information in the patient's file that is not related to the workers' compensation claim.
- Each state may have specific requirements, but at a minimum, the treatment and progress, a statement regarding continued need for treatment, estimate of patient status regarding return to work, and any outside reports (lab, x-ray, or consultants) must be filed on a routine basis, as well as progress reports.
- A final report is usually prepared. This report provides the final medical status regarding permanent disability, expressed as percentage of loss of function.
- Be certain that the CMS-1500 reflects only that care provided for the workers' compensation problem.

Most states use managed care principles to administer workers' compensation, and it is administered differently by each state. For the exam, it is important to know the source of funding for workers' compensation and the basic documentation management principles, regardless of what state you work in. These are outlined in Table 13-3.

Group Plans

A group plan is any health plan sponsored by an organization. Some professional organizations offer group health plan coverage, but typically, group health plans are sponsored by employers.

Before managed care, most group plans were a form of an indemnity plan. An indemnity plan allows the insured the choice of any provider and the plan paid what are referred to as usual, customary, and reasonable (UCR) charges. Other forms of third-party payers may also use UCR. Although indemnity plans still exist, most insurance companies prefer to use at least some form of managed care.

MANAGED CARE

Although different, the terms *managed care plan* and *health maintenance organization* are often used interchangeably. Managed care is a general term referring to any health care plan that has some kind of restrictions on which providers the insured may use. There are four basic types: preferred provider organizations (PPOs), exclusive provider organizations (EPOs), health maintenance organizations (HMOs), and point of service plans (PSPs). All of these types of plans are managed care, but each has different restrictions in place. Table 13-4 describes the differences among the four types of managed care.

Table 13-4 Types of Managed Care

Type of Care Program	Description
Preferred provider organization (PPO)	These are plans that provide coverage through a network of selected health care providers (physicians and hospitals). The insured may go outside the network, but pays more of the costs. Some PPOs have higher deductibles and higher co-insurance payments when the insured goes out of network.
Exclusive provider organization (EPO)	These plans are a more restrictive type of PPO. The insured must use providers from a specified network of physicians and hospitals to receive any coverage. Unless it is an emergency, there is no coverage for care received from a non-network provider.
Health maintenance organization (HMO)	This is a health care system that assumes the financial risk associated with providing comprehensive medical services (the insurance) as well as the responsibility for health care delivery in a particular geographic area (the care). Thus, an HMO is both an insurer and a provider.
Point of service (POS)	This type of plan is an HMO/PPO hybrid; it is sometimes referred to as an "open-ended" HMO when offered by an HMO. POS plans resemble HMOs for in-network services. Services received outside of the network are usually reimbursed in a manner similar to conventional indemnity plans (e.g., provider reimbursement based on a fee schedule or usual, customary, and reasonable charges).

PROCESSING CLAIMS

Manual and Electronic Claims

The CMS-1500 is the accepted claim form for outpatient services. This form was developed by the federal government to ensure that information from all providers was uniform. In today's electronic environment, most claim forms are submitted electronically; in fact, Medicare requires an electronic submittal. The medical office's practice management system is usually set up to create a CMS-1500 once the appropriate CPT (Current Procedural Terminology) and ICD-9 (International Classification of Disease, 9th edition) codes have been submitted. Depending on your office, electronic claims may be sent daily, while paper claims are processed on a weekly or monthly basis.

Tracing Claims

It is critical for the physician's office to have a process in place that monitors for payment of claims. Simply because the claim has been submitted (either electronically or by paper) does not mean that payment is automatic. Managing the accounts receivable is an important part of some medical assistants' job. The process will depend on your physician's office, but any claim not paid within 30 days should be followed up by contacting the payer. The practice management systems in place in most offices will organize the unpaid claim information by payer, so that the medical assistant may contact the same insurance company for several unpaid claims.

Sequence of Medicare Filing

For Medicare claims, it is important to remember that there is a sequence in the filing of the claim. First, the claim should be filed with Medicare. After Medicare has made a determination of payment, then filing with the secondary plan is appropriate. For those patients who have approved Medigap plans, the Medicare payer will automatically submit the claim to the secondary insurance on record. However, if the patient is not participating in a Medigap plan, but has supplemental insurance, many offices file the secondary claim after receiving payment or explanation of nonpayment from Medicare. This is a courtesy only.

Reconciling Payments/Rejections

Insurance companies submit either a remittance voucher or payment advice to the providers. Sometimes the form is called an explanation of benefits. This may be received electronically or by U.S. mail. It is important that the appropriate payment be posted to the patient's account promptly. Depending on the payer, the remaining balance may be adjusted, sent to the secondary payer, or sent to the patient.

If the total claim is denied, the medical assistant should determine the reason for denial. If it is because there was an error on the CMS-1500, then the error should be corrected and the claim refiled. The common reasons that claims are denied because of provider error are:

- Wrong policy or group number
- Provider not listed
- Procedure code or diagnostic code not properly submitted
- Wrong date of birth for patient
- Information missing

However, often a claim is denied for other reasons. If the patient has not met their deductible or is no longer insured by the company, the claim will be denied. Additionally, if the services provided were not covered by the insurance plan, the claim will be denied. The medical assistant should follow up immediately with the patient in these cases.

Inquiry and Appeal

Insurance companies and Medicare and Medicaid have appeal processes in place. Each one requires extensive documentation and timely submittal. This is just one more reason that it is important to actively "work" the accounts receivable. For many insurance companies, inquiries and appeals can be done only within a short time frame from the date of denial—sometimes as little as 30 days.

APPLYING MANAGED CARE POLICIES AND PROCEDURES

Referrals

Most patients have managed care plans to cover their health care costs. Depending on the type of managed care plan, it may be necessary to seek approval of the insurance company before a referral to a specialist is made. In general, most preferred provider and point of service plans do not require approval before sending the patient to a specialist. However, health maintenance organization–type insurance almost always requires an approval before the patient is seen by a specialist. Medical assistants must be aware of the different types of insurance and make sure to seek approval if necessary. If approval is not obtained, and the patient sees the specialist without approval, the patient could be responsible for the entire cost of the care provided by the specialist.

Precertifications

Sometimes confused with pre-authorization and predetermination, precertification is a process initiated by the physician with the insurance company to see if the treatment necessary is covered by the insurance plan. This is critically important for the medical assistant to do, because without a precertification, the patient is liable for the entire bill. A pre-authorization determines the medical necessity of the treatment and whether services are paid. A predetermination defines the amount of money the insurance company will pay for a specific service.

FEE SCHEDULES

The federal government, beginning in 1992, began determining payment of physician services by using a method known as the Resource-Based Relative Value Scale (RBRVS). Because most insurance companies follow the lead of Medicare, it is important to understand the fundamentals of RBRVS. Studies done in the 1980s established a Relative Value Scale (RVS) that assigned a unit value to each procedure performed by a physician or other provider. The cost of resources to perform the individual procedures was established and is reviewed annually. The RBRVS for each CPT code is determined using three separate factors: physician work, practice expense, and malpractice expense. The RBRVS system assigns a relative value that is adjusted by geographic region, so, for example, a procedure performed in Chicago is worth more than a procedure performed in Topeka. This value is then multiplied by a fixed conversion factor, which changes annually, to determine the amount of payment.

The other term that may be on the exam is diagnostic related groups or DRGs. A DRG is a method of reimbursing hospitals for each case in a given category with a fixed fee regardless of the actual costs incurred. A DRG is based on the principal diagnosis, surgical procedure used, age of patient, and expected length of stay in the hospital. It is used by Medicare and many managed care insurance companies.

CONTRACTED FEES

Very few health insurance companies pay the provider's charges in full. Most insurance companies have negotiated with physicians, hospitals, and group practices for a contracted fee to be reimbursed based on the CPT code. Different insurance companies reimburse at different rates, but all reimbursements are established in advance if the physician is a participating provider (a PAR) in the plan. Non-participating providers (non-PARs) expect patients to pay the full bill at the time of service or to work out payment arrangements with the physician.

Some other terms that may appear on the exam include:

- *Assignment of benefits:* This term refers to the process in which a patient "assigns" payment to the physician for direct payment from the insurance company to the physician. In many health insurance plans where the physician is participating, this is an automatic process; however, the patient still signs an approval for assignment of benefits.
- *Balance billing:* This is the process that occurs after the insurance payment has been applied and any required adjustments are made. The patient is billed for the balance owed. Depending on the insurance plan, there may be a zero balance.
- *Capitation:* This is a form of payment to the provider by an HMO for a predetermined fixed amount per member per month (PMPM). The provider must provide all appropriate care for that patient, regardless of cost. However, if the patient is not seen, the provider gets to keep the monthly premium.
- *Clean claim:* An insurance claim filed without any errors is referred to as a clean claim. Something as simple as reversing two numbers within a group plan number can result in the claim being rejected. Clean claims are paid more quickly.
- *Co-insurance:* A sharing of the costs between the patient and the insurance company is called co-insurance. The plan might be an 80-20 plan, which means the insurance company will pay 80% of the covered charges and the patient pays the remaining 20%.
- *Coordination of benefits (COB):* Sometimes patients have more than one health insurance plan that covers services rendered. When that occurs, the payments are coordinated so the total amount of the bill is not exceeded. For example, if an employee is over 65 and enrolled in Medicare as well as their company's health insurance, Medicare is the primary coverage in most cases. After Medicare has paid its share, the employee's health plan usually pays the balance of the approved charges.
- *Co-payments:* Flat fees that are expected to be paid by the patient for each visit or service are called co-payments. Depending on the service, the co-payment may vary. As an example, the co-pay for an x-ray and a prescription may be different. Some services may have no co-pay. Co-payments are not a part of the co-insurance.
- *Deductible:* A deductible is the out-of-pocket costs the patient is expected to pay before the health insurance begins. Most insurance plans, whether an insurance company or Medicare, have a deductible. Most deductibles are on an annual basis, based on a calendar year. The amount of the deductible is specified in the insurance plan. Some services may be exempt from the deductible. For example, some insurance plans cover well baby care regardless of whether the deductible has been met. The deductible can be as low as $500 or as high as $5000, depending on the plan. To keep premium costs down, most individual plans have high deductibles.

- *Explanation of benefits (EOB), also known as remittance voucher or remittance advice:* All third-party payers generate documents that explain how the reimbursement was determined or why the reimbursement was denied. Patients know them as EOBs and practices know them as either EOBs, remittance vouchers, or remittance advice.
- *Pre-existing conditions:* A medical condition the patient had before insurance coverage began is called a pre-existing condition. Services provided to treat that pre-existing condition may or may not be covered by the insurance plan.
- *Premium:* The premium is the amount paid on a monthly, quarterly, or annual basis for health insurance. The cost of the premium is usually shared by the employer and employee in the workplace.

QUESTIONS

13-1. A written authorization by the patient that allows direct reimbursement to the physician for billed charges is called

    A. capitation.
    B. permission.
    C. co-payment.
    D. assignment of benefits.

13-2. The person who is covered by a health plan is the

    A. insured.
    B. covered.
    C. employee.
    D. carrier.

13-3. A bill is never sent to a patient with the following coverage

    A. Medicaid.
    B. preferred provider plan.
    C. workers' compensation.
    D. Medicare.
    E. health maintenance plan.

13-4. The insurance company pays a certain percentage of the approved amount, with the patient paying the balance due for medical services. The portion that each pays is called the

    A. assignment of benefits.
    B. usual, customary, and reasonable charges.
    C. deductible.
    D. co-insurance.
    E. co-payment.

13-5. Indigent or low income people may be covered for health benefits by a government-sponsored program. This program is called

    A. Blue Cross and Blue Shield indigent plan.
    B. TRICARE.
    C. Medicaid.
    D. Medicare.
    E. Medmal Plan.

13-6. Part A of Medicare provides coverage for

    A. services received in physicians' offices.
    B. hospitalization.
    C. x-rays and other diagnostic services.

D. laboratory services.

E. primary care physician services while the patient is in the hospital.

13-7. The mandated claim form to be used for all health insurance claims is the

    A. CMS-1450.

    B. CMS-1500.

    C. HCFA-1450.

    D. HCFA-1500.

13-8. The term that describes a fixed payment per month to the physician, regardless of the services rendered, is called a

    A. fee for service plan.

    B. preferred provider plan.

    C. health maintenance plan.

    D. capitation plan.

    E. indemnity plan.

13-9. Before a health plan begins to pay benefits, the patient must pay a certain amount of eligible charges each calendar year. This is called the

    A. co-payment.

    B. co-insurance.

    C. eligible charges.

    D. capitation.

    E. deductible.

13-10. A person is diagnosed with a disease before the effective date of the insurance plan. The insurance plan may determine that under the terms of its contract with the patient, it is not required to pay for any charges associated with the disease. This is called a(n)

    A. pre-existing condition.

    B. exclusion.

    C. inclusion.

    D. deductible.

    E. precondition.

13-11. Medicare is a federal health insurance program for

    A. anyone over 62 years of age.

    B. anyone over 65 years of age.

    C. disabled workers who are 65 years of age.

    D. low income individuals of any age.

    E. children covered under SCHIP.

13-12. Medicare Part B covers

    A. physician office visits.

    B. nursing home care.

    C. prescriptions.

    D. hospitalizations.

    E. all of the above.

13-13. The process of determining whether a service or procedure is covered by the insurance provider is called

    A. assignment of benefits.

    B. precertification.

    C. review of systems.

    D. coordination benefits.

13-14. The medical bills of spouses and children of veterans with total, permanent, service-connected disabilities are covered under

    A. CHAMPUS.

    B. TRICARE.

    C. HCFA.

    D. MEDISERV.

    E. CHAMPVA.

13-15. To purchase health insurance, the policy holder pays a

    A. premium.

    B. fee.

    C. payment.

    D. capitation.

    E. deduction.

13-16. A primary care physician, or PCP, is

    A. a physician who agrees to oversee a patient's care in a managed care plan.

    B. a physician who is paid by capitation.

    C. a physician who works in an HMO.

    D. a physician who is always a family practitioner.

13-17. When an insurance plan will not cover a specific condition or circumstance, this is called a(n)

    A. preauthorization.

    B. precertification.

    C. exclusion.

    D. capitation.

    E. pre-existing condition.

13-18. Medicare Part C covers

    A. prescriptions.

    B. psychiatric care.

    C. managed care plans in Medicare.

    D. capitation plans in Medicare.

    E. coordination with Medicaid.

13-19. Prescription drug coverage is covered under Medicare

    A. Part A.

    B. Part B.

    C. Part C.

    D. Part D.

    E. None of the above; there is no prescription drug coverage in Medicare.

13-20. Parents may purchase health insurance for their children under which federal plan administered by the individual states?

    A. Medicaid

    B. Medicare Part D

    C. TRICARE

    D. CHAMPVA

    E. SCHIP

ANSWERS

13-1. The correct answer is D. Most insurance companies require that a patient authorize or "assign" the payments to the physician.

13-2. The correct answer is A. Although a person is "covered" by insurance, they are referred to as the insured.

13-3. The correct answer is C. If a workers' compensation claim is approved by the employer, no bills are sent to the patient

13-4. The correct answer is D. Co-insurance is always a percentage of the approved charges. Co-payment is always a specific amount.

13-5. The correct answer is C. Funded by both the federal and individual state governments, Medicaid is the health benefits plan that covers indigent or low income people. Medicare is a federally sponsored plan that covers individuals over the age of 65, as well as certain other people with disabilities.

13-6. The correct answer is B. Part A of Medicare covers hospitalization. Physician services are normally covered under Part B of Medicare.

13-7. The correct answer is B. The correct form number is CMS-1500. The form used to be known as the HCFA-1500 before the Health Care Financing Administration changed its name to Centers for Medicare and Medicaid Services.

13-8. The correct answer is D. The payment per member per month plan is the capitation plan. Many health maintenance plans use a capitation plan to pay physicians, but a health maintenance plan may also employ physicians on a full-time basis with a salary.

13-9. The correct answer is E. The deductible is the amount a patient must pay before the insurance plan begins to pay any charges. A co-payment is a certain amount the patient must pay for each service, and is often not considered a part of the deductible. Co-insurance is the percentage of the charges the insurance company will pay for each service.

13-10. The correct answer is A. A pre-existing condition is one that was diagnosed before the insurance plan took effect. Depending on the type of insurance the patient has, it may or may not be covered under the terms of the contract.

13-11. The correct answer is B. Medicare is available to all U.S. citizens over the age of 65. You may still work full time and have Medicare as your primary insurance coverage.

13-12. The correct answer is A. Medicate Part B covers physician visits and some other outpatient services. Services provided in the in-patient setting, as well as hospice services, are covered by Part A.

13-13. The correct answer is B. In the precertification process, the insurance company makes a determination of whether the service or procedure is "certified" for payment. This usually occurs for surgery, but may also be in place for other expensive procedures.

13-14. The correct answer is E. The Civilian Health and Medical Program of the Veterans Administration, or CHAMPVA, is the program that covers spouses and children of a veteran who has been permanently disabled for a service-connected disability. TRICARE is for active duty and retired members of the military.

13-15. The correct answer is A. To purchase health insurance, a person pays a premium. This premium may be deducted from their paycheck, but not all health insurance is purchased through an employer.

13-16. The correct answer is A. A PCP agrees to oversee a patient's care—they do not necessarily deliver all the care, but in many health plans, a patient must first go to their PCP before seeing a specialist.

13-17. The correct answer is C. When an insurance plan does not cover a specific condition or procedure, it is called an exclusion. For example, plastic surgery for purely cosmetic reasons is an exclusion on almost all insurance contracts.

13-18. The correct answer is C. Medicare Part C covers a variety of managed care plans. Recipients may elect to join a Part C provider instead of the usual Part B and sometimes Part D.

13-19. The correct answer is D. Part D of Medicare covers prescription drugs. Part A is for hospitalization, Part B covers outpatient services, and Part C is the managed care portion of Medicare.

13-20. The correct answer is E. SCHIP is the State Children's Health Insurance Program, which is provided by the federal government and run by the individual states under their Medicaid plans.

Coding Systems

Medical coding is a process that assigns a set of numeric and alphabetic identifiers to medical services, procedures, illnesses and injuries, prescription drugs, and medical equipment. There are two major types of coding—procedural and diagnostic. The two systems are linked. When a medical assistant is coding the physician's services, it is important to make sure that the procedure provided makes sense for the diagnosis given. For example, if the procedure is a chest x-ray, the diagnosis should be one that is linked to the respiratory system.

PROCEDURAL CODING: LEVEL I OR CPT CODES

The system for coding services, procedures, drugs, supplies, and equipment is called procedural coding. The original system was developed by the Health Care Finance Administration (HCFA), now known as the Centers for Medicare and Medicaid Services (CMS). The coding system is used for all billing and coding, not just for Medicare and Medicaid. The Health Insurance Portability and Accountability Act (HIPAA) required a national standard code set for procedures. This was done to ensure consistency across the United States, and to hopefully help eliminate fraud. Accurate coding helps in getting proper payment for health care services provided. Coding is important because incorrect or inaccurate coding can lead to investigations of fraud and abuse. There are two levels of procedural coding.

Level I Health Care Procedural Coding Systems (HCPCS) codes are more commonly referred to as Current Procedural Terminology (CPT). CPT codes are used to identify what services or procedures were done by the provider of service, whether it is a physician, physical therapist, radiology technician, or other health care provider. A CPT code may be for an office visit, surgery, an x-ray, or another diagnostic procedure or test. Each service or procedure is identified with a five-digit code. Understanding how codes are formatted is important for the exam. Codes may also be modified with two more digits—more on that later.

The CPT code book is updated and published annually by the American Medical Association and released in October. The book is called *Current Procedural Terminology,* fourth edition, and is sometimes referred to as CPT-4. Every medical office should purchase the new edition each year because codes may change.

The CPT-4 is divided into six sections. Each of those sections is divided into subsections with anatomic, procedural, condition, or descriptor headings. Table 14-1 illustrates the six areas of the CPT manual. A good review for all students preparing for the exam is to read the introductory pages of each of the six sections of the CPT manual.

The Evaluation and Management (E&M) section of the CPT is unique. First, in most cases it covers services (not procedures). Table 14-2 illustrates some important visit types to remember. Second, there are specific levels of services based on the provider's assessment and judgment of the patient's medical condition and whether the patient is a new or established patient. The focus of the office visit

Table 14-1 CPT Coding Chapters

- Evaluation and Management (99201–99499)
- Anesthesiology (00100–01999, 99100–99140)
- Surgery (10021–69990)
- Radiology (includes nuclear medicine and diagnostic ultrasound) (70010–79999)
- Pathology and Laboratory Services (80048–89356)
- Medicine (except anesthesiology) (90281–99199, 99500–99902)

Table 14-2 Common Visit Types in E&M Coding

Visit Type	Description
New patient	A person who has not received care from the physician or another physician of the same specialty in the same group practice within 3 years.
Established patient	A person who has received care from the physician or another physician of the same specialty in the same group practice within 3 years.
Concurrent care	Similar services provided to the same patient on the same day by more than one physician.
Counseling	(Used for professional services.) The discussion with patient or family members concerning diagnosis, recommendations, risks, benefits, prognosis, options, and necessary condition-related education.
Consultation	Services rendered by a physician whose opinion or advice is requested by another physician or agency in the evaluation or treatment of a patient's illness or suspected problems.
Critical care	(Used for professional services.) Intensive care in acute life-threatening conditions requiring constant bedside attention by the physician.

level is in three areas: history, examination, and complexity of decision making. Table 14-3 lists the definitions of the evaluation and management components. Last, it should not be assumed that the level of care for a new patient, when using the definitions found in Table 14-3, are the same as for an established patient. Confused about levels? For purposes of CPT coding, an office visit is coded based on one of five levels and whether the patient is an established patient or a new patient. The level is the last digit of the CPT code. Table 14-4 shows the five levels. Keep in mind that when a new patient is seen by a provider, that provider has to obtain more information about the patient than they will in subsequent visits.

Table 14-3 Definitions of E&M Components

Component	Description
Problem focused	Minimal; involves only affected body area or one organ system
Expanded problem focused	Low; involves an affected body area or one organ system and symptoms related to other body areas
Detailed	Moderate; involves the affected body area or areas and related body systems(s)
Comprehensive	Moderate to high or high; involves multiple systems or complex involvement of one organ system

Table 14-4 CPT Codes/Levels of Service

CPT Code/Level of Service	Key Components
99201 new patient 99212 established patient	Problem-focused history Problem-focused examination Straightforward decision making
99211 established patient	This is a 5-minute visit, where physician supervision may or may not be necessary (e.g., a blood pressure check)
99202 new patient	Expanded problem-focused history Expanded problem-focused examination Straightforward decision making
99203 new patient	Detailed history Detailed examination Medical decision making of low complexity
99204 new patient	Comprehensive history Comprehensive examination Medical decision making of moderate complexity
99213 established patient	Expanded problem-focused history Expanded problem-focused examination Medical decision making of low complexity
99214 established patient	Detailed history Detailed examination Medical decision making of moderate complexity
99205 new patient 99215 established patient	Comprehensive history Comprehensive examination Medical decision making of high complexity

Reviewing the introductory pages of the manual for E&M codes is important, because there are often several questions about E&M codes on the exam.

The CPT-4 is usually at least 900 pages long. To find a correct code, you first go to the alphabetic index found in the back of the coding book. Usually over 200 pages long, this index is organized alphabetically by four main types of terms, as shown in Table 14-5.

All CPT codes contain five digits; however, they may be modified. Two-digit modifiers are used to give a more accurate description of the services provided. You will find a complete list of

Table 14-5 CPT Index Terms

Term	Example
Procedure or service	Appendectomy, enterectomy
Organ or other anatomic site	Heart, esophagus
Condition	Enterocolitis, prostate cancer
Synonyms, eponyms, and abbreviations	EKG, Cushing's disease, McBurney's incision

modifiers in Appendix A of your CPT-4. Modifiers usually appear at the end of the five-digit code, preceded by a dash. For example, the modifier -25 is used when there is a significant, separate, identifiable evaluation and management code by the same physician on the same day. For example, if a patient was seen in the morning for a follow-up on high blood pressure and then again the same afternoon for an injury to their hand, the second visit would be coded 99213-25.

Proper CPT coding is important. Claims that are improperly coded could mean inappropriate or no reimbursement. More importantly, inappropriate CPT coding on insurance claims could lead to an investigation by CMS or other third-party reimburser as well as possible loss of insurance plan participation privileges and possibly even a felony conviction. Table 14-6 lists the most common fraudulent claim terms or practices.

There may be some questions on the exam about good coding practices. Table 14-7 lists some of the most important things to remember.

Table 14-6 Fraudulent Claims Practices

- Down coding—A provider submits a lower level code for a service that should have been coded at a higher level.
- Phantom billing—Billing for services or supplies never provided.
- Ping-ponging—Unnecessary or excessive referrals of the patient to other providers and back to the primary care provider.
- Split billing—Billing for several visits when all services were provided at one visit.
- Unbundling—Using several CPT codes to identify procedures normally covered by a single CPT code.
- Upcoding—Submitting a higher level code of service than was actually provided to obtain a higher reimbursement.
- Altering dates of service
- Altering the diagnosis so that the insurance company will pay the claim
- Altering the diagnosis so that there is no record of the illness
- Falsifying any part of the medical record to justify higher payment

Table 14-7 Good CPT Practices

- Use the latest edition of the CPT code book.
- Even if you have been coding for years, do not code from the index. Always check the guidelines.
- Make sure the diagnosis code(s) link to the CPT code. If the patient's diagnosis was sinusitis and the procedure code linked to the diagnosis is a mammogram, you aren't going to get paid.
- Never change the diagnosis code without consulting the provider.
- Ask the provider of care to clarify whenever you have questions.
- Pay attention to the need for CPT modifiers. Use them appropriately.

PROCEDURAL CODING: LEVEL II OR HCPCS CODES

Level II HCPCS codes are alpha-numeric codes not covered in Level I CPT. Level II HCPCS codes are commonly referred to as HCPCS codes. These codes are used to identify materials used or given to the patient. For example, some medications, orthotics, or durable medical equipment codes are found in the HCPCS. HCPCS codes are also used for services like dental care. Many of the codes are used only by specific contractors with Medicare or Medicaid. Some of the most commonly used HCPCS codes in the medical office are for injections and supplies. HCPCS codes are published in a separate book from CPT-4 books.

The index for HCPCS codes is usually found in the front of the book, so that is the first place to look for the appropriate code. HCPCS code books also have color coding to aid in determining whether the service is covered by Medicare or other third-party payers. The HCPCS Level II books often contain a variety of appendices to assist in determining the proper code. Table 14-8 illustrates the main areas of HCPCS chapters.

Usually there are only one or two questions on the exam about HCPCS coding. The most important thing to remember is the purpose of HCPCS Level II codes.

Table 14-8 HCPCS Chapter Headings

- Chapter A: Transportation Services Including Ambulance and Medical/Surgical Supplies

  A0021–A0999: Transportation Services

  A4000–A8999: Medical and Surgical Supplies

- Chapter B: Enteral and Parenteral Therapy (B4034–B9999)

- Chapter C: Outpatient Prospective Payment System (C1000–C9999)

  These codes are to be used only in outpatient surgery centers.

- Chapter D: Dental Procedures (D0000–D9999)

- Chapter E: Durable medical equipment (E0100–E9999)

- Chapter G: Procedures/Professional Services (G0000–G9999)

  Temporary: used in lieu of CPT codes

- Chapter H: Alcohol and Drug Abuse Treatment Services (H0001–H2037)

  The H codes are used by state Medicaid agencies that are mandated by state law to establish separate codes for identifying mental health services associated with alcohol and drug treatment.

- Chapter J: Drugs Administered Other than Oral Method (J0000–J9999)

- Chapter K: Temporary Codes (K0000–K9999)

  Used in conjunction with durable medical equipment administrators contracted with Medicare; these are often changed.

- Chapter L: Orthotic Procedures and Devices (L0000–L4999)

- Chapter M: Medical Services (M0000–M0301)

  These are mostly physician office services not listed elsewhere and are either obsolete services or services whose effect has not been proven.

- Chapter P: Pathology and Laboratory Services (P2028–P9999)

- Chapter Q: Temporary Codes (Q0000–Q9999)

  Another miscellaneous section used by local contractors.

- Chapter R: Diagnostic Radiology Services (R0000–R5999)

  R codes fall under the jurisdiction of the local contractors.

- Chapter S: Temporary National Codes (non-Medicare) (S0000–S9999)

  S codes are used by Blue Cross/Blue Shield to report drugs and other services for which there are no national codes. Medicaid also uses these codes, but Medicare does not.

- Chapter T: Codes for State Medicaid Agencies (T1000–T9999)

- Chapter V: Vision Services (V2100–V2999)

  V codes include vision-related supplies such as glasses and contact lenses as well as intraocular lenses.

INTERNATIONAL CLASSIFICATION OF DISEASES, 9TH EDITION (ICD-9) CODES

Diagnostic codes are called ICD-9 codes. The World Health Organization has overall responsibility for determining the codes used worldwide. The code book used is the *International Classification of Diseases,* 9th edition, Clinical Modifications, also referred to as ICD-9 or sometimes ICD-9-CM. The codes identify the reason for the visit, providing the diagnoses associated with the services provided. The ICD-9 also classifies illness (morbidity) and death (mortality) information for statistical purposes.

The U.S. version of ICD-9 is updated every year in October. Four organizations cooperate in putting the update together: the American Hospital Association (AHA), National Center for Health Statistics (NCHS), Centers for Medicare and Medicaid Services (CMS), and American Health Information Management Association (AHIMA).

Diagnoses must be coded based on the primary diagnosis. In the outpatient setting, the primary diagnosis is the main reason that a patient came to see a physician or other health care provider. This could be a symptom like fever, vomiting, or diarrhea; an acute problem such as a back injury while exercising; or a chronic illness such as diabetes. Patients often have more than one diagnosis, but it is critical to identify the primary diagnosis for billing purposes.

ICD-9 codes contain up to five digits; however, unlike CPT codes, the five digits are separated by a period after the third digit. ICD-9 codes may contain only three or four digits or may start with the letter E or V. Cancer registries use M codes or morphology codes to further identify the behavior of a neoplasm. M codes are not used when submitting claims to a third-party payer.

The ICD-9 code book consists of three volumes. Volume 1 lists all the diseases and injuries numerically. There are 17 chapters. Each chapter organizes diagnoses by cause (etiology) or anatomical site. See Table 14-9 for a complete list. Additionally, there are several appendices and tables at the end of Volume 1.

Volume 2, the Index to Diseases, appears first in all ICD-9 books because it is necessary to start with the index to find the correct diagnostic code. There are three sections in Volume 2. Section 1 is the alphabetic listing of symptoms, signs, diagnoses, and conditions. Section 2 is an alphabetic index to poisoning and external causes of adverse effects of drugs and other chemical substances. Section 3 is an alphabetic index to external causes of injury.

Volume 3 is a combined tabular and alphabetic listing of procedures and is used primarily in the hospital setting.

Volumes 1 and 2 are used by physicians and other providers of care who are able to bill for their services. Like the CPT books, it is important to get the update for ICD-9 every year.

Each chapter is divided into sections of similar diseases. As an example, Chapter 9, Diseases of the Digestive System, is divided into seven sections according to organs within the digestive system. Within each section, a three-digit code identifies the general disease category affecting the specific organs. If you look at the second section of the diseases of the digestive system, you will see it contains diseases of the esophagus, stomach, and duodenum. This section is divided into seven categories:

- 530 Diseases of the esophagus
- 531 Gastric ulcer
- 532 Duodenal ulcer
- 533 Peptic ulcer
- 534 Gastrojejunal ulcer
- 536 Disorders of function of the stomach
- 537 Other disorders of stomach and duodenum

Within each category of disease, a fourth and sometimes a fifth digit are necessary to identify the diagnosis correctly. These digits provide more specific information than just a three-digit code can. These digits are placed after the first three digits. Here are two examples:

- 531.0 is gastric ulcer, acute with hemorrhage.
- 531.01 is gastric ulcer, acute with hemorrhage with and without obstruction.

It is important to include fourth and fifth digits where indicated in the ICD-9 code book. Claims will go unpaid for failure to use fourth and fifth digits in ICD-9 coding. Again, the example of gastric ulcer illustrates the need for a fourth or fifth digit. Look at the code 531.0 in the ICD-9 code book.

Table 14-9 ICD-9 Volume 1 Chapters, Appendices, and Tables

- Chapter 1: Infections and Parasitic Diseases (001–139)
- Chapter 2: Neoplasms (140–239)
- Chapter 3: Endocrine, Nutritional and Metabolic, Immunity (240–279)
- Chapter 4: Blood and Blood-Forming Organs (280–289)
- Chapter 5: Mental Disorders (290–319)
- Chapter 6: Nervous System and Sense Organs (320–389)
- Chapter 7: Diseases of the Circulatory System (390–459)
- Chapter 8: Diseases of the Respiratory System (460–519)
- Chapter 9: Diseases of the Digestive System (520–579)
- Chapter 10: Genitourinary System (580–629)
- Chapter 11: Complications of Pregnancy, Childbirth and the Puerperium (630–677)
- Chapter 12: Skin and Subcutaneous Tissue (680–709)
- Chapter 13: Diseases of the Muscoloskeletal System and Connective Tissue (710–739)
- Chapter 14: Congenital Anomalies (740–759)
- Chapter 15: Certain Conditions Originating in the Perinatal Period (760–779)
- Chapter 16: Symptoms, Signs and Ill-Defined Conditions (780–799)
- Chapter 17: Injury and Poisoning (800–999)

V Codes: Supplementary classification of factors influencing health status and contact with health services (V01–V83)

E Codes: Supplementary classification of external causes of injury and poisoning (E800–E999)

Appendix A: Morphology of Neoplasms

Appendix B: Glossary of Mental Disorders

Appendix C: Classification Drugs by AHFS List

Appendix D: Industrial Accidents According to Agency

Appendix E: List of Three-Digit Categories

Tables

  Valid three-digit code table

  Abortion table

  Burn table

  Burn table: Complications

  Diabetes table

  Hernia table

  Ectopic pregnancy table

  Normal pregnancy table

  Antepartum pregnancy table

  Postpartum pregnancy table

It shows "check 5th digit" in front of the code. That means that unless a fifth digit is added, the coding is not correct.

Professional coders will tell you that the cardinal rule in coding is to code to the highest or most specific code. Called "coding to the highest level of specificity," it is a given when coding diagnoses.

As noted in Table 14-9, following the 17 chapters are the V codes and the E codes. V codes are used to identify those patient encounters in which the circumstances are other than an actual disease or injury. For example, the only reason for the office visit may be to receive an immunization. Or the reason for the visit may be that the patient has been exposed to a communicable disease such as meningitis, but is not yet ill. V codes are also used to code supervision of pregnancy. Table 14-10 contains a list of the major V code headings. V codes may be used as a primary diagnosis when appropriate.

Table 14-10 V Codes

V Codes	Definitions
V01–V06	Persons with potential health hazards related to communicable diseases
V07–V09	Persons with need for isolation, other potential health hazards, and prophylactic measures
V10–V19	Persons with potential health hazards related to personal and family history
V20–V28	Persons encountering health services in circumstances related to personal and family history
V30–V39	Healthy live-born infants according to type of birth
V40–V49	Persons with a condition influencing health status
V50–V59	Persons encountering health services for specific procedures and after care
V60–V68	Persons encountering health services in other circumstances
V70–V83	Persons without reported diagnosis encountering during examination and investigation of individuals and populations

V codes are separated into three main categories—problems, services, and factual findings. A problem is something that affects the patient's health status, such as a history of disease; for example, V10.3 is personal history of breast cancer. This is not the primary diagnosis code, but would be important to record if the patient was being assessed for another possible cancer. A service is when a patient is seen for something other than illness or injury. An example would be V26.33, which is the code for genetic counseling. Finally, factual findings are used to describe facts for statistical purposes. The most commonly used are codes related to reproduction and development; for example, V33.01 is the code for twins delivered in the hospital by cesarean delivery.

Like the other diagnostic codes, V codes may have five digits. Using the V33.01 code as an example, the last two digits help to specify the conditions. If the V code was V33.10, that would indicate that the twins (V33) were born before admission to the hospital (1) and without mention of cesarean section (0). As you can see, specificity is important.

The last type of diagnostic coding is E coding. E codes identify the external causes of injury and poisoning and are used to code the events or circumstances surrounding the cause of injury, poisoning, or other adverse effect. For example, the patient may have been thrown off their snowmobile while on duty as a park ranger and comes to the office because his or her neck is strained. The diagnostic code for the neck strain is 847.0. However, it will be important to code for the circumstances as well (nontraffic accident involving motor driven snow vehicle: E820.0). E codes are never used alone. They are always at least secondary to the primary diagnosis.

It is important to do E coding. It is possible that there may be many different payers involved in a patient's care, particularly if the care is needed because of an accident. In the example above, workers' compensation is responsible for payment of the costs associated with care. However, if the patient had been out on his or her personal snowmobile with family, then the patient's general health insurance would be the primary insurance. E coding assists the payers in sorting out who is responsible for paying the costs of care. Table 14-11 illustrates some of the major E codes.

Two abbreviations with special importance are used throughout the ICD-9 code book, and it is possible that there will be at least one question about each of the abbreviations on the exam. NEC stands for not elsewhere classified. This is used when the ICD-9 book does not provide a code specific for the patient's condition. NOS stands for not otherwise specified. This abbreviation is the same as unspecified and is used only when the coder lacks the information necessary to code to a more specific four- or five-digit category.

Diagnostic coding is not easy. To code the diagnosis for an office visit or other outpatient procedure, there are steps that should be routinely followed. Table 14-12 provides you with a list of those

Table 14-11 E Code Divisions

At the beginning of the chapter on E codes, there are specific instructions regarding the coding of accidents involving vehicles with a motor.

- E800–E807 Railway accidents
- E810–E819 Motor vehicle accidents
- E820–E825 Vehicle non-traffic accidents
- E826–E829 Other road vehicle accidents
- E830–E838 Water transport accidents
- E840–E845 Air and space transport accidents
- E846–E848 Vehicle accidents not elsewhere classifiable
- E849 Category used to identify the place of occurrence for E800–E848
- E850–E858 Accidental poisoning by drugs, medicinal substances, and biologicals
- E860–E869 Accidental poisoning by other solid and liquid substances, gases, and vapors
- E870–E876 Misadventures to patients during surgical and medical care
- E878–E879 Surgical and medical procedures as the cause of abnormal reaction of patient or later complication, without mention of misadventure at the time of procedure
- E880–E888 Accidental falls
- E890–E899 Accidents caused by fire and flames
- E900–E909 Accidents due to natural and environmental factors
- E910–E915 Accidents caused by submersion, suffocation, and foreign bodies
- E916–E928 Other accidents
- E930–E949 Drugs, medicinal and biological substances causing adverse effects in therapeutic use
- E950–E959 Suicide and self-inflicted injury
- E960–E969 Homicide and injury purposely inflicted by other persons
- E970–E978 Legal intervention
- E979 Terrorism
- E980–E989 Injury undetermined whether accidentally or purposely inflicted
- E990–E999 Injury resulting from operations of war

Table 14-12 Steps to Code Diagnosis (ICD-9)

1. Identify the reason for the visit—the sign, symptom, diagnosis, or condition.
2. Look up the main term or disease in the alphabetic index (Volume 2). The main term is what is wrong with the patient. The main term is printed in bold in Volume 2. Examples of main terms are abnormal, disorder, fracture, pain, and sprain. Also, the name of the disease or condition (i.e., carcinoma, diabetes, Parkinsonism) is a main term and is used to find the area to check in Volume 1. Do not code by simply using the code found in the alphabetic index.
3. Identify the subterms. Below the main terms are subterms that further describe the main term. For example, under the disease hypertension, there are over 100 subterms.
4. Select a code from the alphabetic list. In the numeric list (Volume 1), locate the code.
5. Have you selected the code at the highest level of specificity? To code to the highest level of specificity means that you select the three-digit code only if there are no four- or five-digit codes within that code category. Fifth-digit coding must be used when available. Most ICD-9 code books clearly label main terms that need a fourth or fifth digit by placing a box or a check mark in front of the main tern that says Check 4th digit or Check 5th digit.
6. Determine the code.

steps. If an incorrect or inappropriate code is submitted for payment the practice may not be paid. You could also be inadvertently labeling a patient with an illness they do not have. It is important to code signs and symptoms if you do not have a confirmed diagnosis. Headache, fever, chills, and muscle aches are all symptoms of Rocky Mountain spotted fever, but they are also symptoms of the flu. In a case like this, the medical professional who may suspect Rocky Mountain spotted fever will be sure to do a detailed patient history and exam looking for whether a tick bite was a possibility. For purposes of coding the first visit, the signs and symptom mentioned above would be coded, not Rocky Mountain spotted fever.

There may be a question about the coding of written diagnoses like "suspected" or "probable" on the exam. Do not code conditions when the provider has said "suspected," "rule out," "questionable," or "probable." It is important to remember that in these cases, the signs and symptoms are coded. Until you have a confirmed diagnosis, you should not code a disease.

To prepare for the exam, students should do a basic review of the setup of the ICD-9 manual and know the differences between the volumes and the importance of coding specificity. As the United States moves to ICD-10 in 2013, it will be important for the medical assistant to learn this new system. It is dramatically different than ICD-9. However, it is not anticipated that there will be ICD-10 questions on the exam until ICD-10 is implemented in 2013.

LINKING CPT AND ICD-9 CODES

Another principle to remember for the exam is that CPT and ICD-9 codes should always be linked. As an example, a patient comes in for her annual physical exam. A part of her annual exam is a pap smear as well as other screening tests done in the office. While there, the patient may complain of a rapid heartbeat. The physician does not yet know what the cause of the rapid heartbeat is. The physician may have an EKG done in the office the same day the pap smear is done. The symptom tachycardia (fast heartbeat) would be linked to the EKG procedure code and not linked to the CPT code for a pap smear.

For the exam, it is usually not expected that you know the specific CPT code for a pap smear or the ICD-9 code for tachycardia. The questions will probably test your ability to recognize that among the five choices only one choice has a CPT and ICD-9 code.

RESOURCE-BASED RELATIVE VALUE SCALE (RBRVS)

In 1992, Medicare established a method of predetermining values for physician services. These values are units based on services performed, practice expenses, and professional liability insurance. These units are then used to help determine reimbursement for physicians billing Medicare. Refer to Chapter 13 for more on RBRVS.

CODING FOR SERVICES PROVIDED BY A HOSPITAL

The exam may have a question or two that asks about how coding is done for hospital services. When a patient is in the hospital, the services provided by the hospital are billed using a system called Diagnostic Related Groups or DRGs. The DRG system determines a specific amount that will be paid to the hospital for services provided based on the diagnosis or diagnoses. Medicare, Medicaid, and some private health insurance plans use this system. When physicians provide services in the hospital, they use CPT codes to bill for their inpatient services or procedures.

QUESTIONS

14-1. A modifier has been attached to a CPT code. This indicates

    A. where the services or procedures were performed.
    B. the amount of time utilized for the services or procedures.
    C. why the services or procedures were performed.
    D. the services or procedures were altered from the standard.
    E. None of the above.

14-2. Which of the following is the coding system used to categorize diseases and injuries?

    A. *U.S. Classifications of Diseases*
    B. *Current Procedural Terminology*
    C. *International Classification of Diseases*
    D. *Physician's Desk Reference*
    E. *Physician's Diagnostic Reference*

14-3. The coding system used by hospitals to bill for services is known as

    A. DRG.
    B. UCR.
    C. CPT.
    D. HCPCS.
    E. H-codes.

14-4. The proper code for the term used to describe a cancer that has not invaded neighboring tissues is

    A. metastatic.
    B. in situ.
    C. carcinoma.
    D. benign.
    E. metacentric.

14-5. CPT stands for

    A. Current Procedure Terms.
    B. Common Procedure Terminology.
    C. Current Procedural Terminology.
    D. Common Procedural Treatments.
    E. Current Procedural Treatments.

14-6. The primary reason that AMA updates CPT codes annually is

    A. inclusion of annual statistics for physician services.
    B. addition of new and revised codes for services rendered.
    C. adjustment of amount of time allowed for services rendered.
    D. amendments to physician fee schedules.
    E. identification of additional diagnoses.

14-7. When is the coding abbreviation NEC used?

    A. When information is not known for specific category coding
    B. To describe internal injuries caused by accident
    C. To identify causes for the disease
    D. When the patient is a new patient
    E. When the patient has extensive injuries requiring surgery

14-8. The appropriate level of E&M coding is determined by all of the elements listed below EXCEPT

    A. patient history.
    B. level of examination.
    C. level of presenting problem.
    D. number of procedures ordered for the patient.
    E. complexity of medical decision making.

14-9. All of the following are associated with procedural coding systems, EXCEPT

- **A.** RBRVS.
- **B.** HCPCS.
- **C.** ICD-9.
- **D.** CPT.
- **E.** E&M.

14-10. The concept of RBRVS is used to determine

- **A.** the value of the hospital services provided to the patient.
- **B.** the value of all the resources used by the physician to provide care.
- **C.** the value of one physician's services for a Medicare patient.
- **D.** the value of prescription drugs provided to the patient in the hospital.
- **E.** the values of services performed, practice expenses, and professional liability insurance.

14-11. Dr. Maple is a pediatrician. A patient comes to his office with an ear infection. The patient is also due for a childhood vaccination. The diagnostic codes to be used are

- **A.** 99201 and 382.9.
- **B.** 382.09 and V03.81.
- **C.** 99214 and V03.81.
- **D.** 38209 and J5675.
- **E.** 38209 and V03.81.

14-12. The purpose of medical coding includes

- **A.** tracking procedures.
- **B.** tracking diseases.
- **C.** identifying disease trends.
- **D.** providing data to medical researchers.
- **E.** All of the above.

14-13. The number of coding sections in the CPT-4 code book is

- **A.** three.
- **B.** four.
- **C.** five.
- **D.** six.
- **E.** seven.

14-14. The term for the cause of a disease is

- **A.** eponym.
- **B.** etiology.
- **C.** causation.
- **D.** classification.
- **E.** etymology.

14-15. A patient has been diagnosed with acute appendicitis. The medical assistant coded the insurance form with the number 540.9. The medical assistant was using which of the following systems of coding?

- **A.** Medicaid
- **B.** CPT-4
- **C.** HCPCS
- **D.** CHAMPUS
- **E.** ICD-9

14-16. Which organization is responsible for producing the CPT code book?

    A. International Medical Association
    B. World Health Organization
    C. Health Care Financing Administration
    D. International Classification of Diseases Organization
    E. American Medical Association

14-17. A disease or procedure named for a person or place is an

    A. eponym.
    B. etiology.
    C. anonym.
    D. abbreviation.
    E. upcode.

14-18. Select the most appropriate reference source for locating a code for chronic arthritis.

    A. Relative Value Scale (RVS)
    B. Healthcare Common Procedure Coding System (HCPCS)
    C. *International Classification of Diseases*, 9th edition, Clinical Modification (ICD-9-CM)
    D. *Current Procedural Terminology* (CPT)
    E. Evaluation and Management System (EMS)

14-19. ICD-9 code books are revised annually to

    A. improve reimbursement for physicians.
    B. allow for faster claims processing.
    C. rebundle codes.
    D. improve specificity of diagnoses.
    E. improve specificity of procedures done.

14-20. Dr. Banyon requests the services of Dr. Oak to assist in the evaluation of a patient's illness. When Dr. Oak bills for services, the code section to be used is

    A. concurrent care.
    B. counseling.
    C. consultation.
    D. co-care.
    E. co-consultation.

14-21. How many times must a patient visit the physician within a 3-year period for a patient evaluation and management examination to be coded as an established visit, according to Current Procedural Terminology (CPT) coding rules?

    A. One
    B. Two
    C. Three
    D. Four
    E. Five

14-22. During an office visit, the patient receives an immunization. Where is the appropriate code most likely to be found in the ICD-9-CM book?

    A. Tabular list
    B. E codes
    C. Alphabetical index
    D. V codes
    E. Appendix A

14-23. Which of the following sections of the CPT code book refers to Evaluation and Management?

    A. 99201–99499
    B. 99501–99901
    C. 80000–89399
    D. 70000–79999
    E. 92201–92499

14-24. The coding system used to document the procedure for removing a gallstone is

    A. Diagnostic-Related Groups (DRGs).
    B. Current Procedural Terminology (CPT).
    C. *International Classification of Diseases*, 9th edition, Clinical Modification (ICD-9-CM).
    D. Resource-Based Relative Value Scale (RBRVS).
    E. Relative Value Studies (RVS).

14-25. The largest of the six major sections of the CPT manual that contains codes from 10000 to 69999 is

    A. anesthesia.
    B. medicine.
    C. surgery.
    D. radiology.
    E. evaluation and management.

ANSWERS

14-1. The correct answer is D. A modifier is used with a CPT code to indicate that the standard was altered. Some examples of modifiers are -51 (multiple procedures at the same session by the same provider) and -62 (two surgeons).

14-2. The correct answer is C. The *International Classification of Diseases,* 9th edition, is used to categorize diseases and injuries. Current Procedural Terminology is used to categorize the services provided or the procedure done. The *Physician's Desk Reference* provides information on all prescription drugs.

14-3. The correct answer is A. The Diagnostic Related Groups system is used to bill for hospital services paid for by Medicare and other third-party payers. UCR means usual, customary, and reasonable and refers to the level of charges. CPT is the Current Procedural Terminology code book used to assign a code for outpatient services. HCPCS is the Healthcare Common Procedure Coding System and has both Level I codes (CPT codes) and Level II codes (durable medical equipment and prescriptions are two examples).

14-4. The correct answer is B. In situ means in place. Metastatic cancer is one that has spread from one organ to another organ or organs. Carcinoma means cancer. Benign means nonmalignant.

14-5. The correct answer is C. CPT stands for Current Procedural Terminology.

14-6. The correct answer is B. The CPT is revised annually to add new codes and revise current codes. The other choices are not reasons for the annual revision.

14-7. The correct answer is A. NEC is the abbreviation for Not Elsewhere Classified, which is to be used when the ICD-9 book does not provide a code specific for the patient's condition.

14-8. The correct answer is D. Each E&M code refers to an office visit, not the number of procedures done.

14-9. The correct answer is C. ICD-9 is a coding system for diagnoses, not procedures. All the other options are part of procedural coding.

14-10. The correct answer is E. The Resource Based Relative Value Scale establishes the value of services performed, practice expenses, and professional liability insurance to determine a scale used to set physician payment in Medicare.

14-11. The correct answer is B. In these types of exam questions, it is not expected that you actually know the specific codes. What is important in this question is that you understand the difference between a procedural code and a diagnostic code. Only answer B has diagnostic codes. The other answers all contain a CPT code. CPT codes never contain a period (.)

14-12. The correct answer is E. All of the listed items are purposes for medical coding—both procedural and diagnostic.

14-13. The correct answer is D. The CPT code book has six sections: Evaluation and Management, Anesthesia, Surgery, Radiology, Pathology, and Medicine.

14-14. The correct answer is B. Etiology is the cause of a disease. An eponym is when a disease or a procedure is named after someone, such as Cushing's disease or cesarean section. Etymology is the study of the history of linguistic forms and is not pertinent to coding.

14-15. The correct answer is E. Diagnoses are coded by using the ICD-9 codes.

14-16. The correct answer is E. The American Medical Association is responsible for the CPT codes. The AMA does work with other organizations such as the American Hospital Association and the Health Insurance Association of America.

14-17. The correct answer is A. An eponym is when a disease or a procedure is named after someone, such as Cushing's disease or Cesarean section. Etiology is the cause of a disease.

14-18. The correct answer is C. Chronic arthritis is a condition/disease. It should be coded from the ICD-9.

14-19. The correct answer is D. ICD-9 code books are revised annually so that more specific information can be provided to both third-party payers and researchers about the nature and occurrence of disease and injury.

14-20. The correct answer is C. Within the Evaluation and Management section of the CPT code book, there are codes for office visits and for consultations. A consultation is considered a higher level of care so it is important to distinguish between an office visit and a consultation. Concurrent care is when the same patient is seen by more than one physician in one day and is usually seen only in hospital care.

14-21. The correct answer is A. A returning patient may be considered a new patient only if the physician has not seen the patient in 3 years. There are E&M codes for both established and new patients. The assumption is that a new patient (or one who hasn't been seen in 3 years) will require more evaluation and management then a patient seen regularly by the physician. Also, it is important to remember that in the group practice, if a patient is seen by more than one doctor in the specialty, the second doctor cannot consider the patient a new patient for billing purposes.

14-22. The correct answer is D. An immunization is a V code within ICD because it pertains to a factor influencing health status and contact with a health service provider that is not because the patient is ill.

14-23. The correct answer is A. 99201–99499 are E&M codes. The other selections do not represent the code range for the other five sections of CPT.

14-24. The correct answer is B. Removing a gallstone is a procedure. Therefore, the only correct answer can be CPT.

14-25. The correct answer is C. The surgery section of the CPT code book is the largest.

Clinical Knowledge

Asepsis and Infection Control

Asepsis refers to the practice of eliminating contaminants in the medical or surgical environments. Even though intact skin is a good barrier against microbial contamination, a patient can become colonized with microbes if appropriate precautions are not taken. Education and training are critical elements of asepsis and infection control because they facilitate appropriate decision making. Thus, many of the aseptic techniques will be asked about on the exam.

PRINCIPLES OF DISEASE

Diseases are caused by pathogens. Most pathogens belong to one of four groups—bacteria, fungi, protozoa, or viruses. Table 15-1 describes each pathogen.

Although all four types of pathogens live in our environment, they don't always cause disease. The chain of infection in Figure 15-1 illustrates the six elements (or links) necessary for disease to occur and to spread. By understanding each link, a medical assistant may apply the principles of asepsis and infection control to eliminate the transmission of disease.

Diseases that are spread via respiratory droplets, such as influenza (the flu), are probably the most difficult to prevent. Questions on the exam might ask about some common infectious diseases and their mode of transmission, as outlined in Table 15-2. Pathogens may cause acute, chronic, or latent infection, as described in Table 15-3.

ASEPTIC TECHNIQUE

Aseptic technique includes medical asepsis and surgical asepsis. The principle behind aseptic technique is to prevent the spread of disease. In the medical office, aseptic technique is referred to as medical asepsis; in the surgical environment, aseptic technique is referred to as surgical asepsis.

Medical Asepsis

In the medical office, the methods and practices designed to prevent the spread of disease are referred to as medical asepsis. Methods used in medical asepsis include handwashing, sanitization, and chemical disinfection. Medical asepsis reduces the number of microorganisms in the environment.

Handwashing

The single most important way to prevent the spread of infection is by frequent handwashing. In the medical environment, everyone should wash his or her hands before and after patient contact, after

Table 15-1 Pathogens

Pathogen	Description	Example
Bacteria	One-celled microorganisms, defined by their shape (spherical, rod, spiral, or spore) and whether or not air is required for survival (aerobic or anaerobic)	*Escherichia coli (E. coli):* Most strains are harmless and found normally in the colon, but some strains cause diarrhea. *Staphylococcus aureus:* May cause minor skin infections or life-threatening illnesses like meningitis or septicemia.
Fungi	Microbes that grow on other organisms	*Tinea* causes ringworm, athlete's foot, and jock itch. *Candida* causes oral thrush and yeast infections.
Protozoa	Tiny parasites that live in another organism	*Plasmodium falciparum* (Malaria protozoa) causes anemia, fever, and flu-like illness. *Giardia* causes debilitating diarrhea.
Viruses	Tiny pieces of DNA coated by protein that require another living organism's cells to reproduce	Human immunodeficiency virus (HIV) causes AIDS. Hepatitis virus (A, B, C, D, and E) causes inflammation and infection of the liver. Influenza causes the flu.

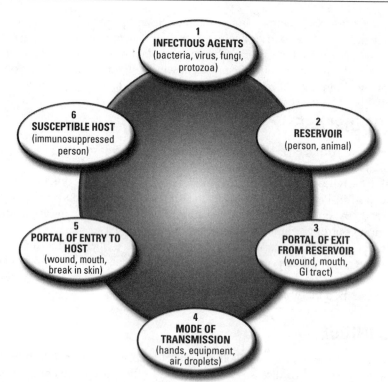

Figure 15-1 The Six Elements Needed for Disease to Occur and Spread

any contact with contaminated material, before and after any contact with food, and after coughing, sneezing, blowing their nose, or using the restroom. There is much evidence to suggest that correct handwashing is essential in preventing infection.

Proper medical handwashing is outlined in the following steps:

1. Remove jewelry. (Simple wedding bands may remain.)
2. Avoid contact with the faucet by using a paper towel to turn on the faucet or by using a foot-controlled sink.
3. Wash both hands and wrists for 2–3 minutes.

Table 15-2 Transmission of Infectious Diseases

Infectious Disease	Mode of Transmission
Varicella zoster virus (chicken pox)	Direct contact or respiratory droplets
E. coli bacteria (food poisoning)	Contaminated food
Giardiasis	Contaminated water (fecal-oral transmission)
Hepatitis A and E	Contaminated water (fecal-oral transmission)
Hepatitis B and C	Blood, sexual, maternal-fetal transmission
HIV/AIDS	Blood, sexual, maternal-fetal transmission
Influenza virus (flu)	Respiratory droplets (airborne droplets)
Malaria	Mosquito bite
Measles	Respiratory droplets (airborne droplets)
Mononucleosis	Saliva
Pneumonia	Respiratory droplets (airborne droplets)
Rabies	Animal bite
Tuberculosis	Respiratory droplets (airborne droplets)
Viral meningitis	Saliva or sputum

Table 15-3 Duration of Infection

Pathogen	Description	Example
Acute	Infection develops quickly and lasts for a variable amount of time	Influenza virus (flu)
Chronic	Infection lasts for a long period of time (even a lifetime)	Hepatitis C virus
Latent	Infection may not be active all the time, may lie dormant in the body and become active when the immune system is weakened (immunocompromised state)	Tuberculosis (bacteria)

4. Use a nailbrush to clean cuticles and nails.
5. Rinse and hold hands in a *downward* position.
6. With water still running, dry hands with a clean towel, and use a paper towel to turn off the faucet.

Sanitization

Sanitization removes contaminants and debris from the surface of various medical office items by scrubbing them (using a scrub brush) with warm, soapy water. Enzymatic detergents can be used as the soap and are specially designed for use on medical instruments because they contain enzymes that will break down proteins found in body fluids and tissues. Effective sanitization should be performed as soon as possible after contamination because once debris dries on an instrument, it is more difficult to remove. Sanitization can be used to clean items such as the stethoscope, ophthalmoscope, otoscope, blood pressure cuff, reflex hammer, and penlight.

Chemical Disinfection

Chemical disinfection goes one step further than sanitization, although disinfectants are more effective if the items have been sanitized first. A common chemical disinfectant is bleach. Chemical disinfection is used to clean medical instruments, lab glassware, and countertops.

Surgical Asepsis

In the surgical setting, the methods and practices designed to eliminate all microorganisms in the environment are called surgical asepsis. Surgical asepsis is also referred to as sterile technique. When using sterile technique (performing surgical asepsis), it is essential that the sterilization steps are done in the correct order and that nothing interrupts the process. If there is any question of contamination, then one needs to start the process over again. It is important that surgical asepsis be maintained throughout the preparation and performance of surgical procedures. Methods used in surgical asepsis include scrubbing, gowning, gloving, preparing equipment, preparing items for autoclave, and performing sterilization techniques.

Scrubbing

Scrubbing in surgical asepsis is analogous to handwashing in medical asepsis. Proper scrubbing is outlined in the following steps:

1. Remove all jewelry.
2. Use a foot- or knee-controlled faucet.
3. Wash both hands, wrists, and forearms with a sterile scrub brush. (The first surgical scrub of the day is longer and depends on the protocol of the facility with a range from 5–10 minutes; thereafter, the surgical scrub can be between 2–5 minutes.)
4. All planes of the fingers and hands should be scrubbed multiple times. Use a sterile nail-brush to clean cuticles and nails.
5. Rinse and hold hands in an *upward* position. (Water cannot be allowed to run from unwashed areas to already sterile, washed areas.)
6. With water still running, dry hands with a sterile towel.
7. Turn off faucet with foot or knee.
8. Do not touch anything and proceed to gowning and gloving.

Gowning

After finishing the surgical scrub, sterile persons are gowned and gloved immediately. Self-gowning and gloving should be done from a separate sterile field in order to avoid contamination of sterile supplies. The technique is very specific and outlined in the following steps:

1. Lift the folded gown directly up from the sterile package.
2. Step away from the sterile surface (into an open area) to provide a wide margin of safety.
3. Locate the neckline of the folded gown.
4. Allow the gown to unfold, keeping the inside of the gown toward the body. Do not touch the outside of the gown.
5. Slip both arms into the armholes simultaneously while not extending one's hands beyond the cuffs of the gown.
6. The circulator or operating room assistant pulls the gown over the shoulders, leaving the cuffs of the sleeves extended over the hands. The back of the gown is securely tied.

The back of the gown is considered contaminated. Also, the gown is considered sterile only to the highest level of the sterile tables.

Gloving

After surgical scrubbing and gowning, gloving is the final step to complete the sterile dress. Once complete, a person may handle sterile equipment in a surgical setting. Sterile persons keep their hands in sight at all times and at or above waist level or the level of the sterile field.

The technique of sterile gloving, using the closed glove technique, is outlined in the following steps:

1. Often the circulator opens the sterile pack of gloves and places it on the sterile field.
2. The right hand is used to pick up the left glove and place it on correctly while the left hand is used to pick up the right glove and place it on correctly.

3. Grasp the first glove at the top edge of the folded-down cuff and partially slip in first hand.
4. Grasp the back of the cuff and turn it over the end of the sleeve. The cuff of the glove is now over the stockinette cuff of the gown, with the hand still inside the sleeve. The hand can now be removed from the sleeve of the gown and inserted into the glove. The stockinette cuffs of the gown are enclosed beneath the sterile gloves. The stockinette is absorbent and retains moisture, but does not provide a microbial border.
5. Slip gloved fingers into cuff of second glove and slip in second hand without contaminating. The outer aspect of the glove must remain sterile.
6. If contamination occurs, start again with new pair of gloves.

There is also an open glove technique in which either a gown is not worn but the hands are scrubbed, or a gown is worn but the hands are pushed all the way through the cuffs of the gown before gloving. Prior to gloving, only the outside of the glove package may be touched with bare (but scrubbed) hands. The inside of the package, in which the gloves are places, is considered sterile. This method of scrubbing used a skin-to-skin, glove-to-glove technique. The first glove is put on using the skin-to-skin technique which means bare hands may only touch the inside of the first glove. Once the first hand is gloved, the sterile fingers of that glove may touch the sterile exterior of the second glove, which is the glove-to-glove technique.

Preparing Equipment

The surgical assistant helps the surgeon carry out a safe operation with optimal results for the patient. The surgical assistant has preoperative duties (prepares the sterile field, preps the patient), intraoperative functions (exposure, hemostasis, closure), and finally postoperative duties (assists the patient after surgery, performs terminal care of room and equipment).

The following points should be remembered when preparing the sterile field:

1. Open the sterile drape package correctly—top flap unfolds first (place away from you so as not to reach over sterile field), right and left sides next, and last flap unfolds toward you.
2. Open sterile packages of instruments and supplies. (They are packaged in a manner so that surgical sterility is not compromised.)
3. Sterile instruments can only come into contact with other sterile supplies.
4. All sterile instruments and equipment need to be kept above the waistline.
5. Dry, sterile transfer forceps may be used to add sterile items to the sterile field or rearrange items on a tray.
6. Any member of the surgical team should not lean or reach over the sterile field.
7. Any member of the surgical team should not turn their back to the sterile field.
8. Contaminated or non-sterile instruments cannot be passed over the sterile field.
9. Coughing and sneezing over a sterile field will contaminate the sterile field.

The following points should be remembered when preparing the patient for surgery:

1. Remove all hair at the surgical site.
2. Cleanse the skin with an antiseptic cleansing solution (e.g., Betadine, Hibiclens); use a circular motion from the point of the incision outward. Repeat with a clean sponge.
3. Paint the patient's operative site with an antiseptic solution. Let dry and repeat with another sterile sponge.
4. Drape the patient with a fenestrated drape (a drape with a hole for the surgical site).

Preparing Items for Autoclave

Autoclaving uses high-pressure steam heat for sterilization. Because of their ease of use, autoclaves also are frequently used for sterilization in medical offices. An autoclave device forces the temperature of steam above water's boiling point. This high temperature allows for sterilization. The water temperature must be 212 degrees Fahrenheit, which will achieve a steam temperature between 250 and 254 degrees Fahrenheit. Steam pressure is equivalent to 15 pounds of pressure. Only distilled water should be used, to prevent mineral buildup in the machine.

The time required for the process to work is between 20 and 40 minutes, and depends on how loosely or tightly items are wrapped. Unwrapped items should be sterilized for 20 minutes, loosely wrapped items for 30 minutes, and tightly packed items for 40 minutes. Instruments that must remain sterile after autoclaving should be wrapped in special sterilization bags, disposable paper wraps, or surgical towels before being placed in the autoclave. Instruments that will be in the sterile field should be double-wrapped. The double-wrapped procedure allows for the inner sterile package to be placed in the surgical tray (field). Hinged surgical instruments should be placed in the open position.

Sterilization indicators (also called sterilization strips) are used for quality control. These strips contain a dye that darkens (changes color) when exposed to steam at the proper temperature and pressure.

When wrapping items for autoclaving (using the double-wrap method), the following steps should be taken:

1. Sanitize, rinse, and dry instruments.
2. Use two wraps of equal size. Place one wrap like a diamond, with a corner towards you.
3. Place the already-sanitized instrument in the center. Any hinge should be opened as wide as possible or a cotton ball can be placed in the center of hinge.
4. One sterilization indicator is placed with the instrument to ensure sterilization of each package.
5. Make a fan-shape fold with the bottom corner of the wrap and keep the instrument completely covered.
6. Repeat the fan shape with the opposite corner.
7. Fold the package up from the bottom.
8. Fold the top edge down.
9. Place this folded package in the center of the second wrap and repeat the folding procedure.
10. Tape with autoclave tape and label the package with the date, the name of the instrument inside the package, and the initials of the person preparing the package.

After autoclaving, packs need to be dry before being put away.

Performing Sterilization Techniques

Sterilization destroys all living microorganisms as well as spores and is the highest level of infection control. Sterilization is required of all instruments that will be used during surgery and kept in the sterile field. Sterilization is also required of all instruments that penetrate the body. Examples of such instruments include curettes, needles, syringes, and vaginal specula. There are four different methods of sterilization: autoclaving (steam sterilization), gas sterilization, dry heat sterilization, and chemical sterilization. Each method is described further in Table 15-4.

Table 15-4 Sterilization Methods

Method	Description
Steam sterilization (autoclave)	Uses high-pressure steam heat for sterilization. Steam temperature is between 250 and 254 degrees Fahrenheit; steam pressure is equivalent to 15 pounds of pressure.
Gas sterilization	Uses gas ovens large enough for wheelchairs and beds. It takes hours for gases to sterilize; only practical in a hospital setting.
Dry heat sterilization	Uses even higher temperatures than steam sterilization and requires longer exposure times (at least 1 hour at 320 degrees Fahrenheit). It is used for instruments that will corrode easily (would be damaged by steam or chemicals).
Chemical sterilization (cold sterilization)	Equipment is soaked in large, closed containers with chemicals. It is used for instruments that are either too large or too heat sensitive for autoclaving; fiber-optic endoscopes are frequently sanitized using this method because they are unable to withstand the heat of an autoclave.

THE OCCUPATIONAL SAFETY AND HEALTH ADMINISTRATION (OSHA)

The Occupational Safety and Health Administration (OSHA) is the federal agency that establishes general guidelines to address asepsis. OSHA has a set of standards that apply to medical offices. (Each state may have additional guidelines.) The Bloodborne Pathogen Standard aims to reduce the medical assistant's (or any health care worker's) exposure to bloodborne diseases such as HIV and hepatitis B and C. This standard contains many regulations including the use of universal precautions, the use of safe needles and sharps with their proper identification and disposal, the proper containment of regulated waste, the use of personal protective equipment (gloves, masks, gowns), medical follow-up after an exposure incident, no-cost hepatitis B vaccines, an updated written exposure control plan, and employee training.

OSHA has another standard concerned with hazards. Under this standard, The Occupational Exposure to Hazardous Chemicals in the Laboratory, OSHA has regulations that cover workers exposed to hazardous chemicals, require employers to have a chemical hygiene plan with hazard identification, and requires employers to provide training to everyone who potentially may be exposed. Failure to comply with OSHA standards could result in a large monetary penalty.

DISPOSAL OF BIOHAZARDOUS MATERIAL

Biohazardous materials include blood and body fluids in addition to clothing, gloves, masks, gauze, wipes, aprons, or needles that may be contaminated with blood or infectious agents. Biohazardous material needs to be handled in a safe, secure manner so that it is disposed of properly.

Important requirements for biohazardous material include:

- Red biohazard bags are used for biohazardous material.
- Double bag biohazard containers with two red bags to ensure safety.
- Place only biohazardous material in this container.
- Make sure the international biohazard symbol is on the bag or container.
- Keep the lid on the container or the bag closed except for when it is specifically in use.
- Sharps (e.g., needles, glass pipettes, blades) belong only in a sharps container.
- A sharps container must be a rigid, tamper-proof container labeled with the international biohazard symbol.
- When the container is approximately two thirds full, close and tie off the inside bag; close and tie off the outside bag before removing the bag from the container.
- All biohazardous material must be decontaminated prior to disposal, either by autoclaving, by chemical disinfection, or by being transported off-site for treatment by an approved medical waste vendor.

STANDARD PRECAUTIONS

Standard precautions were established after the Centers for Disease Control and Prevention (CDC) spent several years researching ways to protect health care providers, patients, and their visitors from infectious and communicable diseases. The guidelines for standard precautions were released in 1996 after revising the old universal precautions that were established in 1985. Standard precautions include a group of infection-prevention practices that apply to all patients, regardless of suspected or confirmed infection status, in any setting in which health care is delivered. Standard precautions assume all bodily fluids, blood, nonintact skin, and mucous membranes are contaminated. Standard precautions protect you from the patient and protect the patient from you. All health care professionals should use standard precautions.

Standard precautions include the use of personal protective equipment. Personal protective equipment includes:

- Gloves
- Goggles or eye shields
- Masks
- Gowns
- Possibly aprons

Standard precautions for infection control are further described in Table 15-5.

Table 15-5 Standard Precautions

Standard Precaution	Notes
Hand hygiene	One of the most important methods in preventing and controlling spread of infection; hand hygiene refers to either handwashing or surgical scrubbing.
Gloves	Use gloves often, including in these situations: potentially touching blood, handling body fluids, mouth care, perineal care, providing care of broken skin, providing care if there are cuts on your own hands.
Mask, eye protection, face shield	Intended to protect the face (and mucous membranes) during procedures that may generate splashes or while examining patients with diseases that can spread via airborne droplets.
Gown	Provides protection from procedures that may generate splashes or sprays of body fluids.
Safe injection practices	Includes the use of a sterile, single-use, disposable needle and syringe for each injection.
Safe handling of equipment	Anything in the patient environment that may have been contaminated with infectious body fluids must be handled in a manner to prevent transmission of infectious agents.
Environment control	Follow procedures/policies in place for care of environment—includes cleaning of linen and disinfection of environmental surfaces.
Patient placement	The use of a private room for a patient who is at risk of contaminating others.

The CDC has also issued a second tier of precautions called transmission-based precautions. These precautions are supposed to be used in addition to standard precautions when caring for a patient with a specific communicable disease. Thus, when examining a patient with tuberculosis, airborne precautions (use of a private room, respiratory protection during patient contact, and limited patient transport) are necessary because of the method of transmission of the disease. Other second-tier precautions include contact precautions and droplet precautions.

QUESTIONS

15-1. What does the term "asepsis" mean?

    A. Weekly autoclaving
    B. The absence of or the control of microorganisms
    C. Disinfecting surgical equipment
    D. Standard precautions
    E. Proper immunization

15-2. Which process is a common method used in medical offices to destroy all living organisms?

    A. Autoclaving
    B. Cleansing
    C. Disinfecting
    D. Sanitizing
    E. Immunization

15-3. When achieving medical asepsis, which of the following techniques is used as the first line of defense against microorganisms?

    A. Disinfecting countertops
    B. Autoclaving
    C. Handwashing

D. Sanitizing

E. Immunization

15-4. Which of the following organizations has established standards for safe working medical environments?

A. American Medical Association (AMA)

B. National Institutes of Health (NIH)

C. Ambulatory Health Care Standards (AHCS)

D. Occupational Safety and Health Administration (OSHA)

E. Food and Drug Administration (FDA)

15-5. How is tuberculosis spread from person to person?

A. Sexual contact

B. Fecal contamination

C. Dirty needles

D. Respiratory droplets

E. Mosquito bites

15-6. _____ is a technique that uses disinfectants on countertops to remove or inhibit growth of bacteria.

A. Sanitization

B. Surgical asepsis

C. Autoclaving

D. Scrubbing

E. Chemical disinfection

15-7. All of the following are personal protective equipment EXCEPT

A. gloves.

B. gowns.

C. masks.

D. hairnets.

E. goggles.

15-8. Which of the following techniques is used to eliminate all microorganisms in the environment?

A. Standard precautions

B. Isolation

C. Reverse isolation

D. Chemotherapy

E. Surgical asepsis

15-9. Which of the following describes all of the elements necessary for disease to spread?

A. Portal of entry

B. Means of transmission

C. Nosocomial infection

D. Epidemiology

E. Chain of infection

15-10. During proper autoclaving, what is the temperature and pressure of the steam?

A. Steam temperature at 250 degrees Fahrenheit; steam pressure of 10 lb

B. Steam temperature at 250 degrees Fahrenheit; steam pressure of 15 lb

C. Steam temperature at 150 degrees Fahrenheit; steam pressure of 10 lb

    D. Steam temperature at 150 degrees Fahrenheit; steam pressure of 15 lb

    E. All of the above would be appropriate for autoclaving.

15-11. What is the process of washing and removing debris from medical instruments called?

    A. Surgical asepsis

    B. Chemical disinfection

    C. Sanitization

    D. Autoclaving

    E. Handwashing

15-12. Before applying sterile surgical gloves, which of the following steps is most important to do first?

    A. Wash hands with warm, soapy water

    B. Disinfect wounds

    C. Put on surgical apron

    D. Apply moisturizer to hands

    E. Surgical scrub

15-13. When using an autoclave, how does one know that sterilization has been achieved?

    A. Dry autoclave wraps

    B. Color change on indicator strip

    C. Steam when opening up the autoclave

    D. Shiny instruments

    E. Bacterial spores on culture test

15-14. To which of the following pathogen groups would *Candida* belong?

    A. Bacteria

    B. Fungi

    C. Protozoa

    D. Viruses

    E. None of the above

15-15. In the chain of infection, which link would an elderly patient with poor nutrition fall under?

    A. Reservoir

    B. Portal of exit from reservoir

    C. Mode of transmission

    D. Portal of entry to host

    E. Susceptible host

15-16. A patient is bleeding from a wound. Transmission of infection could be prevented if which link in the chain of infection is managed first?

    A. Reservoir

    B. Portal of exit from reservoir

    C. Mode of transmission

    D. Portal of entry to host

    E. Susceptible host

15-17. Which sterilization method is most appropriate for a fiber-optic endoscope?

    A. Steam sterilization

    B. Gas sterilization

    C. Dry heat sterilization

   D. Chemical sterilization
   E. All of the above would be appropriate.

15-18. Which of the following instruments can be used to set up a sterile field?

   A. Dry transfer forceps
   B. Wet transfer forceps
   C. Sponge forceps
   D. Scalpel
   E. Towel clamp

15-19. The main objective of medical asepsis is to

   A. maintain standard precautions.
   B. use steam sterilization to eliminate spores.
   C. reduce the number of microorganisms.
   D. isolate pathogens.
   E. facilitate transmission to susceptible hosts.

15-20. Which liquid should be used for autoclaving?

   A. Distilled water
   B. Tap water
   C. Alcohol
   D. Bleach
   E. Soapy liquid

ANSWERS

15-1. The correct answer is B. Asepsis refers to the practice of eliminating contaminants in the medical or surgical environments.

15-2. The correct answer is A. Because of their ease of use, autoclaves are frequently used for sterilization in medical offices. Autoclaving uses high-pressure steam heat for sterilization.

15-3. The correct answer is C. Methods used in medical asepsis include handwashing, sanitization, and chemical disinfection. The single most important way to prevent spread of infection is by frequent handwashing. In the medical environment, everyone should wash his or her hands before and after patient contact, after any contact with contaminated material, before and after any contact with food, and after coughing, sneezing, blowing their nose, or using the restroom. There is much evidence to suggest that correct handwashing is essential in preventing infection.

15-4. The correct answer is D. OSHA, the Occupational Safety and Health Administration, is the federal agency that establishes general guidelines to address asepsis. OSHA has a set of standards that apply to medical offices. (Each state may have additional guidelines.)

15-5. The correct answer is D. Tuberculosis is spread by breathing in infectious droplets that have been expelled from the respiratory tract of infected persons.

15-6. The correct answer is E. Chemical disinfection goes one step further than sanitization, although disinfectants are more effective if the items have been sanitized first. A common chemical disinfectant is bleach. Chemical disinfection is used to clean medical instruments, lab glassware, and countertops.

15-7. The correct answer is D. Standard precautions include the use of personal protective equipment, including gloves, goggles or eye shields, masks, gowns, and aprons.

15-8. The correct answer is E. The methods and practices designed to eliminate all microorganisms in the environment is called surgical asepsis. Surgical asepsis is also referred to as sterile technique.

15-9. The correct answer is E. The chain of infection includes the five elements necessary for disease to occur and to spread. By understanding each link, a medical assistant may apply the principles of asepsis and infection control to eliminate the transmission of disease.

15-10. The correct answer is B. An autoclave device forces the temperature of steam above water's boiling point. This high temperature allows for sterilization. The steam temperature must be between 250 and 254 degrees Fahrenheit. Steam pressure is equivalent to 15 pounds of pressure.

15-11. The correct answer is C. Sanitization removes contaminants and debris on the surface of various medical office items by scrubbing them (using a scrub brush) with warm, soapy water. Enzymatic detergents can be used as the soap and are specially designed for use on medical instruments because they contain enzymes that will break down proteins found in body fluids and tissues.

15-12. The correct answer is E. The surgical scrub is essential before applying sterile gloves. Scrubbing in surgical asepsis is analogous to handwashing in medical asepsis. After finishing the surgical scrub, sterile persons are gowned and gloved immediately.

15-13. The correct answer is B. Sterilization indicators (also called indicator strips or sterilization indicator strips) are used for quality control. Sterilization indicator strips contain a dye that darkens when exposed to steam at the proper temperature and pressure.

15-14. The correct answer is B. *Candida* is a fungus that causes oral thrush and yeast infections. (Yeasts are unicellular fungi.)

15-15. The correct answer is E. An elderly patient with poor nutrition is immunosuppressed and cannot fight the infectious agent. This patient would be a susceptible host.

15-16. The correct answer is D. A break in the skin is a good portal of entry to a host. Appropriate treatment of the wound could prevent transmission of infection.

15-17. The correct answer is D. Fiber-optic endoscopes are frequently sanitized using chemical sterilization because they are unable to withstand the heat of an autoclave. Chemical sterilization uses chemicals to soak equipment in large, closed containers. It is used for instruments that are either too large or too heat sensitive for autoclaving.

15-18. The correct answer is A. Dry, sterile transfer forceps may be used to add sterile items to the sterile field or rearrange items on a tray, especially if sterile gloves have been removed. Wet transfer forceps are no longer recommended.

15-19. The correct answer is C. Medical asepsis reduces the number of microorganisms in the environment.

15-20. The correct answer is A. Only distilled water should be used in an autoclave machine to prevent mineral buildup in the machine.

Patient Preparation and Assisting the Physician

The exam will contain a variety of questions about preparing the patient for examination by the physician. This chapter outlines the basic concepts, but it is also a good idea to review your main textbooks and your completed competencies to help you prepare for the exam.

VITAL SIGNS AND ANTHROPOMETRIC MEASUREMENTS

When a patient comes to the medical office to see the physician, the first step for the medical assistant is taking vital signs. Vital comes from the Latin *vita*, meaning life. The vital signs of the patient, combined with the information from the patient history, physical examination, and test results, allow the physician to complete a diagnosis.

Generally, the temperature of the patient is the first vital sign taken by the medical assistant. Temperature will show the balance between body heat gained through metabolism and the normal heat loss of the body. Temperature is normally taken with an oral thermometer; however, rectal or aural thermometers may also be used. The average adult body temperature is 98.6 degrees Fahrenheit, but may be affected by factors such as the environment the patient has been in, recent physical activity, and normal changes during the course of the day.

The pulse of the patient is an indicator of the health of the cardiovascular system, and is generated by contractions of the left ventricle of the heart, resulting in the alternating relaxation and expansion of the walls of the artery. Pulse is monitored by counting the number of heartbeats per minute. The average pulse rate for adults will be 60 to 100 beats per minute; it will be higher in infants and lower in the elderly and well-conditioned athletes. The pulse of the patient may be taken from a number of sites, most commonly the radial pulse located on the thumb side of the inner wrist. Other pulse sites include the carotid pulse at the groove of the neck, the brachial pulse located at the fold of the elbow, and the femoral pulse at the groin. A rapid pulse in excess of 100 beats per minute is called tachycardia. A slow pulse of less than 60 beats per minute is called bradycardia.

Respiration is controlled by the brain, based on the need to replace carbon dioxide with oxygen. The average respiratory rate for an adult is 12 to 20 cycles per minute; it is significantly higher for an infant, with a normal rate of 30 to 80 cycles per minute, which declines as the infant matures. Respiration may be affected by factors such as medication, stress, disease, and recent physical activity. Respiratory rate may be controlled by the patient; therefore, respiration should be monitored and reported by the medical assistant without noting this action to the patient.

Blood pressure is monitored with the use of a sphygmomanometer. A cuff is placed over the arm of the patient approximately at heart level and inflated. As the cuff is deflated, blood will resume circulating past the cuff. The first beat heard at the start of deflation of the cuff measures the systolic pressure. The last beat heard measures the diastolic pressure. The average adult blood pressure is

120/80, with 120 representing the systolic pressure and 80 the diastolic pressure; it is lower in infants and increases through adulthood. The elderly generally will have a higher average reading. Blood pressure can be affected by stress, medications, disease, gender, and normal changes during the course of the day. Thus, a persons blood pressure can change based on the time of the day.

Hypertension, or high blood pressure, is indicated when the patient has consistently *either* a systolic reading over 140 or a diastolic reading over 90. Most cases of hypertension are classified as essential (or primary) hypertension. Essential hypertension indicates that no specific medical cause can be found to explain the elevated readings. Persistent untreated hypertension is one of the biggest risk factors for stroke, heart disease, and kidney disease.

Korotkoff sounds are sounds heard through the stethoscope during the measurement of blood pressure. There are five phases; each is described in Table 16-1.

Table 16-1 Korotkoff Sounds

Phase	Description
I	The first Korotkoff sound; it is heard as a tapping sound when the cuff pressure equals the systolic pressure.
II	The second Korotkoff sound; it is characterized by a swishing sound as the cuff is deflated slowly.
III	The third Korotkoff sound in which a tapping sound similar to phase I returns. At this stage, there is increased flow of blood pushing against the artery's wall.
IV	The fourth Korotkoff sound, heard as faded and muffled, before the sounds totally disappear.
V	Phase V of Korotkoff sounds is silence. The blood flow has returned to normal. The blood pressure is deflated entirely and removed.

The medical office will commonly use a combined weight scale and height scale to measure the height and weight of the patient. The patient is requested to stand on the scale after removing shoes. The height scale is lowered until it touches the crown of the patient's head. A large weight indicator and a small weight indicator are used in combination to measure the weight of the patient. The large weight measures in 50-pound increments and is set at the closest level below the patient's actual weight. The small weight is then moved to bring the scale to balance. The reading from the large weight and the small weight are added together for the weight reading. Many offices now use digital scales. Weight measurement is usually faster when taken on a digital scale. When weighing a patient, privacy is an important consideration as many patients are conscious of their weight.

Vital signs and measurements taken by the medical assistant will be recorded on the proper form, which will contain the patient's name and the current date. The form will be included in the patient's chart and used by the physician as part of the examination.

EXAMINATIONS

The physical examination of the patient will be either a general examination performed on a new patient, part of the ongoing care for an established patient, or an examination performed to develop a diagnosis of a specific medical concern raised by the patient. The medical assistant will assist the physician by preparing the patient for the examination by helping with the disrobing, draping, and positioning of the patient based on the type of examination and the preference of the physician. As part of the preparation process, the medical assistant will explain to the patient the reason for the specific examinations to be performed, describe the tools to be used and their function, and provide instruction on the proper positioning of the patient's body for the examination. The patient's need for privacy must be taken into account, and the patient should not be placed into an uncomfortable position before the physician is ready to begin the examination. When the physician and the patient are of different genders, it is preferable to have a medical assistant from the same gender as the patient present during the examination.

To properly position the patient for the examination, the medical assistant will need to know the specific examination to be performed and the positioning preference of the physician. Patients will be unclothed and draped based on the specific examination. Commonly used patient positions are listed in Table 16-2.

Table 16-2 Patient Examination Positions

Position	Description
Sitting	The patient is asked to sit at the edge of the examination table with legs dangling, or using the footrest at the end of the table. The physician examines the upper body and respiration.
Standing	The patient stands with weight balanced on both feet, with palms of hands facing forward. The musculoskeletal and neurological systems are examined from this position.
Supine (recumbent)	The patient is lying flat on the examination table, face up. The physician will use this position for examination of the head, neck, chest areas and heart, abdomen, and arms and legs.
Prone	The physician examines the back and feet with the patient lying flat on the examination table, face down.
Knee-chest	The patient is lying prone but resting on their knees, with their buttocks high in the air and their arms flexed above their head. This position is used for proctoscopic examinations and is difficult for the patient to maintain for any period of time. The patient should not be placed into this position until the physician is in the examination room.
Fowler's	Same as the supine position, except the top portion of the examination table is elevated, most commonly at 45 degrees. Used by the physician to examine the head, neck, and chest areas. This position would be used for examination of a patient with a head injury or one complaining of shortness of breath.
Dorsal recumbent	Same as the supine position, except the legs are flexed so that the bottom of the feet are flat on the examination table. Used for examination of the vaginal and rectal areas.
Lithotomy	This position is used with female patients for examination of the vaginal area. The patient is supine, with the knees flexed and feet resting in stirrups attached to the examination table.
Sim's (lateral)	The physician is able to examine the rectal area with the patient lying on the left side with left leg slightly bent. The right leg has a greater flex and overlaps the left leg.

During the examination, the physician may use some or all of the following examination methods: visual inspection, palpation (the use of the hands for touching or feeling for abnormalities, manipulation (the movement of body parts such as joints), percussion (monitoring vibration and sound caused by the fingers, knuckles, or a percussion hammer), auscultation (using a stethoscope to listen to body sounds), and mensuration (measurement of parts of the body and the makeup of bodily fluids).

The most common piece of equipment in the examination room is the examination table. Examination tables are designed specifically for patient examination, allowing a number of adjustments for the patient to use different positions. The examination table will normally include a roll of paper at the head, allowing for fresh paper to cover the table for each patient. The following instruments will commonly be used by the physician during the physical examination: an ophthalmoscope for the examination of the inner eye, an otoscope for the examination of the inner ear, a reflex hammer to test the reflexes of the patient, a stethoscope for listening to various body sounds, a light source such as a penlight for illumination of the mouth and throat, a nasal speculum and vaginal speculum to allow for examination of these areas, and a tape measure to allow for measurement of body parts.

Disposable supplies in the examination room will include gloves, tissues, cotton balls, disposable needles and syringes, and tongue depressors. Disposable supplies are those used once and then properly disposed of. It is the responsibility of the medical assistant to assure that supplies used by the physician during the examination are always stocked in the examination room.

PATIENT EDUCATION

Patient education is an important tool for the lifetime health of the patient. The medical office can help to reinforce basic health principles such as diet and exercise, limiting alcohol, quitting smoking, and techniques to limit stress in daily life. Information can be provided to patients on early detection of disease through proper screening tests and the dangers of unprotected sexual activity. Patient education may include written materials supplied by the medical office, videotapes/DVDs, and discussions with medical staff. The medical office will find a wide variety of information that may be of value to patients at the local library or through the Internet.

MOBILITY-ASSISTING EQUIPMENT

As a result of the aging process, injuries, or congenital disabilities, patients may need assistance in mobility. The physician is best qualified to make recommendations to the patient on the advantages of the use of a cane, crutches, walker, or a wheelchair. Normally, a physical therapist will provide training to the patient on the use of this mobility-assisting equipment; however, the medical assistant may be asked to be involved in the training process by reviewing patient progress and reinforcing instruction.

A cane needs to be fitted to the individual patient and should come to the top of the patient's femur, with the patient's elbow bent at a 30-degree angle. A tripod cane will provide greater stability than a standard cane. The cane will always be used on the strong side of the body. In walking, the cane is first moved forward approximately 12 inches. The weak-side foot is then moved forward to be level with the cane. The strong-side foot is then moved forward of both the cane and the weak-side foot. Specific directions are also available to help the patient go up and down stairs.

A standard set of crutches will fit 2–3 inches below the patient's axillae and will have handgrips for stability. Proper fitting of crutches is critical to their appropriate use. The patient will be taught to stand erect and to support the weight of their body with their hands, not their armpits. Specific instructions for the use of crutches will depend on the relative strength of both legs of the patient. The person providing instructions will review leg strength and recommend a gait appropriate to the patient's condition.

A walker is made of tubular metal, with two legs ending in wheels and two ending in rubber tips. The patient will step into the walker and grip the sides of the walker. As with other mobility-assisting equipment, a physical therapist will normally provide instruction in proper use to the patient.

For a patient with severe mobility issues, either temporary or permanent, the physician may recommend the use of a wheelchair. Wheelchairs come with a variety of features designed to accommodate the specific needs of the patient.

MEDICATIONS

All patients should be asked to provide the medical office with a complete listing of medications they are taking, both prescription and nonprescription, as well as disclosure of the use of alcohol and recreational drugs. This information will be available to the physician before prescribing medication for the patient's chief complaint at the time of visit to the medical office.

Medications prescribed by the physician come with a variety of proper means of administration. Oral drugs are swallowed. Buccal drugs are placed between the gum and cheek, and sublingual drugs are placed under the tongue; both are left in place until dissolved. Topical drugs are rubbed into the skin, and transdermal drugs are applied as a patch. Other drugs are designed to be inhaled or injected. The medical assistant will review the medications prescribed by the physician and discuss with the patient the proper administration of each medication, frequency of use, and possible side effects.

PATIENT HISTORY INTERVIEW

An appointment for a new patient will be scheduled to provide sufficient time between the time of arrival of the patient and the time when the patient will be seen by the physician. In the majority of medical offices, this time will be used by the patient to complete a series of forms that provide basic information on personal data and the health history of the patient. In other medical offices, this information will be recorded by the medical assistant during an interview with the patient. Under either approach, the information in the patient history will include the items in Table 16-3.

After the patient has completed the forms, office procedures may dictate that the patient be interviewed by the medical assistant. During this interview, the medical assistant will review the information provided by the patient, convert the patient's lay descriptions into proper medical

Table 16-3 Patient History Information

Information	Description
Personal data	Name, address, phone numbers, date of birth, education, occupation and employer, and emergency contact information; health insurance information may be included in this section or provided separately
Health and lifestyle	Tobacco and alcohol use, diet, sleep patterns, and type and frequency of exercise
Family history	Details of the illnesses and diseases of parents and brothers and sisters, including dates and causes of death, if appropriate
Past illnesses and surgeries	A listing of the previous illnesses and surgeries of the patient back to childhood; includes any details on drug reactions and allergies
Female patients	Information on menses, any pregnancies, and the results of the pregnancies
Health statement	A statement in the patient's own words describing their general health
Following the section on personal data and general health history, forms will be used to review each of the major body systems:	
Head	Questions concerning frequency of headaches and stress; details on issues relative to eyes, ears, nose, throat, and mouth
Cardiovascular	Questions about blood pressure issues, chest pain, and irregular heartbeat
Respiratory	Questions about shortness of breath, coughing, asthma, and allergies
Gastrointestinal	Questions about indigestion, bowel movements, nausea, and vomiting
Neurological	Questions about coordination, issues with memory and concentration, vertigo, and tremors
Musculoskeletal	Questions about pain or swelling, deformities, and mobility
Female patients	Questions on menstrual cycle and irregularities

terminology, quantify the data as fully as possible, and fill in any gaps in the patient history. Notations made by the medical assistant should be brief and directly to the point. All notations should be dated and initialed. If the patient is complaining of pain, the medical assistant should question and note the time of onset of pain, region of the pain, type of pain such as dull or throbbing, and any symptoms relating to the pain such as swelling or nausea. The patient should be asked for their view on the cause of the pain.

The interview by the medical assistant may save time for the physician during the examination, but may mean that questions asked by the medical assistant are duplicated by the physician. During this interview process, conducted by either the medical assistant or the physician, the chief complaint of the patient will be thoroughly reviewed and documented in the patient records.

QUESTIONS

16-1. When using clinical thermometers, cross-contamination may BEST be prevented by

    A. using a disposable plastic sheath.
    B. storing in a closed container after drying.
    C. soaking for 20 minutes in commercial disinfectant.
    D. cleaning in cold water.
    E. cleaning in hot water.

16-2. The term for a rapid, regular pulse is

    A. tachycardia.
    B. bradycardia.

    C. fibrillation.

    D. systole.

    E. asystole.

16-3. When the patient history is first taken, which of the following is NOT a physical assessment observed by the medical assistant?

    A. Grooming

    B. Ease of conversation

    C. Appropriate answers to basic questions

    D. Strength

    E. Skin color, pallor, etc.

16-4. A review of which of the following systems will include determination of muscle pain, stiffness in joints, and limits on degree of movement of arms and legs?

    A. Nervous

    B. Musculoskeletal

    C. Gastrointestinal

    D. Respiratory

    E. Cardiovascular

16-5. All of the following are arterial sites at which the pulse may be felt EXCEPT

    A. carotid

    B. femoral

    C. radial

    D. corneal

16-6. Hypernea may be defined as

    A. normal breathing in a standing position.

    B. air in the pericardium.

    C. rapid breathing.

    D. breathing painful to the patient.

    E. gas in the pleura.

16-7. Which of the following is NOT a piece of equipment to assist the patient with mobility?

    A. Wheelchair

    B. Cane

    C. Walker

    D. Arm sling

    E. Crutches

16-8. Sublingual drugs are self-administered by the patient by

    A. placing under the tongue until dissolved.

    B. placing between cheek and gum until dissolved.

    C. swallowing with water.

    D. attaching a patch with the medication to the upper arm.

16-9. Which of the following subjects is appropriate to be discussed with the patient and answers recorded during the patient interview?

    A. Personal data

    B. Family history

    C. Health and lifestyle

    D. Past illnesses and surgeries

    E. All of the above

16-10. Hypertension would be indicated when the patient has which of the following blood pressure readings?

    A. 100/60

    B. 120/80

    C. 120/90

    D. 130/85

    E. 160/100

16-11. The medical assistant should wait until the physician is in the examination room before assisting the patient into which of the following positions for examination?

    A. Knee-chest

    B. Prone

    C. Supine

    D. Dorsal recumbent

    E. Sim's

16-12. The pulse point located at the groove of the neck is the

    A. temporal.

    B. femoral.

    C. popliteal.

    D. carotid.

16-13. All of the following are vital signs EXCEPT

    A. chief complaint

    B. blood pressure

    C. pulse

    D. temperature

    E. respiratory rate

16-14. There are five phases of Korotkoff sounds as the blood pressure cuff is deflated. Which is the stage when the sounds are fading and are muffled?

    A. I

    B. II

    C. III

    D. IV

    E. V

16-15. The primary reason for draping the patient is to

    A. provide for the privacy of the patient.

    B. keep the patient from becoming chilled.

    C. prevent cross-contamination.

    D. allow the physician to examine selected areas.

    E. control the anxiety of the patient.

16-16. Dr. Brown is conducting an examination of a patient's head and neck. The following instruments will be used by the physician

    A. otoscope, ophthalmoscope, flashlight, and percussion hammer.

    B. otoscope, ophthalmoscope, flashlight, and stethoscope.

C. otoscope, ophthalmoscope, flashlight, and tongue depressor.

D. otoscope, ophthalmoscope, flashlight, and vaginal speculum.

16-17. The pulse rate for a normal adult is

A. 90–140 beats per minute.

B. 80–130 beats per minute.

C. 70–125 beats per minute.

D. 60–100 beats per minute.

E. 50–90 beats per minute.

16-18. The blood pressure of a patient is measured by the

A. audiometer.

B. pulse oximeter.

C. tympanometer.

D. doppler.

E. sphygmomanometer.

16-19. A patient arrives at the medical office for an appointment with the physician. The main reason the patient is seeking medical attention is called the

A. patient history.

B. chief complaint.

C. assessment.

D. symptoms.

E. observation.

16-20. The physician's assessment of major body functions is referred to as the

A. medical history questionnaire.

B. diagnosis of illness.

C. review of systems.

D. social history.

E. family history.

ANSWERS

16-1. The correct answer is C. Cross-contamination may best be prevented by soaking the clinical thermometer in a 70% solution of methanol or similar commercial disinfectant, after washing in cool, sudsy water and rinsing in cool water.

16-2. The correct answer is A. A rapid heartbeat, in excess of 100 beats per minute, is termed tachycardia.

16-3. The correct answer is D. In the initial medical history, the medical assistant will make observations of the new patient, including grooming, skin color, and ease of conversation and response to questions. Strength is not a characteristic based on observation.

16-4. The correct answer is B. A review of the musculoskeletal system will include reviewing muscle pain, stiffness in joints, and degrees of movement of arms and legs.

16-5. The correct answer is D. The pulse of the patient may be taken from a number of sites, most commonly the radial pulse located on the thumb side of the inner wrist. Other pulse sites include the carotid pulse at the groove of the neck, the brachial pulse located at the fold of the elbow, and the femoral pulse at the groin. The cornea has no blood supply; hence, the corneal artery is fictitious.

16-6. The correct answer is C. Hypernea is the rapid, deep breathing normal in patients exercising and abnormal in patients with pain or fever.

16-7. The correct answer is D. Of the items listed, only the arm sling is not a piece of equipment for patient mobility.

16-8. The correct answer is A. Sublingual medications are placed under the tongue until dissolved.

16-9. The correct answer is E. Each of the listed subjects, as well as a health statement in the patient's own words and specific information on menses and pregnancies for female patients, are covered during the patient interview.

16-10. The correct answer is E. Hypertension is indicated when the patient has consistently *either* a systolic reading over 140 or a diastolic reading over 90.

16-11. The correct answer is A. The knee-chest position is used for proctoscopic examinations and is difficult for the patient to maintain for any period of time. The patient should not be placed into this position until the physician is in the examination room.

16-12. The correct answer is D. The carotid pulse point is located at the groove of the neck.

16-13. The correct answer is A. When a patient comes to the medical office to see the physician, the first step for the medical assistant is taking vital signs. Vital signs include the patient's temperature, pulse, respiratory rate, and blood pressure. The patient's chief complaint is not considered a vital sign.

16-14. The correct answer is D. The last sounds heard, fading and muffled, before the sounds totally disappear are heard in Phase IV of Korotkoff sounds.

16-15. The correct answer is A. Draping is used to provide for the privacy of the patient during the examination by the physician

16-16. The correct answer is C. An ophthalmoscope is used for the examination of the inner eye, an otoscope is used for the examination of the inner ear, and a flashlight (or penlight) is used for illumination of the mouth and throat. Of the other items listed, only the tongue depressor will be used during the examination of the patient's head and neck. The percussion hammer, stethoscope, and vaginal speculum are used for examination of other parts of the body.

16-17. The correct answer is D. The normal adult pulse rate is 60 to 100 beats per minute.

16-18. The correct answer is E. The sphygmomanometer, consisting of the cuff, pressure bulb, control valve, and manometer, is used to measure blood pressure.

16-19. The correct answer is B. The primary reason that a patient is seeking medical attention is referred to as the chief complaint.

16-20. The correct answer is C. The review of systems is the assessment by the physician of major body functions.

Specimen Collection, Diagnostic Testing, and Medical Equipment

The exam will contain a variety of questions that cover clinical equipment operation, collecting and processing specimens, and diagnostic testing. Medical assistants are responsible for these activities in the physicians office. Basic information on all three areas is covered in this chapter.

TREATMENT

Many questions on the exam cover the proper techniques required for treatment. These will include questions about equipment and its appropriate use, supplies, treatment areas, and safety precautions.

Principles of Equipment Operation

Not only does the medical assistant assist in the examination and treatment of patients, but he or she must also know how to operate numerous pieces of equipment in the medical office. Table 17-1 describes the equipment with which the medical assistant must be knowledgeable.

Restocking Supplies

The medical office needs to be maintained. One of the roles of the medical assistant is to both inventory and restock supplies. Part of this role requires organization. Supplies should be put back in their place with lids replaced properly to prevent any accidents. Supplies that are low in number should be reordered. Medication storage requires special attention. Some medications need to be stored at specific temperatures. All medications, especially narcotics, must be kept out of areas in which patients may have access. The medical assistant is responsible for checking medications' expiration dates and disposing of outdated medicines.

Preparing and Maintaining Treatment Areas

The medical assistant is responsible for maintaining a clean, tidy, and safe treatment area. The medical assistant makes sure that all diagnostic equipment is clean, calibrated, and well maintained. He or she also makes sure that surgical instruments are properly cleaned, wrapped, and sterilized.

The medical assistant may have a quality control log to show the documentation of quality control done on every piece of equipment. Equipment requires maintenance and testing to ensure proper function. Certain equipment needs to be calibrated regularly in accordance with the manufacturer's guidelines.

Table 17-1 Equipment in the Medical Office

Equipment	Indication
Autoclave (steam sterilizer)	Uses high-pressure steam heat for sterilization; most common sterilization technique used in the medical office
Cast equipment and materials	Used to immobilize fractures and sprains; materials include plaster, synthetic and plastic, and air casts
Electrocardiograph (EKG or ECG)	Measures electrical activity of the heart
Endoscope	Instrument used to view within the body via a lighted camera and tube; examples include bronchoscope, gastroscope, colonoscope, sigmoidoscope, anoscope, and esophagogastroduodenoscope
Examination table	Table upon which patients sit during medical assessment; table types vary based on use (e.g., GYN, pediatric)
Microscope	Magnifies very small objects not visible to the naked eye; important in the medical office for examining blood smears, blood cell counts, and body fluid samples
Mobility assistive devices	Devices such as walkers, crutches, canes, and wheelchairs that assist with movement disabilities
Nebulizer	Used to administer medicine via mist inhalation in respiratory diseases such as asthma.
Ophthalmoscope	Allows for visual examination of the retina and interior eye
Otoscope	Used for visual examination of the external ear canal and tympanic membrane
Oxygen	Used to treat patients with hypoxemia; methods of oxygen delivery include nasal cannula, nasal catheter, and mask
Physical therapy modalities	Noninvasive therapeutic procedures used in physiatry, rehabilitation medicine, sports medicine, and preventative health; includes thermotherapy (heat), cryotherapy (cold), hydrotherapy (water), and ultrasound (sound waves)
Pulse oximeter	Measures the percentage of oxygen in the blood
Scales	Used to measure patient height and weight
Sphygmomanometer	Measures blood pressure; also known as a blood pressure cuff
Spirometer	Evaluates lung capacity
Stethoscope	Used for auscultation of heart and lung sounds
Thermometer	Measures body temperature; types include mercury (used infrequently), electronic, tympanic, and disposable; tympanic electronic thermometers are becoming more popular because they are accurate and comfortable and can be used in a patient of any age, even uncooperative patients

Safety Precautions

Safety precautions are taken when using specialized medical equipment, while restocking supplies, and in preparing and maintaining the treatment area. The medical assistant should be aware of and practice standard precautions when needed (see Chapter 16).

COLLECTING AND PROCESSING SPECIMENS

In a medical office, a medical assistant is responsible for collecting many types of specimens. The medical assistant may then perform CLIA-waived tests (based on the Clinical Laboratory Improvement

Act) on the specimens; otherwise, these specimens are sent on to a laboratory for processing. CLIA-waived tests are considered relatively simple procedures with little risk for errors or interpretation of results. CLIA-waived tests include testing for the rapid strep antigen, infectious mono, and *Helicobacter pylori* as well as qualitative urine dipstick testing. Only a small percentage of all laboratory tests are considered waived. It is essential that the medical assistant is careful and responsible while collecting specimens so that the sample is reliable and the test is accurate, regardless of whether or not the test is waived (will be performed by the medical assistant) or is more complex (will be sent elsewhere).

Collecting Specimens

Many questions on the exam focus on the proper methods involved in specimen collection. Specimens may be collected from blood, urine, stool, and sputum. In addition, specimens may be collected so that cultures can be grown. Cultures can be grown from specimens gathered from the throat, vagina, wounds, urine, or blood. In general, no matter what the specimen collected is, the medical assistant should keep the following points in mind:

- Make the patient as comfortable as possible.
- Provide detailed, clear instructions if the patient will collect the specimen on his or her own.
- Avoid contamination.
- Follow aseptic techniques.
- Collect the specimen from the most likely site where the potential pathogen will be found.
- Collect the specimen at the appropriate time.
- Collect the appropriate amount of specimen.
- Collect the specimen before giving antibiotics.
- Use proper specimen containers, transport systems, and culture media to ensure growth.
- Label containers properly and use the proper request forms for further lab testing.

Blood

Phlebotomy is the process of collecting blood for diagnostic purposes. Typically, blood is drawn (or collected) from a vein. This procedure is widely used and an integral part of making a diagnosis and treatment plan for a patient. An alternative method collects blood from a capillary. Capillary puncture is typically used when patient blood volume is a concern, as with infants or with severely burned or scarred patients.

Vein

Drawing blood from a vein is also referred to as venipuncture. The antecubital space, which is found on the anterior surface of the arm, directly in front of the elbow, is used for venipuncture. Veins in this area have wide lumens and thick walls, making them less likely to collapse. In general, there are also fewer nerve endings in this area. The veins found in this area are the cephalic vein, median cubital vein, and basilic vein. The median cubital vein is typically the most frequently used because it tends to be the most prominent. When inserting the needle, the needle's bevel should be face up at a 15- to 30-degree angle.

The formed elements (cells) and the liquid portion (plasma) of the blood are often separated for laboratory testing. A centrifuge is used to spin the blood so it separates based on density, with the red blood cells falling to the bottom of the tube and the serum rising to the top. In between the red blood cells and plasma is the buffy coat, which contains leukocytes and thrombocytes. Thus, un-coagulated (not clotted) blood can be separated into three layers: plasma, a buffy coat, and red blood cells. When collecting both plasma and whole blood, a tube containing anticoagulant is used.

Sometimes blood tests need to be done on serum. The main difference between serum and plasma is that plasma contains fibrinogen (used in clotting) whereas serum does not. In the instance where serum is required for a test, a serum separator vacuum tube with thixotropic gel is used. This process separates the blood into serum and clotted elements; the blood is then considered coagulated (or clotted) blood.

Three methods are used to perform a venipuncture: the syringe method, the vacuum tube method, and the butterfly method. Each method has advantages and disadvantages. Vacuum tubes are used whenever possible for routine collection and when multiple tubes are needed. The butterfly method is used for difficult blood draws on small or fragile veins and in small children and the elderly. The syringe method is used for very inaccessible and fragile veins in children and the elderly. This method is also used for home testing by the patient. Regardless of which method is used, blood will be transferred into a vacuum tube eventually because vacuum tubes contain the required chemicals for the blood tests to be performed.

Vacuum tubes are vacuum-packed plastic test tubes with rubber stoppers. The color of the rubber stopper ensures the correct laboratory test is done. Different tubes have different additives in order to run the appropriate test. Regardless of manufacturer, the stopper colors are universal; they are outlined in Table 17-2.

The order in which blood is drawn is important. Sterile collection needs to be done first to prevent any contamination. After the sterile collection is done, the order of draw into vacuum tubes depends on the additive. You do not want a back flow of additives into the tubes as this could create false results. Table 17-3 outlines the correct order.

Table 17-2 Color Codes for Blood Collection

Color of Tube Top	Lab Use	Additive
Red *Clotting tube*	Serum testing	None or glass particles
Red/gray *Tiger Tops or SST*	Serum testing; speeds clot formation	Serum separator gel
Green/gray *Plasma separator tube (PST)*	Serum testing; coagulation studies	Heparin with separator gel
Light blue *Anticoagulant*	Coagulation studies	Sodium citrate
Green *Anticoagulant*	Coagulation studies, electrolytes, STAT chemistry panels	Heparin
Lavender *Anticoagulant*	Whole-blood specimen; hematology: complete blood count (CBC), white blood cell count (WBC), differentials, sedimentation rate, hemoglobin (Hgb)	Ethylenediamine tetraacetate (EDTA)
Gray *Antiglycolitic*	Blood glucose levels; blood alcohol levels	Potassium oxalate or sodium fluoride
Yellow	Bacteria-blood cultures; viral loads; DNA or paternity testing	Sodium polyanetholesulfonate (SPS); acid citrate dextrose (ACD)
Royal blue	Toxicology studies (lead, copper, iron)	Trace; some may contain heparin

Table 17-3 Order of Blood Draw

Order	Color of Tube Top	Additive
1	Yellow top (or culture bottle) *Sterile procedures*	Sodium, SPS, ACD
2	Light blue top	Sodium citrate
3	Red tops and red/gray tops *Serum tubes*	Glass particles
4	Green top	Heparin
5	Lavender	EDTA
6	Gray *Glycolitic inhibitor*	Sodium fluoride or potassium oxalate

Capillary

Capillary punctures collect a small amount of blood from a superficial capillary. Sites used are typically the fingertip in an adult or the heel in an infant. Glucose levels and hemoglobin can be measure by a capillary puncture. In a neonate, two tests required by law in the United States are capillary puncture for phenylketonuria (PKU) and thyroid hormone. Both tests are done prior to the infant leaving the hospital because if either lab value is abnormal, both conditions (PKU or hypothyroidism) can be treated successfully.

The following techniques should be remembered when performing a capillary puncture:

1. Increase circulation to the area by gentle massage or warm pack/towel. (Do *not* squeeze the fingertip because it forces tissue fluid into the blood sample and may cause erroneous results.)
2. Clean with alcohol, and ensure the area is dry (air-drying is best).
3. Use standard precautions.
4. Puncture the tip of the fleshy part of the finger (adult) using a disposable lancet.
5. Squeeze it lightly to stimulate the flow of blood.
6. Discard the first drop of blood (it may be contaminated with tissue fluid).
7. Only use the second and following drops of blood for testing.
8. Hold the capillary tube horizontally and blood will enter via capillary action.
9. Avoid air bubbles or spaces in the tube.
10. Apply a cotton ball compress to the puncture site.

Urine

There are different methods of collecting urine. Different situations require different urine samples. For a routine urinalysis, a clean-catch midstream urine sample is acceptable. Table 17-4 describes the methods of obtaining various urine samples.

Stool

Stool specimens are obtained for a variety of reasons. Disease such as cancer or colitis may show blood in the stool. Parasites and their ova (eggs) as well as pathological bacteria may also be tested

Table 17-4 Urine Collection

Type of Urine Sample	Method
Catheterized collection	Urine is collected from a catheter bag; the patient may already be catheterized or may not be able to follow cleansing instructions, so may need to be catheterized to obtain a sterile specimen.
Clean-catch midstream collection	Used when a sterile specimen is necessary (to check for bacteria in the urine); the urethral meatus is cleaned with towelettes (twice in males, three times in females); the patient begins urinating, then pulls the cup into the urine stream to collect the sample.
First-voided collection	The first morning void is concentrated and is usually the specimen method of choice for many tests.
24-hour collection	Urine is collected over a 24-hour period; used to determine both the amount of urine produced by the patient and the quantity of certain substances (sodium, potassium, calcium, and creatinine); many containers for 24-hour collection contain preservatives; sample must be refrigerated between voids.
Fasting collection	Used to obtain a urine sample without interference of food (can be used as first voided collection because of fasting overnight).
Timed collection	Patients have a meal and then urine is collected 4 hours later.
Random collection	This is the most common type of collection performed in a medical office; patients give a sample when they are there for their appointment; also used for drug screens.

for in a stool specimen. A specimen that will be checked for ova and parasites is called an O and P specimen. Stool specimens need to be kept at room temperature because refrigeration may destroy any parasites. Patients may collect stool in a clean container; it is not required to be sterile. However, the stool should not be contaminated with urine. Several different samples of stool specimens may be ordered for testing at different times.

Sputum

In order to collect sputum correctly, the patient must cough deeply to get enough mucus into the sterile container. A first morning specimen is the best. The medical assistant should remember to use standard precautions while obtaining this specimen.

Cultures

A culture refers to the process of growing pathogens. Cultures can be obtained from the throat, vagina, wounds, urine, or blood. Table 17-5 describes the method of collecting each culture.

Specimens are grown in a culture medium and maintained at a designated temperature. Culture media are used to promote growth of the bacteria by providing a nutrition source. The culture medium (or agar) in which bacteria will grow is typically placed in a Petri dish. *Plating* refers to the process of placing the bacteria in the Petri dish's culture medium using an inoculating loop. *Transport media* refers to a tube-like structure used temporarily until the bacteria can be grown more permanently.

When any culture is being performed, the primary result can be read in 24–48 hours. The purpose of performing a culture is to identify the specific microorganisms contained in the specimen so the patient can be treated appropriately. Sensitivity tests may be ordered in addition to the culture to determine which antibiotic will effectively treat (kill) the pathogen.

Processing Specimens

There will be questions on the exam concerning specimen processing. It is important to be familiar with the guidelines established by The Clinical Laboratory Improvement Amendments of 1988, commonly called CLIA '88. The medical assistant is not only able to collect specimens but must also be able to process specimens safely, reliably, and accurately.

Centers for Disease Control and Prevention (CDC) Guidelines for Processing Specimens

The Centers for Disease Control and Prevention (CDC) is a division of the U.S. Department of Health and Human Services. The CDC investigates various diseases and makes recommendations on how to prevent their spread. The Clinical Laboratory Improvement Amendments of 1988, commonly called CLIA '88, was established to protect patients by regulating all human body specimen testing (blood, secretions, and excretions). CLIA '88 regulations were passed in response to public outcry about misread

Table 17-5 Cultures

Culture	Method of Collection
Throat	Use a sterile swab to swipe the back of the throat. Use a tongue depressor to hold the tongue down and out of the way. Place the swab with culture in a culturette that contains a moist medium to keep any potential bacteria viable. Rapid strep tests for the detection of Group A *Streptoccocus* may be performed in the medical office (CLIA-waived).
Vagina (cervix)	Do a pelvic exam; cultures may detect sexually transmitted diseases.
Wounds	Use either a sterile swab or a sterile needle to aspirate pus. Don't contaminate the specimen by touching the surrounding skin. Place the specimen in anaerobic transport material.
Urine	Instruct the patient to obtain a clean-catch urine sample (or you may use a catheterized sample). Collect the urine in a sterile container.
Blood	Blood cultures are obtained in the same manner as regular blood collection; culture blood if concerned about sepsis.

Pap smears in 1988. All laboratories, no matter how small or large, including the physician's office lab or an ambulatory care setting, must abide by CLIA '88 regulations. Hence, quality control is established.

CLIA '88 has established three categories of testing:

- Waived tests
- Moderate-complexity tests, including Provider-performed microscopy procedures (PPM)
- High-complexity tests

Most of the tests that a medical assistant will perform fall into the waived category. These tests are the simplest and require a minimal amount of judgment and interpretation. The CDC publishes a list of CLIA-waived tests, and these tests do not have as strict of standards as the other two categories. Moderate-complexity and high-complexity tests use further criteria such as the expertise of the operator, the degree of operator intervention needed, and the amount of maintenance and/or troubleshooting required to perform the test. The moderate complexity tests mostly involve testing that is essential for immediate patient care. Many of the moderate complexity tests may be performed in physician office labs. A subcategory of the moderate-complexity tests is the PPM, which was added to include specific microscopic tests (e.g. urine microscopy or a KOH smear). Typically, a midlevel provider may perform these tests. In general, the more complicated the test, the more stringent the requirements. The high-complexity tests require more knowledge and training to perform and interpret results. These tests are typically performed in specialized labs.

There are many components to the CLIA '88 law, including proper labeling of specimens, avoiding contamination, specimen preservation, good recordkeeping, and quality control. Proper labeling of specimens is essential. Specimens are typically labeled with the patient's name, identification number, date, type of specimen, time of collection, and physician's name. The container should be labeled, not the lid or the wrapping because they may be discarded later. Obtaining the specimen in the proper manner will prevent contamination. The medical assistant is required to collect specimens that will be preserved correctly. This includes being aware of the following aspects of a test: proper temperature, amount of specimen, time limits, and the use of nonexpired chemicals or reagents. The law also mandates documentation or recordkeeping. A procedure manual should be kept. The accuracy of any laboratory test depends on having quality controls in place. CLIA '88 mandates quality assurance and proficiency testing for nonwaived tests in addition to regular testing of equipment, maintaining supplies, and education of personnel.

PERFORMING SELECTED TESTS

The medical assistant is responsible for performing selected tests that assist with diagnosis and treatment. The clinical significance of each test is reviewed here. Many questions on the exam cover these clinical tests.

Urinalysis

A urinalysis studies the urine as an aid in patient diagnosis or in follow-up to prior diagnosis. A routine urinalysis is one of the most commonly performed procedures in a medical office. For a routine urinalysis, a clean-catch midstream urine sample is acceptable. Urine can be examined for its physical, chemical, or microscopic properties. *Physical properties* include specimen volume, color and transparency, odor, and specific gravity. *Chemical properties* include pH, glucose, protein, ketones, bilirubin, blood, leukocyte esterase, nitrite, and urobilinogen. The reagent test strip (dipstick) is useful for measuring the chemical properties of urine. *Microscopic* examination of urine looks for microorganisms and abnormal urinary sediment cells, including red blood cells, white blood cells, renal epithelial cells, crystals, and casts. A drop of urinary sediment is placed on a slide and viewed microscopically. The medical assistant is responsible for properly centrifuging the urine and setting up the slide. Normal values, along with the potential pathology of all urinary properties, are outlined in Table 17-6.

Hematology

Hematology is the study of blood cells and their coagulation in both normal and disease states. Hematologic tests are the second most common tests performed in the medical office, next to urinalysis.

Table 17-6 Urinalysis Properties

Properties of Urine	Normal Value	Potential Pathology
Specimen volume	Half a cup—fill a test tube, leaving at least 10 ml for a chemical reagent strip	Dehydration; lack of kidney function
Urine color	Straw to yellow	Possible abnormal colors result from blood, vitamin intake, drugs
Odor	Not pungent	Sweet = ketoacidosis; Foul = bacterial infection
Specific gravity	1.002–1.030	High specific gravity may mean diabetes or dehydration; may be tested with a reagent test strip, urinometer, or refractometer
pH	4.5–8.0	Some medications, diets high in one food group, renal TB, extremely high fevers, UTI, uncontrolled diabetes
Glucose	Negative	Diabetes; extreme physical and emotional stress
Protein	Negative	Excessive exercise, exposure to extreme heat/cold, extreme emotional stress, renal disease, high blood pressure, diabetes
Ketones	Negative	Diabetes, noncarbohydrate diets
Bilirubin	Negative	Liver and/or gallbladder disease
Blood (RBCs)	Negative	Contaminate from menstruation, UTI, kidney stone, neoplasm
Leukocyte esterase	Negative	Bacteria (UTI)
Nitrite	Negative	Bacteria (UTI)
Urobilinogen	0.2–1.0	Liver disease
Microorganisms	Negative	May see bacteria, yeast, or parasites; a urine culture with sensitivity can be ordered
Red blood cells	Negative	Disease, trauma
White blood cells	Negative	UTI
Renal epithelial cells	Negative	Kidney disease
Crystals	Negative or normal	Uric acid (gout), sulfa drug, or urine that has been refrigerated
Casts	Negative	Kidney disease, fever, emotional stress, strenuous exercise

Hematologic tests can measure hematocrit, hemoglobin, erythrocyte sedimentation rate (ESR), RBC count with indices, WBC count with differential, platelet count, and prothrombin time. A complete blood count, also known as a CBC, is a common test ordered. The CBC includes values for hemoglobin, hematocrit, RBC count, WBC count, WBC differential, and erythrocyte indices. Hematologic tests are described further in Table 17-7.

Blood Chemistry

Blood chemistry tests measure the levels of chemical substances released from the body's tissues. The amounts of these chemicals give an indication of an individual's health in relation to an organ's function. Typically, blood chemistry tests are performed by testing the blood's plasma rather than whole blood.

A general chemistry panel can be ordered or a specific panel can focus on one organ's function. The general chemistry panel is called the Comprehensive Metabolic Panel (CMP) and is used as a broad screening tool to evaluate organ function and check for conditions such as diabetes, liver disease, and kidney disease. The CMP may also be ordered to monitor known conditions, such as

Table 17-7 Hematologic Tests

Cell Type	Normal Range	Notes
Hematocrit (Hct)	Male: 39–52% Female: 35–47%	Ratio of the volume of packed RBCs to that of the whole blood sample
Hemoglobin (Hgb)	Male: 13.5–17.5 g/dL Female: 12.0–16.0 g/dL	Measures amount of Hgb in RBCs (oxygen-carrying capacity of blood); the hemoglobin: hematocrit ratio is normally 1:3
Erythrocyte sedimentation rate	Wintrobe scale (method): Male: 0–9 mm/hr Female: 0–16 mm/hr	Measures the rate at which RBCs settle to the bottom of a well-mixed anticoagulated sample; nonspecific test to screen for inflammation, infection, and disease because RBCs fall faster when their surface membrane is damaged
Red blood cell count (RBCs, erythrocytes)	Male: 4.3–5.7 million cells/mm^3 Female: 3.8–5.2 million cells/mm^3	Decreased in anemia (many causes—bleeding, especially)
RBC indices: mean corpuscular volume (MCV), mean corpuscular Hgb (MCH), and mean corpuscular Hgb concentration (MCHC)	MCV: 80–100 fl MCH: 27–33 pg MCHC: 32–36 g/dL	Measures specifications of the RBCs: MCH = weight of Hgb in an average RBC MCV = average volume of the RBCs MCHC = average concentration of Hgb in a given volume of RBCs
White blood cell count (leukocytes, WBCs)	4500–11,000 cells/mm^3	Increased in viral infections; decreased in stress, burns, trauma, uremia
Leukocyte differential: basophils	0–1%	Increased in polycythemia vera, chicken pox, and ulcerative colitis
Leukocyte differential: eosinophils	1–3%	Increased with allergic reactions, hay fever, and parasitic infections
Leukocyte differential: lymphocytes	20–40%	Increased with infectious mononucleosis, lymphocytic leukemia, and many diseases of viral origin
Leukocyte differential: monocytes	4–10%	Increased in tuberculosis and monocytic leukemia
Leukocyte differential: neutrophils	55–62%	Increased with bacterial infections
Platelet count	150,000–400,000/mm^3	Increased with trauma, fractures, postsurgery; decreased with Disseminated intravascular coagulation (DIC), Idiopathic thrombocytopenic purpura (ITP), and other disorders; platelet function is assessed by using the bleeding time test
Prothrombin time	INR System: Normal: 0.75–1.30 Therapeutic: 2.0–4.5	Evaluates the extrinsic clotting cascade (clotting factors I, II, V, VII, and X); useful when administering warfarin (Coumadin)

hypertension, and to monitor patients taking specific medications for any kidney- or liver-related side effects. This panel measures the blood levels of sodium, potassium, calcium, chloride, carbon dioxide, glucose, blood urea nitrogen, creatinine, protein, albumin, bilirubin, and liver enzymes. The CMP is routinely ordered as part of a blood work-up for a yearly physical. If results of the CMP are abnormal, a more specific blood chemistry panel (or test) will be ordered. Such specific blood chemistry tests and their significance are described in Table 17-8.

Immunology

Immunology is sometimes referred to as serology. Certain diseases can be tested for based on the reactions of antibodies to antigens. Immunologic tests are used to detect for infectious mononucleosis, strep throat, infectious and inflammatory diseases, and pregnancy. Each test and its significance is described in Table 17-9.

Table 17-8 Blood Chemistry Tests

Test	Significance
Blood glucose	Important screening test for diabetes—can do a fasting blood glucose test, a 2-hour postprandial blood glucose, or a glucose tolerance test.
Kidney function	Includes measurement of BUN (blood urea nitrogen) and creatinine to evaluate renal function. BUN measures the amount of urea in the blood, which reflects the excretory function of the kidney; creatinine reflects the glomerular filtration rate at the level of the nephron.
Liver function	Includes measurements of alanine transaminase (ALT), aspartate transaminase (AST), alkaline phosphatase (ALP), total bilirubin (TBIL), direct bilirubin, gamma glutamyl transpeptidase (GGT), albumin, prothrombin, and total protein; taken together these enzymes and proteins detect, evaluate, and monitor liver disease or damage.
Lipid profile	Includes total cholesterol, high-density lipoprotein (HDL), low-density lipoprotein (LDL), and triglycerides; together they help to determine a patient's risk of heart disease and stroke.
Hemoglobin A$_{1c}$	Measures the amount of glycosylated hemoglobin in the blood (hemoglobin that has glucose stuck to it); measuring this determines how well a diabetic patient's glucose has been controlled over the past 4–6 weeks.

Table 17-9 Immunologic Tests

Test	Significance
Mononucleosis	Tests for infectious mononucleosis (IM) caused by the Epstein-Barr virus; must combine the blood test with a serologic test (and patient symptoms) for diagnosis of IM. The blood test looks for a large number of lymphocytes while the serologic test looks for heterophile IgM antibodies. CLIA-waved IM kits may be used by the medical assistant.
Strep	A rapid test done for Group A *Streptococcus* (also known as beta-hemolytic Group A *Streptococcus*), which causes strep throat; a throat swab is placed directly on an antibody-coated slide and the test will be positive if agglutination (clumping) occurs.
C-reactive protein (CRP)	A nonspecific screen for infectious and inflammatory diseases; correlates well with erythrocyte sedimentation rate (ESR); however, CRP appears and then disappears sooner than changes in the ESR.
Pregnancy	Measures the amount of human chorionic gonadotropin (hCG) in either the blood or urine; this hormone is secreted by the placenta and may be detected in the serum as soon as 5 days after conception. A CLIA-waved urine test is commonly used. The over-the-counter kit works via enzyme immunoassay (EIA) for hCG using antibodies and antigens

Microbiology

Microbiology is a vast field and includes the study of bacteria, viruses, fungi, parasites, and protozoa. Each pathogen is described in Table 17-10. A microscope is required to view all of these small, living organisms. When dealing with microorganisms, the medical assistant's role is to obtain specimens, test specimens within the scope of CLIA '88 regulations, and prepare slides and cultures for microscopic examination.

Gram Staining

The Gram stain is used in the identification of Gram-positive and Gram-negative bacteria. Bacteria are considered either Gram-positive or Gram-negative based on their cell wall and their ability to retain or lose color through staining. Gram-positive organisms stain dark blue to purple whereas Gram-negative bacteria stain red. The reagent or stain used is crystal violet, also known as Gram stain. Iodine is used as a mordant to hold the stain in place, and acetone-alcohol solution decolorizes the slide. A counterstain called safranin is then applied and the slide is rinsed to see the final result. Figure 17-1 illustrates the process of Gram staining.

Tuberculosis Testing

Tuberculosis (TB) is caused by a rod-shaped bacteria called *Mycobacterium tuberculosis* and is a major health concern worldwide. The screening test used for tuberculosis is the Mantoux test. This test uses tuberculin, also referred to as purified protein derivative (PPD), which is a filtrate of tuberculin cultures used for skin testing. The PPD is injected intradermally using a 1 ml tuberculin syringe. A short 26- or 27-gauge needle is used to inject the PPD so that a wheal forms. The standard site for injection is the left forearm, 3 or 4 inches below the elbow. A patient who has been exposed to TB will develop a hard, red spot on the skin, known as an induration. This is a hypersensitivity reaction and will be seen within 48–72 hours after the injection.

If a patient has either a questionable PPD reaction (via the Mantoux test) or a positive PPD reaction, a chest x-ray should be obtained to look for lung tubercles. A sputum sample can also be

Table 17-10 Microorganisms

Microorganism	Description	Example
Bacteria	One-celled microorganisms, defined by their shape (spherical, rod, spiral, or spore) and whether air is required for survival (aerobic or anaerobic)	*Escherichia coli (E. coli):* Most strains are harmless and found normally in the colon, but some strains cause diarrhea. *Staphylococcus aureus:* May cause minor skin infections or life-threatening illnesses like meningitis or septicemia.
Viruses	Tiny pieces of DNA coated by protein that require another living organism's cells to reproduce	Human immunodeficiency virus (HIV) causes AIDS. Hepatitis virus (A, B, C, D, and E) causes inflammation and infection of the liver. Influenza causes the flu.
Fungi	Microbes that grow on other organisms	*Tinea* causes ringworm, athlete's foot, and jock itch. *Candida* causes oral thrush and yeast infections.
Parasites	Microorganisms that live within or on another organism at the expense of that organism	*Enterobius vermicularis* causes pinworm. *Trichomonas vaginalis* infects the urogenital tracts of men and women.
Protozoa	One-celled microorganisms that may be divided into four groups: amoebae, flagellates, ciliates, and sporozoans	*Plasmodium falciparum* (Malaria protozoa) causes anemia, fever, and flu-like illness. *Giardia lamblia* causes debilitating diarrhea.

Step	Time	Procedure	Result
1	Wait 1 minute.	Apply crystal violet stain (Gram stain). ↓ Wash slide with water.	All bacteria stain purple.
2	Wait 1 minute.	Apply iodine solution. ↓ Wash slide with water.	All bacteria remain purple.
3	Wait 3–5 seconds.	Apply acetone-alcohol solution (decolorizes slide). ↓ Wash slide with water.	Purple stain is removed from Gram-negative bacteria.
4	Wait 1 minute.	Apply safranin stain (counterstains the slide). ↓ Wash slide with water.	Gram-negative bacteria stain red while Gram-positive bacteria remain purple.

Figure 17-1 The Process of Gram Staining

stained to look for the actual acid-fast rods. The reason for obtaining a chest x-ray and sputum sample is to distinguish whether the patient has active TB. Active TB is a serious and contagious condition that is treated differently from inactive TB.

Guaiac Testing

The guaiac test, also called the Hemoccult test, measures occult or hidden blood in stool. A small amount of stool is applied to the test site on a Hemoccult card. Two to three drops of developer are added to the test and positive control panels. The result can be read in 30 seconds. A blue color typically indicates a positive result. This test detects less than 5 mg hemoglobin per gram of feces. The guaiac test is used as a screening test for early indication of colorectal cancer or any ulceration of the GI tract. However, further evaluation of the patient is necessary because the test misses many cases of undiagnosed colon polyps and colon cancers.

Electrocardiography (EKG/ECG)

The EKG or ECG provides a graphic representation of the electrical activity as it flows through the heart. This graphic representation is sometimes referred to as an ECG tracing. An ECG is an easy, non-invasive test to perform; it is an extremely useful tool both to establish a patient's baseline and to diagnose and monitor heart diseases.

Waves seen on an ECG correspond to the cardiac cycle. A cardiac cycle consists of the systole (contraction) and diastole (relaxation) of both atria, rapidly followed by the systole and diastole of both ventricles. During a cardiac cycle, atria and ventricles alternately contract and relax, forcing blood from areas of high pressure to areas of lower pressure. Table 17-11 describes the major waves, complexes, intervals, and segments that can be examined on an ECG. Figure 17-2 shows a normal tracing.

If a patient has cardiac symptoms that are not seen on the ECG done in the office, a Holter monitor can be ordered. A Holter monitor is a portable ECG device worn by a patient to monitor heart activity for 24 hours. The patient is also instructed to keep a diary of activities to help in diagnosis.

The role of the medical assistant is not to interpret the fine details of an ECG; rather, a medical assistant places the electrodes in the correct place, ensuring an accurate reading of the heart. In

Table 17-11 ECG

Wave	Significance
P wave	Depolarization (contraction) of the atria.
QRS complex	Depolarization (contraction) of the ventricles.
T wave	Repolarization (relaxation) of the ventricles.
PR interval	The time taken for the electrical impulse to travel from the SA node to the AV node.
QT interval	Measures the time between the start of the QRS complex and finish of the T wave; it is heart rate dependent, with faster heart rates having a shorter QT interval. Drugs also may affect the QT interval.
ST segment	Measures the time between the contraction of ventricles and their relaxation.

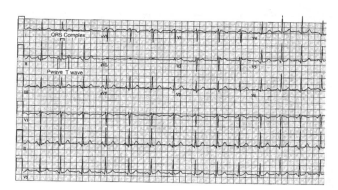

Figure 17-2 A Normal ECG Tracing

addition, a medical assistant should be able to distinguish a normal ECG from a completely abnormal ECG and notify the physician.

The 12-lead ECG uses 10 electrodes. Table 17-12 describes the correct placement of the electrodes. Electrodes should not be placed over clothing or bony prominences. When set up correctly, the ECG will produce leads (12 in a standard setup) that record electrical activity between two electrodes and allow the physician to view the heart's function from various angles. The physician might order an ECG tracing of Lead II only as opposed to a complete ECG. This is called a single-lead ECG; Lead II measures electrical activity through the heart from the right arm to the left leg.

Vision Testing

The medical assistant is commonly asked to screen a patient's visual acuity. The commonly used chart to measure distance vision is the Snellen eye chart, which consists of letters in various combinations starting with a large E at the top. The last line that the patient is able to read is recorded. Near vision is commonly checked using the Jaeger card, a small card held by the patient between 14 and 16 inches from the eye. The card has written material printed on it in which the letters gradually become smaller. The last line that the patient is able to read is recorded.

Patients should be screened in both eyes separately and together. If the patient already wears glasses, results should be recorded with and without the glasses.

Normal vision is recorded as 20/20, which means that at 20 feet the eye is seeing what the normal eye sees at 20 feet. If a patient's vision is 20/30, this means that the patient's eye is seeing at 20 feet what the normal eye is capable of seeing at 30 feet.

Checking for color vision is not part of the routine examination. The Ishihara color test may be used if there is a question of color blindness. A patient is typically referred to an ophthalmologist for this test.

An ophthalmoscope is used to view the interior of the eye, such as the retina, optic disc, and vitreous humor. Typically, the physician performs this part of the exam.

Table 17-12 Electrode Placement on a 12-Lead EKG

Electrode Number	Placement
V1	Fourth intercostal space at right margin of sternum
V2	Fourth intercostal space at left margin of sternum
V3	Midway between V2 and V4
V4	Fifth intercostal space at left midclavicular line
V5	Midway between V4 and V6
V6	Fifth intercostal space at left midaxillary line
RA	Right arm
LA	Left arm
RL	Right leg
LL	Left leg

Hearing Testing

There are various methods to screen for hearing loss. The audiometry test uses an audiometer. The patient is seated facing away from the medical assistant with earphones covering his or her ears. The audiometer tests for various sound wavelengths and wave intensity.

Tympanometry is used commonly in children to test for the ability of the middle ear to conduct sound waves. Some children suffer from frequent cases of otitis media and thus, their hearing may be affected.

Vibrating tuning forks can also be used. Tuning forks can help to distinguish nerve or conduction deafness.

Respiratory Testing

If a primary concern for a patient is respiratory-related, further tests might be ordered. There may be questions on the exam that cover pulmonary function tests, spirometry, pulse oximetry, and nebulizer treatment.

Pulmonary Function Tests

The measurements of air flow, different lung volumes, and lung capacities are known as pulmonary function tests (PFTs). These measurements are based on a patient's age, sex, height, and weight. PFTs are also done before and after administration of a bronchodilator medication to assess its efficacy. Pulmonary function tests may include any of the following: spirometry, gas diffusion tests, body plethysmography, inhalation challenge tests, exercise stress tests, and arterial blood gases. Table 17-13 summarizes the lung measurements that can be obtained from performing PFTs.

Table 17-13 Pulmonary Function Test Measurements

Measurement	Definition
Tidal volume	Volume of air moved in one normal breath
Inspiratory reserve volume	Inspiration beyond resting
Expiratory reserve volume	Expiration beyond resting (active)
Residual volume	Air left in lungs after a maximum expiration
Inspiratory capacity	Tidal volume + Inspiratory reserve volume
Functional residual capacity	Residual volume + Expiratory reserve volume
Vital capacity	Expiratory reserve + Tidal volume + Inspiratory reserve volume
Total lung capacity	Vital capacity + Residual volume

Spirometry

Spirometry is the most common of the PFTs, and is used to measure the volume and/or speed of air that can be inhaled and exhaled. In a spirometry test, you breathe into a mouthpiece that is connected to an instrument called a spirometer. The spirometer records the amount and the rate of air that you breathe in and out over a period of time. Table 17-14 describes three important components of lung function that are measured. The ratio between your FEV_1 and FVC is important clinically and is known as FEV_1/FVC. This ratio can help to diagnose obstructive versus restrictive diseases. The patient may be given instructions about the use of bronchodilators and/or smoking prior to the test. Also, loose clothing and a light meal make it easier and more comfortable for the patient to follow instructions.

Pulse Oximetry

Pulse oximetry is a noninvasive test used to evaluate oxygen saturation levels in the blood. Pulse oximetry uses a small probe with an infrared light. The probe is placed on the earlobe, toe, finger, or bridge of the nose. The infrared light is able to measure the amount of hemoglobin in the blood, which is a reflection of blood oxygen levels. A reading less than 95% typically indicates hypoxemia.

Nebulizer Treatment

A nebulizer is a device that delivers a fine mist of medication to the respiratory tract, including the lungs. There are a variety of types of nebulizers, but the handheld metered-dose nebulizer is the most prescribed because it is convenient and portable. It consists of a canister that holds the medicine and a mouthpiece. The patient places his or her mouth around the mouthpiece and inhales while releasing the medicine from the canister. The medication in a metered-dose inhaler may be a bronchodilator, a corticosteroid, or a combination of the two.

Medical Imaging

Medical imaging refers to the techniques used to create images of the human body, and the results. Table 17-15 describes some of the more common techniques used in medical imaging.

Safety Principles

Safety must be taken into consideration for both the patient and the health care provider when dealing with medical imaging. Radiation, which is used in x-rays and CT scans, is especially harmful. Radiation can damage tissues and cause harm to a developing fetus. Providers are educated to be certain that patients receive as low a dose of radiation as possible. Health care workers exposed to x-rays on a regular basis must wear a dosimeter. The dosimeter contains a strip of film that measures the amount of x-ray to which a person has been exposed. The dosimeter is monitored on a regular basis by a supervisor. Health care workers must also shield themselves from the x-ray beams during a test by standing behind a lead wall or by wearing a lead apron. When a test is in progress, a red light will alert others not to enter the room. Rooms in which x-rays are taken are lined with lead walls to absorb any scattering rays.

Table 17-14 Spirometry

Measurement	Definition
Forced vital capacity (FVC)	Measures the amount of air you can exhale with force after you inhale as deeply as possible
Forced expiratory volume in 1 second (FEV_1)	Measures the amount of air you can forcefully blow out in the first second of the FVC
Peak expiratory flow (PEF) or peak flow (PF)	Measures the fastest flow rate reached at any time during an FVC; measured on a volume-time curve

Table 17-15 Medical Imaging Techniques

Medical Image	Definition
Projection radiographs (x-rays)	Uses a wide beam of x-rays; used to view bones and lungs; through the use of a radio-opaque contrast medium (barium), they can also be used to visualize the GI tract
Fluoroscopy	Uses a constant input of x-rays at a low dose rate to produce real-time images of tissues; used to look at the GI tract and blood vessels
Magnetic resonance imaging (MRI)	Uses a combination of radio waves and a strong magnetic field to produce images of any plane through the body; used for the study of the heart, blood vessels, brain, spinal cord, joints, muscles, and internal organs
Nuclear medicine	Uses energetic photons emitted from radioactive nuclei for viewing various tissues
Computed tomography (CT)	Uses radiation (x-rays) with computer assistance to produce multiple cross-sectional views; used for the study of the brain and skull, lungs, and abdominopelvic organs
Ultrasound	Uses high-frequency sound waves that are reflected by tissue to produce three-dimensional images; used in imaging the fetus, abdominal organs, heart, breast, muscles, tendons, arteries, and veins

Prior to preparing a female patient for x-ray, always ask about the possibility of pregnancy. If there is any possibility of pregnancy, most likely the test will not be done. Regardless of gender, lead shields are used to cover reproductive organs and any other organs not involved in the exam.

Patient Preparation

Most medical imaging requires patient preparation. The role of the medical assistant is to prepare and educate the patient. Regardless of the test being done, the medical assistant should always ask about allergies, especially if contrast materials will be used. The patient may be anxious and have questions. The medical assistant should have a thorough knowledge of the procedure that the physician has ordered.

Positioning the patient is important for obtaining the best study possible. Also, proper positioning avoids repetition of the test. There are many ways to position the patient for x-ray. The physician usually orders an x-ray based on the view(s) he or she wants. The medical assistant must know the meaning of the positions to properly set up the patient. X-ray views are named for the direction of the beam through the body. It is also important to note where the x-ray tube is placed in order to get the proper setup. Figure 17-3 illustrates the standard positions for specific x-ray views.

Patient Instruction

The medical assistant gives the patient instructions both prior to and after having a medical imaging test. Table 17-16 outlines some specific instructions and preparation for commonly performed tests.

QUESTIONS

17-1. If a specimen of urine is refrigerated, which of the following is likely to occur?

    A. Crystals will form.
    B. Bacteria will grow.
    C. Ketones will appear.
    D. Red blood cells will undergo hemolysis.
    E. Nitrates will be converted to nitrites.

17-2. Which of the following lab values best measures kidney function?

    A. Hemoglobin A_{1c}
    B. Cholesterol

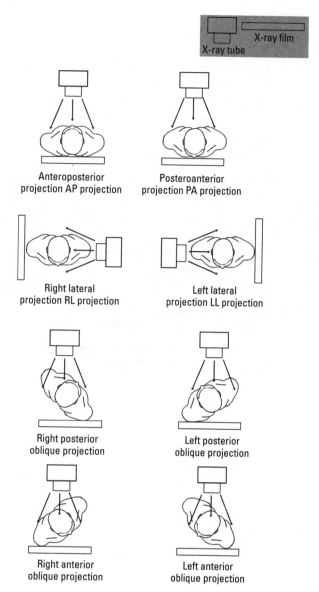

Figure 17-3 Standard Positions for Specific X-ray Views

    C. AST

    D. Creatinine

    E. Nitrates

17-3. Which of the following blood levels is considered a liver function test?

    A. Potassium

    B. BUN

    C. Aspartate transaminase (AST)

    D. High-density lipoprotein (HDL)

    E. C-reactive protein (CRP)

17-4. In a diabetic patient, which of the following lab values shows the patient's control of blood sugar over the past month?

    A. BUN

    B. Cholesterol

Table 17-16 Common Imaging Instructions

Test	Instructions
Angiography	No food or drink (NPO) for 8 hours prior; ask about blood thinning medication (aspirin, etc.).
Barium enema	Only clear liquids the day before the test with instructions for NPO 8 hours prior; give instructions about bowel cleansing. After the test, have the patient report if he or she does not have a bowel movement in 24 hours.
Barium swallow	NPO for 8 hrs prior; increase fluids after test; recommend a laxative.
Cholangiogram	Fat-free meal prior to test; 2 hours after eating, take color contrast tablets, NPO after the tablets. Bowel cleansing might be required.
Computed tomography (CT)	Explain contrast media (if used) and describe the sound and motion of the CT machine.
Intravenous pyelogram (IVP)	Only clear liquids the day before; NPO for 8 hrs prior. Bowel cleansing might be required.
Mammography	Instruct patient not to use lotions and powders above the waist.
Magnetic resonance imaging (MRI)	Check the patient for internal metals (clips, pacemaker); instruct the patient not to wear any metal for the test.
Ultrasound	A full bladder may or may not be necessary; describe the gel and transducer used in the procedure.

    C. Hemoglobin A_{1c}

    D. Sodium

    E. Albumin

17-5. The Holter monitor measures the activity of which organ?

    A. Heart

    B. Liver

    C. Kidney

    D. Bladder

    E. Pancreas

17-6. The standard order for a blood draw is

    A. yellow top (culture), green, gray, lavender, red or red/gray, light blue

    B. light blue, green, red or red/gray, gray, yellow top (culture), lavender

    C. yellow top (culture), light blue, red or red/gray, green, lavender, gray

    D. light blue, yellow top (culture), green, red or red/gray, gray, lavender

    E. green, red or red/gray, gray, yellow top (culture), light blue, lavender

17-7. Which type of thermometer is convenient to use for a patient of any age who does not cooperate?

    A. Oral thermometer

    B. Tympanic membrane thermometer

    C. Rectal thermometer

    D. Mercury thermometer

    E. Disposable oral thermometer

17-8. The most commonly performed test in the physician's office laboratory is

    A. Pathology

    B. Urinalysis

    C. Chemistry

    D. Microbiology

    E. Hematology

17-9. After obtaining a clean-catch urine sample, you perform a urine culture. After how many hours of incubation can the result be read?

    A. 3

    B. 6

    C. 9

    D. 12

    E. 24

17-10. What does the QRS complex represent in an ECG tracing?

    A. Atrial depolarization

    B. Atrial repolarization

    C. Ventricular depolarization

    D. Ventricular repolarization

    E. None of the above

17-11. Which of the following is used to measure distance vision?

    A. Snellen eye chart

    B. Jaeger card

    C. Ishihara color test

    D. Ophthalmoscope

    E. All of the above

17-12. Which lab work would be helpful prior to prescribing warfarin (Coumadin)?

    A. Liver function tests

    B. Prothrombin time

    C. Hematocrit

    D. Erythrocyte sedimentation rate

    E. Leukocyte differential

17-13. Which microorganism stains dark blue or purple with Gram staining?

    A. Gram-positive bacteria

    B. Gram-negative bacteria

    C. Parasites

    D. Viruses

    E. Protozoa

17-14. While performing a spirometry test, you ask the patient to inhale as deeply as possible and then exhale forcefully into a spirometer. You then measure the amount of air that the patient blows out in the first second. This is called

    A. expiratory reserve volume.

    B. tidal volume (TV).

    C. forced vital capacity.

    D. forced expiratory volume in 1 second (FEV_1).

    E. peak expiratory flow (PEF).

17-15. Which vein is typically the most frequently used for a venipuncture?

    A. Median cubital vein

    B. Basilic vein

    C. Cephalic vein

    D. Subclavian vein

    E. Brachiocephalic vein

17-16. The presence of which of the following in a urinalysis would be indicative of an infection?

    A. Nitrite

    B. Leukocyte esterase

    C. Hemoglobin

    D. A and B

    E. All of the above

17-17. Which test is used as a screening test for tuberculosis?

    A. Gram stain

    B. Mantoux test

    C. Guaiac test

    D. Spirometry

    E. Magnetic resonance imaging (MRI)

17-18. Which patient is most at risk if exposed to radiation?

    A. Elderly man

    B. Middle-aged woman

    C. Pregnant woman

    D. Teenager

    E. Patient with TB

17-19. In adults, which of the following is the usual site for capillary puncture?

    A. Nose

    B. Ear lobe

    C. Heel

    D. Toe

    E. Fingertip

17-20. Which of the following organizations is responsible for quality control of laboratory tests and CLIA '88 regulations?

    A. Centers for Medicare and Medicaid Services

    B. Centers for Disease Control and Prevention

    C. U.S. Department of Labor

    D. Occupational Safety and Health Administration

    E. Food and Drug Administration

17-21. What is the normal ratio of hemoglobin to hematocrit for a healthy adult?

    A. 1:1

    B. 1:2

    C. 1:3

    D. 1:4

    E. 1:5

17-22. The pattern of an ECG is commonly called a(n)

    A. base.

    B. deflection.

    C. crescendo.

    D. tracing.

    E. electrode.

17-23. Which way should the patient face during an audiometry test?

    A. Away from the medical assistant

    B. Towards the medical assistant

    C. Next to the medical assistant

    D. At an angle to the medical assistant

    E. Position does not matter

17-24. While performing a capillary puncture, which of the following is TRUE?

    A. Squeeze the fingertip to increase blood flow.

    B. Do not use alcohol for cleaning.

    C. Perform the test while the finger is still wet.

    D. Discard the first drop.

    E. Standard precautions do not apply.

17-25. Which of the following hematologic tests is used as a nonspecific screening test for inflammation?

    A. RBC indices

    B. Red blood cell count

    C. Erythrocyte sedimentation rate

    D. Prothrombin time

    E. Platelet count

ANSWERS

17-1. The correct answer is A. If urine is refrigerated, amorphous (without any clear shape) crystals will form. This is not part of any disease process.

17-2. The correct answer is D. Creatinine and BUN are considered kidney function tests. Creatinine reflects glomerular filtration rate at the level of the nephron. BUN measures the amount of urea in the blood, which reflects the excretory function of the kidneys.

17-3. The correct answer is C. Liver function tests include measurements of alanine transaminase (ALT), aspartate transaminase (AST), alkaline phosphatase (ALP), total bilirubin (TBIL), direct bilirubin, gamma glutamyl transpeptidase (GGT), albumin, prothrombin, and total protein. Taken together these enzymes and proteins detect, evaluate, and monitor liver disease or damage.

17-4. The correct answer is C. Hemoglobin A_{1c} is useful in long-term monitoring of diabetic blood sugar control. This test measures glycosylated hemoglobin in the blood, which is hemoglobin that has glucose stuck to it.

17-5. The correct answer is A. A Holter monitor is a portable ECG device worn by a patient to monitor heart activity for 24 hours.

17-6. The correct answer is C. The order of the draw is important. Sterile collection (yellow top) needs to be done first to prevent any contamination. After the sterile collection is done, the order of draw into vacuum tubes depends on the additive. You do not want a back flow of additives into the tubes as this could create false results.

17-7. The correct answer is B. A thermometer measures body temperature. Many types of thermometers exist including mercury (used infrequently), electronic, tympanic, and disposable. Tympanic electronic thermometers are becoming more popular because they are accurate and comfortable and can be used in a patient of any age, even uncooperative patients.

17-8. The correct answer is B. Urinalysis is the most common test performed in the office setting. This test is easy to instruct the patient to complete and the results may be read by the medical assistant.

17-9. The correct answer is E. When any culture is being performed, the primary result can be read in 24–48 hours. Some organisms take longer to grow. Thus, the final results are typically not available until later.

17-10. The correct answer is C. The QRS complex represents depolarization or contraction of the ventricles.

17-11. The correct answer is A. The commonly used chart to measure distance vision is the Snellen eye chart. The Snellen chart consists of letters in various combinations starting with a large E at the top. The last line that the patient is able to read is recorded.

17-12. The correct answer is B. Prothrombin time (PT) is a hematologic test used to measure how long it takes blood to clot. A prothrombin time test can be used to check for bleeding problems. PT is also used to check whether medicine such as warfarin (Coumadin) that is used to prevent blood clots is working.

17-13. The correct answer is A. The Gram stain is used in the identification of Gram-positive and Gram-negative bacteria. Bacteria are considered either Gram-positive or Gram-negative based on their cell wall and the ability to retain or lose color through staining. Gram-positive organisms stain dark blue to purple whereas Gram-negative bacteria stain red.

17-14. The correct answer is D. Forced vital capacity measures the amount of air a person can exhale with force after inhaling as deeply as possible. Forced expiratory volume in 1 second (FEV_1) measures the amount of air a person can forcefully blow out in the first second of the FVC. The ratio between FEV_1 and FVC is important clinically and is known as FEV_1/FVC. This ratio can help to diagnose obstructive versus restrictive diseases.

17-15. The correct answer is A. The median cubital vein is typically the most frequently used because it tends to be the most prominent.

17-16. The correct answer is D. Leukocyte esterase detects an enzyme that is released by white blood cells. A positive nitrite test indicates that bacteria may be present in significant numbers in urine. When leukocyte esterase is combined with the nitrite test, it has an extremely high predictive value of a patient having a urinary tract infection.

17-17. The correct answer is B. The screening test used for tuberculosis is the Mantoux test. This test uses tuberculin, also referred to as PPD, which is a filtrate of tuberculin cultures that are used for skin testing.

17-18. The correct answer is C. Radiation, used in x-rays and CT, is especially harmful to a developing fetus. Prior to preparing a female patient for x-ray, always ask about the possibility of pregnancy. If there is any possibility of pregnancy, most likely the test will not be done.

17-19. The correct answer is E. Capillary punctures collect a smaller amount of blood from a superficial capillary. Sites used are typically the fingertip in an adult or the heel in an infant.

17-20. The correct answer is B. The Centers for Disease Control and Prevention (CDC) is a division of the U.S. Department of Health and Human Services. The Clinical Laboratory Improvement Amendments of 1988, commonly called CLIA '88, was established to protect patients by regulating all human body specimen testing. All laboratories, no matter how small or large, including the physician's office lab or an ambulatory care setting, must abide by CLIA '88 regulations.

17-21. The correct answer is C. The ratio of hemoglobin to hematocrit is normally 1:3.

17-22. The correct answer is D. The EKG or ECG is the graphic representation of the electrical activity as it flows through the heart. This graphic representation is sometimes referred to as an ECG tracing.

17-23. The correct answer is A. The audiometry test uses an audiometer. The patient is seated facing away from the medical assistant with earphones covering his or her ears. The audiometer tests for various wavelengths and wave intensity.

17-24. The correct answer is D. Discard the first drop of blood in a capillary puncture because it may be contaminated with tissue fluid. Only use the second and following drops of blood for the test. All of the other choices are false.

17-25. The correct answer is C. Erythrocyte sedimentation rate measures the rate at which RBCs settle to the bottom of a well-mixed anticoagulated sample. It is a nonspecific test to screen for inflammation, infection, and disease because red blood cells fall faster when their surface membrane is damaged.

Pharmacology and Medication Administration

The exam will include a variety of questions about basic pharmacology and administering medications, prescriptions, and immunizations. For a list of the most commonly used medications, go to http://www.pharmacytimes.com and search for "top 200 drugs." It is possible that there may be very basic questions about some of the most frequently used prescription drugs on the exam.

PHARMACOLOGY

Each drug has four names that apply to it. The two names which you should be most familiar with are the generic name and the trade name. A pharmaceutical company identifies its product by the trade name, which is always capitalized. It is copyrighted and used exclusively by that company. The generic name is the common name assigned to each drug. When 17 years have passed and the pharmaceutical company's original patent on the drug has expired, other companies may begin to combine the same chemicals from that specific generic product for marketing. The drugs may differ in color, cost, and ingredients that are used to hold the drug together. They may not differ in the actual content of the drug. See Table 18-1 for the definitions.

Each drug also can be categorized under a broad category called a classification. Drugs that affect the body in similar ways are listed in the same classification. Table 18-2 lists some of the major classifications of drugs and gives specific examples of each. You should become familiar with the examples given. Table 18-3 lists commonly used pharmacology-related abbreviations.

Table 18-1 Names of Drugs

Name	Meaning	Example
Generic name	The general name assigned to a drug Always written with a lowercase letter	ibuprofen
Trade name	The pharmaceutical company's name for the drug Copyrighted and used exclusively by that company The first letter is capitalized; often used with a registered trademark symbol®	Motrin®
Chemical name	The exact molecular formula of a drug	2-(p-isobutylphenyl) propionic acid
Official name	The name of the drug as it appears in the official reference Generally the same as the generic name	ibuprofen

Table 18-2 Drug Classifications

Classification	Therapeutic Use	Examples: Generic (Trade Name)
Adrenergic	Mimics the action of the sympathetic nervous system: elevating blood pressure, restoring rhythm in cardiac arrest	epinephrine (Adrenalin chloride)
Analgesic	Lessens pain	ibuprofen (Motrin), acetaminophen (Tylenol)
Anesthetic	Causes lack of feeling or awareness; produces the sensation of numbness	lidocaine (Xylocaine)
Antacid	Neutralizes gastric acid	calcium carbonate (Tums), aluminum-magnesium (Maalox)
Antiarrhythmic	Prevents cardiac irregularities	digoxin (Lanoxin)
Antiasthmatic	Asthma prophylaxis and treatment of chronic asthma; helps to control the inflammatory process of asthma	montelukast (Singulair), cromolyn sodium (Intal)
Antibiotic	Destroys or inhibits bacterial growth	ciprofloxacin (Cipro), cephalexin (Keflex), ampicillin (Amcill, Principen), amoxicillin (Amoxil), gentamicin (Garamycin), trimethoprim-sulfamethoxazole (Septra), azithromycin (Zithromax)
Anticholinergic	Blocks the action of the parasympathetic nervous system: dries all secretions, decreases GI motility, dilates pupils	atropine (Atreza)
Anticoagulant	Prevents formation of clots; decreases the formation of existing clots	warfarin (Coumadin), heparin (Hep-Lock or Heparin Lock Flush)
Anticonvulsant	Reduces the number and severity of seizures in patients with epilepsy	phenytoin (Dilantin), gabapentin (Neurontin)
Antidepressant	Elevates mood	amitriptyline (Elavil), sertraline (Zoloft), fluoxetine (Prozac), bupropion (Wellbutrin)
Antidiarrheal	Inhibits or decreases diarrhea	kaolin/pectin (Kaopectate), loperamide hydrochloride (Imodium)
Antidiabetic	Oral medications to control sugar levels in patients with type II, non-insulin-dependent diabetes	glyburide (Micronase), glipizide (Glucotrol), metformin (Glucophage)
Antiemetic	Controls nausea, vomiting, and motion sickness	dimenhydrinate (Dramamine), meclizine (Antivert), metoclopramide (Reglan), promethazine (Phenergan), ondansetron (Zofran)
Antihistamine	Relieves symptoms of allergies like sneezing, itchy and watery eyes, and a runny nose; can also relieve itchiness caused by insect bites and stings	cetirizine (Zyrtec), fexofenadine (Allegra), loratadine (Claritin), diphenhydramine (Benadryl)
Antihypertensive	Prevents or controls high blood pressure	lisinopril (Zestril, Prinivil), amlodipine (Norvasc), metoprolol tartrate (Lopressor), propranolol (Inderal)

(continues)

Table 18-2 Drug Classifications (Continued)

Classification	Therapeutic Use	Examples: Generic (Trade Name)
Anti-inflammatory	Reduces inflammation	celecoxib (Celebrex), ibuprofen (Motrin)
Antilipemic agent	Lowers LDL cholesterol	simvastatin (Zocor), pravastatin (Pravachol), atorvastatin (Lipitor)
Antipsychotic	Reduces delusions and hallucinations seen in schizophrenia	haloperidol (Haldol), olanzapine (Zyprexa), risperidone (Risperdal)
Antipyretic	Reduces fever	ibuprofen (Motrin), acetaminophen (Tylenol)
Antiseptic	Used for surgical scrubs and applied to the skin as a bacteriostatic skin cleanser	povidone-iodine (Betadine), chlorhexidine (Hibiclens), hydrogen peroxide, isopropyl alcohol, 70%
Antitussive	Relieves or prevents cough	dextromethorphan, (Robitussin)
Antiulcer	Agent for ulcer and GERD prevention (blocks acid and proton pump)	cimetidine (Tagamet), famotidine (Pepcid), ranitidine (Zantac), lansoprazole (Prevacid), esomeprazole (Nexium), omeprazole (Prilosec)
Anxiolytic	Antianxiety medication; used for short-term treatment of anxiety	diazepam (Valium), alprazolam (Xanax), clonazepam (Klonopin)
Bronchodilator	Dilates the bronchi	albuterol inhalation (Ventolin, Proventil)
Cardiotonic	Strengthens the heartbeat	digoxin (Lanoxin)
Cholinergic	Mimics the action of the parasympathetic nervous system: increased GI motility, increased secretions, constriction of pupils, slowed heartbeat	bethanechol (Urecholine), neostigmine (Prostigmin), pilocarpine (Isopto Carpine)
Contraceptive	Used to prevent pregnancy	norgestimate/ethinyl estradiol (Ortho Tri-Cyclen)
Decongestant	Decreases nasal congestion	pseudoephedrine (Sudafed)
Diuretic	Decreases body fluid by increasing urination	hydrochlorothiazide (Dyazide), furosemide (Lasix)
Electrolyte	A mineral dissolved in body fluids that is required for the body's activities	potassium chloride (K-dur)
Expectorant	Increases secretions, helps to expel sputum	guaifenesin (Mucinex, Robitussin)
Hypnotic/Sedative	Controlled substance to promote sedation or sleep	temazepam (Restoril), zolpidem (Ambien), zaleplon (Sonata)
Laxative	Promotes evacuation of the intestine	bisacodyl (Dulcolax, Correctol), docusate (Colace), senna (Senokot), psyllium (Metamucil), magnesium hydroxide (Phillips' Milk of Magnesia)

(continues)

Table 18-2 Drug Classifications (Continued)

Classification	Therapeutic Use	Examples: Generic (Trade Name)
Muscle relaxant	Short-term treatment of muscle pain, spasm, and impaired mobility	cyclobenzaprine (Flexeril)
Platelet inhibitor	Decreases platelet clumping	clopidogrel (Plavix)
Steroid	Relieves swelling and inflammation	prednisone (Deltasone), dexamethasone (Decadron)
Vasoconstrictor	Constricts blood vessels to increase blood pressure	norepinephrine (Levophed)
Vasodilator	To treat angina; dilates coronary arteries immediately or for long-term prophylactic management	nitroglycerin (Nitrostat tabs, Nitrolingual spray)

Table 18-3 Commonly Used Prescription and Pharmacology-Related Abbreviations

Abbreviation	Meaning
a	before
a.c.	before meals
AD	right ear
ad lib	as desired, as needed
AS	left ear
AU	each ear or both ears
b.i.d.	twice a day
$\bar{c}$	with
Fe	iron
g	gram
gtt	drop
h.s.	at bedtime (hour of sleep)
IM	intramuscular
IV	intravenous
K	potassium
KCl	potassium chloride
kg	kilogram
L	liter
mcg	microgram
mg	milligram
ml	milliliter
mm	millimeter
Na	sodium
NaCl	sodium chloride
NPO, npo	nothing by mouth

(continues)

Table 18-3 Commonly Used Prescription and Pharmacology-Related Abbreviations (Continued)

Abbreviation	Meaning
OD	right eye
oint	ointment
OR	operating room
OS	left eye
OU	each eye (or both eyes)
$\bar{p}$	after
p.c.	after meals
p.o., PO	by mouth, orally
PRN, prn	whenever necessary
q	every
q.d	every day
q.h	every hour
q.2h	every 2 hours
q.4h	every 4 hours
q.i.d.	four times a day
Rx	prescription
$\bar{s}$	without
sig	write
sol	solution
subq, SubQ	subcutaneous
susp	suspension
Tab	tablet
t.i.d.	three times a day

Factors that Affect Drug Action

Pharmacokinetics refers to the four processes that drugs must undergo in the body: absorption, distribution, metabolism, and excretion. These four factors can affect drug action, along with the individual patient, the form and chemical composition of the drug, and the method of administration. Absorption refers to the process in which the drug passes into the body's fluids and tissues. Distribution is the process in which the drug is transported from the blood to the intended site of action. Metabolism is the physical and chemical alterations that a substance undergoes in the body. The liver is the primary site of this process. Finally, elimination refers to the process in which the drug is excreted. Although it is possible for some drugs to be eliminated through perspiration, feces, bile, breast milk, or exhaled through the lungs, *most* drugs are excreted by the kidneys.

Side Effects/Adverse Reactions

Drug side effects are regarded as undesirable symptoms that occur in addition to the desired therapeutic effect of a drug. Every medication contains chemicals that may potentially cause side effects. Side effects may vary for each individual depending on the person's overall health, age, weight, gender, and ethnicity. Some side effects are considered minor whereas, others are more severe and potentially life-threatening. Table 18-4 lists some of the more serious adverse reactions and the drugs that have been found to cause them.

Table 18-4 Adverse Reactions

Adverse Reaction	Causal Agent
Anaphylaxis	Penicillin antibiotics
Aplastic anemia	Antiepileptic (carbamazepine); antineoplastic (methotrexate)
Birth defects (teratogens)	Isotretinoin (Accutane); retinoic acid (Retin-A)
Bleeding	Heparin, warfarin
Carcinogenic effects	Aflatoxin; tobacco
Crystalluria	Antineoplastic (methotrexate); antibacterial (sulfonamide)
Cutaneous flushing	Niacin (vitamin B_3)
Gynecomastia	H2-antagonist—acid blocker (cimetidine); diuretic (spironolactone)
Hepatic necrosis	Acetaminophen (Tylenol); antidepressant (valproic acid); anesthetic (halothane)
Hepatitis	Isoniazid (INH)
Hot flashes	Antineoplastic (Tamoxifen)
Hypertensive crisis	Antidepressants (combination of MAOIs and tricyclic antidepressants)
Increased digitalis levels	Antiarrhythmic (combination of quinidine and digitalis)
Increased risk of breast/endometrial cancer	Estrogens
Lupus-like syndrome	Antiarrhythmic (procainamide); antihypertensive (hydralazine)
Malignant hyperthermia	Anesthetic (succinylocholine)
Nephritis	Antibacterial (sulfonamides)
Ototoxicity and nephrotoxicity	Aminoglycoside antibiotics (neomycin, amikacin, streptomycin, gentamicin); antineoplastics (cisplatin); loop diuretics (furosemide, bumetanide)
Photosensitivity	Retinoic acid (Retin-A); antibacterial (tetracyclines); antiarrhythmics (amiodarone)
Pulmonary fibrosis	Antineoplastics (bleomycin; busulfan) antiarrhythmics (amiodarone)
Respiratory depression	Pain modulator (opioids)
Stevens-Johnson syndrome	Antibacterial (sulfonamides)
Tendonitis, tendon rupture	Antibacterial (fluoroquinolones)
Thrombosis (with complications)	Oral contraceptives
Toxic sedation	CNS depressants with alcohol

Sometimes a drug may have contraindications associated with it. A contraindication is any circumstance in which the drug is inappropriate to use. For example, many drugs are contraindicated in pregnant woman because of the risk to the developing fetus. Yet another adverse reaction to be wary of is a paradoxical drug reaction. A paradoxical effect is an unexpected response to a drug. It is the opposite effect from that expected. For example, if a medicine is intended to cause drowsiness and it causes excitement instead, it is having a paradoxical effect.

Emergency Use

Sudden disturbances in cardiac rhythm, cardiogenic shock, cardiopulmonary arrest, and severe allergic reactions are the most serious medical emergencies. In addition to supportive measures, quick therapeutic interventions are essential in most cases and codes. Therefore, access to the right medication to resolve the problem is critical. A selection of drugs that are most effective and appropriate in these situations are kept in a special cart known as a *crash cart* in all hospital departments responsible for patient care. The pharmacy departments are responsible for providing these medications and regularly checking them for stability, replacement, and expiration dates. Some physician offices may have a modified crash cart available, depending on the type of practice. However, because potential liability exists if a crash cart is in a physician's office, many offices do not have a crash cart. Table 18-5 lists the drugs most commonly found on a crash cart.

Table 18-5 Common Drugs on a Crash Cart

Drug	Indication
Atropine	Restore cardiac rate and arterial pressure (in cardiovascular collapse)
Bretylium tosylate (Bretylol)	Prophylaxis and therapy of ventricular fibrillation and life-threatening ventricular arrhythmias
Calcium chloride	Treatment of hypocalcemia in conditions requiring a prompt increase in blood plasma calcium levels; treatment of magnesium intoxication due to overdose of magnesium sulfate; combat the deleterious effects of hyperkalemia; for cardiac resuscitation when weak or inadequate contractions return following defibrillation
Dextrose	Treatment of insulin hypoglycemia to restore blood glucose levels.
Diazepam (Valium)	Treatment of seizures and anxiety disorders or the short-term relief of symptoms of anxiety; treatment of acute alcohol withdrawal
Diphenhydramine (Benadryl)	Antihistaminic for amelioration of allergic reactions; in anaphylaxis as an adjunct to epinephrine
Dopamine (dopamine hydrochloride in 5% dextrose injection)	Correction of hemodynamic imbalance present in shock due to myocardial infarction, trauma, endotoxic septicemia, open heart surgery, renal failure, and chronic cardiac decompensation (as in refractory congestive failure)
Epinephrine	Acute hypersensitivity reactions to drugs, animal serum, and allergens; acute anaphylactic shock; acute asthmatic attacks to relieve bronchospasm
Furosemide (Lasix)	Treatment of edema associated with congestive heart failure
Isoproterenol (Isuprel)	Mild or transient episodes of heart block that do not require electric shock; use in cardiac arrest until electric shock, pacemaker therapy, or the treatment of choice is available
Lidocaine	Life-threatening arrhythmias, particularly those of ventricular origin, such as during acute myocardial infarct
Magnesium sulfate	Effective antiarrhythmic
Midazolam (Versed)	Preoperative sedation and to impair memory of perioperative events

PREPARING AND ADMINISTERING ORAL AND PARENTERAL MEDICATIONS

One of the medical assistant's most important jobs is the preparation and administration of medication. If an error does occur, the patient's life is in jeopardy. Thus, the exam will test on one's ability to calculate and measure medications accurately.

Oral Administration

Oral medications are given by mouth and come in various forms, including tablet, capsule, liquid, and gel. Oral is the most common medication route. Typically, oral medications are given because of their convenience, ease, and safety. Oral medications are absorbed into the bloodstream via the small intestine, which means that drug absorption is slower than the parenteral method and may be altered by the presence of food.

Parenteral Administration

The parenteral method of drug administration refers to taking medicine into the body in some manner other than through the digestive tract. The most common parenteral methods are intravenous, intramuscular injection, subcutaneous injection, and intradermal injection.

Calculation of Dosage

The medical assistant is expected to do simple calculations to determine correct dosage. The dosage depends on the patient's age, weight, sex, as well as other variable factors such as presence of more than one disease process, physical and emotional condition, and the safest method, route, and time to achieve the desired result. The exam typically contains at least one of these problems. Set the problem up as a ratio equation in which each side of the equation is equal. Always label each term in the equation. Your units on each side of the equation should be the same.

For example, acetaminophen solution 650 mg is ordered. The container is labeled 325 mg/5 ml. How many ml would you administer?

$$\frac{\text{Dose ordered (in mg)}}{\text{Unknown dose (in ml)}} = \frac{\text{Dose on hand (in mg)}}{\text{Dose on hand (in ml)}}$$

$$\frac{650 \text{ mg}}{? \text{ ml}} = \frac{325 \text{ mg}}{5 \text{ ml}}$$

Solve for the unknown value by cross-multiplying:

$$(325 \text{ mg})(? \text{ ml}) = (650 \text{ mg})(5 \text{ ml})$$
$$? = 10 \text{ ml}$$

Types of Injections and Injection Sites

Depending on the type of medication, injections may be delivered into various tissues—muscle, subcutaneous tissue, or skin. Regardless of the type of injection, the medical assistant should follow basic guidelines. The angle of insertion as well as the gauge and length of the needle varies with the injection type. Once the needle is inserted, the medical assistant should gently aspirate the plunger (pull back on the plunger) to ensure that the needle is not in a blood vessel. If blood does appear, the needle must be withdrawn immediately and a new site should be prepared for injection.

Common intramuscular sites are the deltoid muscle, dorsogluteal area, ventogluteal area (gluteus medius muscle and now the preferred site in adults), and vastus lateralis muscle (lateral part of thigh and a preferred site in infants and young children). Common subcutaneous sites include the upper arms, upper thighs, upper medial back, and abdominal external oblique muscles. These subcutaneous sites are good because they are located away from bones, joints, nerves, and large blood vessels. A common intradermal site is the inner forearm. Figure 18-1 illustrates the three main types of injections and the angle at which the needle is inserted. Table 18-6 provides the corresponding information you need to know about the types of injections and injection sites.

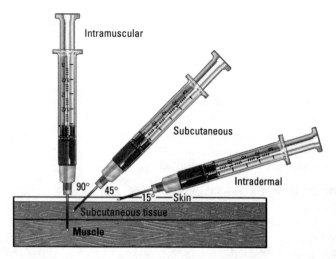

Figure 18-1 Needle Angles for Administration of Intramuscular, Subcutaneous, and Intradermal Injections

Gauge of Needle

The gauge of a needle is the size (diameter) of the lumen or hole. The gauge is numbered in reverse order: a thinner needle with a smaller diameter has a larger number (26–27, for intradermal injections) than a thicker needle with a larger opening (18–21) that is used for IM injections.

Length of Needle

The length of the needle is also important. Longer needles (1 1/2 to 2 inches) are used for intramuscular injections. Insulin needles are typically 1/2 inch in length and tuberculin needles are typically 5/8 of an inch. The length of the needle depends on the type of injection and the size of the patient.

The Z-Track Method

The Z-track method is a type of intramuscular injection that is used when medications are given that contain chemicals that would cause irritation if they leaked into the subcutaneous tissue through the path made by the needle. Haloperidol (Haldol) and hydroxyzine (Atarax, Vistaril) are examples of medications that cause irritation to the tissues.

The technique involves pulling the skin to one side and inserting the needle at a 90-degree angle. When the skin returns to the normal position, the needle track is sealed off. The Z-track

Table 18-6 Types of Injections and Injection Sites

Injection Type	Angle of Insertion	Tissue	Gauge of Needle	Example
Intramuscular injection	90 degrees	Injected into the muscle	18–21	Depo-Provera
Subcutaneous injection	45 degrees	Injected into the fatty layer just beneath the skin but above the muscle	25	Insulin
Intradermal injection	10 to 15 degrees	Injected just beneath the skin within the dermis	26–27	Allergy skin testing PPD testing (also called Mantoux screening test, tuberculin sensitivity test, purified protein derivative test)

method is also used when giving dark-colored medication solutions, such as iron solutions, that can stain the subcutaneous tissue or skin.

PRESCRIPTIONS

Prescriptions are the written legal documents for preparing, distributing, and administering medications. Legislation allows licensed physicians, licensed nurse practitioners, registered certified physician assistants, clinical pharmacists, dentists, and veterinarians to write prescriptions for their specific field of work, within limitations. A medical assistant may never prescribe medications (write a prescription). A prescription contains the following information:

- Physician's name, address, and phone number
- Date of prescription
- Patient's name, address, and phone number
- Drug, dose, and form
- Number of doses to be dispensed
- Patient instructions
- Number of refills
- Physician's signature
- DEA number

Qualified medical practitioners who prescribe and/or administer drugs must comply with the federal and state laws. The Federal Food, Drug, and Cosmetic Act passed in 1938 controls all drugs available for legal use. This set of laws protects the public by ensuring the quality (purity, strength, and composition) of food, drugs, and cosmetics. The U.S. Food and Drug Administration (FDA) is responsible for enforcement of this act.

Safekeeping and Recordkeeping

It is critical that medical assistants store drugs safely and maintain accurate inventory records. Some medications, such as antibiotics, need to be refrigerated. All medications should remain in their original bottles or containers. Any out-of-date medication or medication without a label should be discarded. Controlled substances must be stored in a locked cabinet. The key to this locked cabinet must be kept in a secure place away from the locked drug storage area. Different states have different guidelines as to how best to keep controlled substances safe.

Schedule of Controlled Substances

Controlled substances are classified into five levels based on abuse potential. Drugs that have the highest potential for abuse are classified as schedule I. Drugs that have the lowest potential for abuse are classified as schedule V. The Drug Enforcement Administration (DEA) enforces the schedule. Each prescriber of these substances must register with the DEA and obtain a DEA number to present on their prescriptions. Controlled substances should be locked securely when kept in an office. Table 18-7 summarizes the DEA schedule.

IMMUNIZATIONS

There will be questions about immunizations on the exam. Table 18-8 reflects the 2009 Immunization Schedule for Children as published by the Centers for Disease Control and Prevention. The Adult Immunization Schedule can be found in Table 18-9. You should check the Centers for Disease Control and Prevention website for updates. The web address is http://www.cdc.gov/vaccines.

Storage and Recordkeeping

Vaccines need to be stored correctly at the proper temperature. Certain vaccines require refrigeration whereas others require freezing temperatures. Inattention to vaccine storage conditions can contribute to

Table 18-7 DEA Schedule of Drugs

Schedule	Use	Example
I	Highest abuse potential Not approved for medical use in the U.S.	Heroin, LSD, marijuana
II	Second highest abuse potential Medical use with precaution and limitations Written prescription only by a physician	Morphine, codeine, methadone, Percocet, oxycodone, Ritalin, cocaine
III	May lead to dependence May be refilled up to five times in 6 months Written, faxed, or verbal prescription by physician	Tylenol with codeine, and other preparations in combination with codeine
IV	Lower abuse potential May be refilled up to five times in 6 months Prescription may be written by a health care worker but must also be signed by physician	Valium, Ativan, Xanax, Librium, Darvocet, Restoril, Ambien
V	Lowest abuse potential Over-the-counter purchase Consists primarily of preparations for cough suppressants	Robitussin, Benadryl

vaccine failure. A refrigerator/freezer should be organized and set up solely for the purpose of storing vaccines. Expiration dates should be noted on the vaccines. Expired vaccines must never be used, so appropriate arrangement of the vaccines in the refrigerator by date is a good practice. The refrigerator should be plugged into an outlet from which it cannot be disconnected accidentally. Old vaccine materials should be disposed of using medical waste disposal procedures outlined by the state health department.

Optimal recordkeeping requires maintaining patient histories and adhering to a recommended schedule of vaccine administration. This good practice ensures that needed vaccines will not be missed and unnecessary vaccines will not be given. Immunization providers are required by law to record what vaccine was given, the date the vaccine was given (month, day, year), the name of the manufacturer of the vaccine, the lot number, the signature and title of the person who gave the vaccine, and the address where the vaccine was given. Good practice also recommends that the patient (or parent/guardian) receive a record to bring to office visits for updates.

THE SIX RIGHTS OF MEDICATION ADMINISTRATION

A medical assistant should know and follow the six rights of medication administration for safe drug administration.

1. *The right medication:* Comparison of the medication to the medication order is imperative. The medical assistant must only give medications they have prepared themselves and be present when they are taken.
2. *The right dose (amount):* To ensure that the right dose is given, the medical assistant should compare the drug dosage ordered to the dose listed on the package or bottle. The medical assistant should triple check any calculations and have another team member check the calculation as well.
3. *The right patient:* The medical assistant must identify the patient by checking the identification band and asking the patient to confirm his or her name in order to ensure that the right patient is receiving the right medication.
4. *The right route:* The medical assistant must give the medication via the right route. The route of administration is important because of its effect on degree of absorption, speed of drug action, and side effects.

Table 18-8 Childhood Vaccinations

Vaccine ▼ Age ▶	Birth	1 month	2 months	4 months	6 months	12 months	15 months	18 months	19–23 months	2–3 years	4–6 years
Hepatitis B[1]	HepB	HepB		see footnote1		HepB					
Rotavirus[2]			RV	RV	RV[2]						
Diphtheria, Tetanus, Pertussis[3]			DTaP	DTaP	DTaP	see footnote3	DTaP				DTaP
Haemophilus influenzae type b[4]			Hib	Hib	Hib[4]	Hib					
Pneumococcal[5]			PCV	PCV	PCV	PCV					PPSV
Inactivated Poliovirus			IPV	IPV		IPV					IPV
Influenza[6]						Influenza (Yearly)					
Measles, Mumps, Rubella[7]						MMR		see footnote7			MMR
Varicella[8]						Varicella		see footnote8			Varicella
Hepatitis A[9]						HepA (2 doses)				HepA Series	
Meningococcal[10]										MCV	

Legend:
- Range of recommended ages
- Certain high-risk groups

This schedule indicates the recommended ages for routine administration of currently licensed vaccines, as of December 1, 2008, for children aged 0 through 6 years. Any dose not administered at the recommended age should be administered at a subsequent visit, when indicated and feasible. Licensed combination vaccines may be used whenever any component of the combination is indicated and other components are not contraindicated and if approved by the Food and Drug Administration for that dose of the series. Providers should consult the relevant Advisory Committee on Immunization Practices statement for detailed recommendations, including high-risk conditions: http://www.cdc.gov/vaccines/pubs/acip-list.htm. Clinically significant adverse events that follow immunization should be reported to the Vaccine Adverse Event Reporting System (VAERS). Guidance about how to obtain and complete a VAERS form is available at http://www.vaers.hhs.gov or by telephone, 800-822-7967.

Vaccine ▼ Age ▶	7–10 years	11–12 years	13–18 years
Tetanus, Diphtheria, Pertussis[1]	see footnote 1	Tdap	Tdap
Human Papillomavirus[2]	see footnote 2	HPV (3 doses)	HPV Series
Meningococcal[3]	MCV	MCV	MCV
Influenza[4]	Influenza (Yearly)		
Pneumococcal[5]	PPSV		
Hepatitis A[6]	HepA Series		
Hepatitis B[7]	HepB Series		
Inactivated Poliovirus[8]	IPV Series		
Measles, Mumps, Rubella[9]	MMR Series		
Varicella[10]	Varicella Series		

Legend:
- Range of recommended ages
- Catch-up immunization
- Certain high-risk groups

This schedule indicates the recommended ages for routine administration of currently licensed vaccines, as of December 1, 2008, for children aged 7 through 18 years. Any dose not administered at the recommended age should be administered at a subsequent visit, when indicated and feasible. Licensed combination vaccines may be used whenever any component of the combination is indicated and other components are not contraindicated and if approved by the Food and Drug Administration for that dose of the series. Providers should consult the relevant Advisory Committee on Immunization Practices statement for detailed recommendations, including high-risk conditions: http://www.cdc.gov/vaccines/pubs/acip-list.htm. Clinically significant adverse events that follow immunization should be reported to the Vaccine Adverse Event Reporting System (VAERS). Guidance about how to obtain and complete a VAERS form is available at http://www.vaers.hhs.gov or by telephone, 800-822-7967.

Table 18-9 Adult Vaccinations

VACCINE ▼ / AGE GROUP ▶	19–26 years	27–49 years	50–59 years	60–64 years	≥65 years
Tetanus, diphtheria, pertussis (Td/Tdap)[1,*]	Substitute 1-time dose of Tdap for Td booster; then boost with Td every 10 yrs				Td booster every 10 yrs
Human papillomavirus (HPV)[2,*]	3 doses (females)				
Varicella[3,*]	2 doses				
Zoster[4]				1 dose	1 dose
Measles, mumps, rubella (MMR)[5,*]	1 or 2 doses		1 dose		
Influenza[6,*]	1 dose annually				
Pneumococcal (polysaccharide)[7,8]	1 or 2 doses				
Hepatitis A[9,*]	2 doses				
Hepatitis B[10,*]	3 doses				
Meningococcal[11,*]	1 or more doses				

*Covered by the Vaccine Injury Compensation Program.

Legend:

☐ (light gray) For all persons in this category who meet the age requirements and who lack evidence of immunity (e.g., lack documentation of vaccination or have no evidence of prior infection)

■ (dark) Recommended if some other risk factor is present (e.g., on the basis of medical, occupational, lifestyle, or other indications)

☐ (white) No recommendation

(continues)

273

Table 18-9 Adult Vaccinations (Continued)

VACCINE ▼ / INDICATION ▶	Pregnancy	Immuno-compromising conditions (excluding human immunodeficiency virus [HIV])[13]	HIV infection[3,12,13] CD4+ T lymphocyte count <200 cells/µL	HIV infection[3,12,13] CD4+ T lymphocyte count ≥200 cells/µL	Diabetes, heart disease, chronic lung disease, chronic alcoholism	Asplenia[12] (including elective splenectomy and terminal complement component deficiencies)	Chronic liver disease	Kidney failure, end-stage renal disease, receipt of hemodialysis	Health-care personnel
Tetanus, diphtheria, pertussis (Td/Tdap)[1,*]	Td	Substitute 1-time dose of Tdap for Td booster; then boost with Td every 10 yrs							
Human papillomavirus (HPV)[2,*]		3 doses for females through age 26 yrs							
Varicella[3,*]	Contraindicated	Contraindicated	Contraindicated		2 doses				
Zoster[4]	Contraindicated	Contraindicated	Contraindicated		1 dose				
Measles, mumps, rubella (MMR)[5,*]	Contraindicated	Contraindicated	Contraindicated		1 or 2 doses				
Influenza[6,*]	1 dose TIV annually				1 dose TIV annually				1 dose TIV or LAIV annually
Pneumococcal (polysaccharide)[7,8]		1 or 2 doses							
Hepatitis A[9,*]		2 doses							
Hepatitis B[10,*]		3 doses							
Meningococcal[11,*]		1 or more doses							

Legend:

- For all persons in this category who meet the age requirements and who lack evidence of immunity (e.g., lack documentation of vaccination or have no evidence of prior infection)
- Recommended if some other risk factor is present (e.g., on the basis of medical, occupational, lifestyle, or other indications)
- No recommendation

*Covered by the Vaccine Injury Compensation Program.

5. *The right time:* For maximum effectiveness, drugs must be given on a prescribed schedule. Some medications like antibiotics are more effective on an empty stomach, so they are prescribed before meals (a.c.). Some medications are irritating to the stomach, so they are prescribed after meals (p.c.).

6. *The right documentation:* An essential part of safe drug administration is documentation. Every medication given must be recorded on the patient's record, along with the dose, time, route, and location of injection (if appropriate). The medical assistant must initial the record after administration.

QUESTIONS

18-1. Which agency is responsible for the approval of drugs and the removal of unsafe medications from the market?

A. FDA
B. DEA
C. CDC
D. HMA
E. DAG

18-2. Which is NOT a regulation established by the Federal Food, Drug, and Cosmetic Act?

A. All labels must include generic names.
B. Only physicians can write prescriptions.
C. All drugs must be approved by the FDA before release.
D. Warning labels must be present on certain preparations.
E. All labels must be accurate.

18-3. The DEA (Drug Enforcement Administration) regulates all of the following EXCEPT

A. stimulants.
B. vitamins.
C. narcotics.
D. depressants.
E. anabolic steroids.

18-4. The Controlled Substances Act of 1970 classified drugs into schedules based on their abuse potential. Which schedule includes drugs with the highest abuse potential, including drugs that are not approved for medical use in the United States?

A. Schedule I
B. Schedule II
C. Schedule III
D. Schedule IV
E. Schedule V

18-5. The common name that begins with a lowercase letter and is assigned to every drug is called the

A. chemical name.
B. drug company name.
C. trade name.
D. generic name.

18-6. Generic and trade name drugs may differ in all of the following ways EXCEPT

A. color.
B. cost.
C. drug contents.

     D. fillers.

     E. capitalization of first letter.

18-7. If a drug is contraindicated in pregnancy, it should be

     A. given only in the last trimester.

     B. given only to men.

     C. administered carefully.

     D. omitted while pregnant.

     E. used with caution.

18-8. Adverse reactions to a medication might include

     A. photosensitivity.

     B. tinnitus.

     C. headaches.

     D. urinary problems.

     E. All of the above.

18-9. Which variable affects the speed and efficiency of drug processing by the body?

     A. Age

     B. Weight

     C. Sex

     D. Psychological state

     E. All of the above

18-10. What does the term "loading dose" refer to?

     A. The smallest amount of a drug that will produce a therapeutic effect

     B. The largest amount of a drug that will produce a therapeutic effect

     C. The initial maximum dose used to quickly elevate the level of a drug in the blood

     D. The dose required to keep the drug blood level at a steady state

     E. The dose that is customarily given

18-11. After administering an injection, the needle should be

     A. cut or broken.

     B. recapped immediately.

     C. thrown out.

     D. put in the sharps box uncapped.

     E. put in a recycle container.

18-12. Which of the following is a parenteral route of administration for a drug?

     A. Oral (PO)

     B. Nasogastric (NG)

     C. Rectal (R)

     D. Intravenous (IV)

     E. None of the above

18-13. Signs of an anaphylactic reaction to a drug include all of the following, EXCEPT

     A. urticaria.

     B. laryngeal edema.

     C. shock.

     D. bloodshot eyes.

     E. hyperemia.

18-14. What is a paradoxical effect of a drug?

    A. An allergic response
    B. A psychological dependence
    C. A tolerance to the medicine
    D. The opposite effect from that expected
    E. Nausea, vomiting, and diarrhea

18-15. What is the primary site in which drugs are metabolized in the body?

    A. Stomach
    B. Small intestine
    C. Liver
    D. Kidney
    E. Circulatory system

18-16. Drug processing in the body is described by four main processes: absorption, distribution, metabolism, and excretion. These are known as

    A. pharmacochanges.
    B. pharmacotherapeutics.
    C. pharmacodynamics.
    D. pharmacokinetics.
    E. pharmacoeffects.

18-17. What is the primary site from which drugs are excreted from the body?

    A. Stomach
    B. Small intestine
    C. Liver
    D. Kidneys
    E. Circulatory system

18-18. Which method of administering drugs is the most rapid-acting?

    A. Oral
    B. Topical
    C. Buccal
    D. Rectal
    E. Intravenous

18-19. The abbreviation that means whenever necessary is

    A. DC.
    B. SL.
    C. NPO.
    D. BID.
    E. PRN.

18-20. Medication orders must contain all of the following EXCEPT

    A. date.
    B. patient's name.
    C. medication name.
    D. dosage.
    E. reason for prescription.

18-21. What does the gauge of the needle refer to?

    A. Quantity
    B. Brand
    C. Length
    D. Diameter
    E. None of the above

18-22. Lasix is available in 40 mg tablets. The order reads Lasix 60 mg PO qAM. How many tablets should you give each morning?

    A. 1
    B. 1.5
    C. 2
    D. 2.5
    E. 3

18-23. Phenergan 12.5 mg is ordered. Vials of Phenergan are available as 25 mg/1 ml. How many ml would you administer?

    A. 0.5
    B. 1
    C. 1.5
    D. 2
    E. 2.5

18-24. According to the six rights of medication administration, all of the following should be checked carefully before administering medicine, EXCEPT

    A. right price.
    B. right route.
    C. right medication.
    D. right time.
    E. right patient.

18-25. Medical assistants have a responsibility to do all of the following, EXCEPT

    A. assess patient response to medication.
    B. provide patient education.
    C. deliver medication accurately.
    D. be familiar with the medication to be administered.
    E. diagnose the patient.

18-26. Correct documentation of an injection given for pain should include all of the following, EXCEPT

    A. insurance.
    B. time.
    C. route.
    D. dose.
    E. location.

18-27. Before administering medication, a medical assistant has the responsibility to question all of the following, EXCEPT

    A. manufacturing process of the medicine.
    B. significant allergies to the medicine.
    C. conflicting interactions of other medicines.
    D. incorrect medicine.
    E. inappropriate dosage.

18-28. All of the following are true about giving medication orally (in comparison to parenteral administration), EXCEPT

    A. faster onset of action.
    B. more economical.
    C. easier for patient.
    D. absorption rate varies.
    E. more convenient.

18-29. When a medical assistant administers oral medications, all of the following are appropriate, EXCEPT

    A. identify patient.
    B. leave medicines at patient's bedside.
    C. provide a glass of water and assist as necessary.
    D. give the most important medicines first.
    E. document the patient's record.

18-30. When administering medication by nasogastric tube, all of the following are true EXCEPT

    A. medication should flow through the tube by gravity.
    B. the medication should be cold.
    C. the patient's head should be elevated.
    D. placement of the NG tube should be verified.
    E. the procedure should be stopped with any sign of discomfort.

18-31. At what angle are intradermal injections given?

    A. 90 degrees
    B. 60 degrees
    C. 45 degrees
    D. 15 degrees
    E. It doesn't matter.

18-32. Which is an appropriate gauge for an intradermal needle?

    A. 18–19
    B. 20–21
    C. 22
    D. 23–25
    E. 26–27

18-33. Which is the preferred site for an intramuscular injection in adults?

    A. Deltoid
    B. Dorsogluteal
    C. Ventrogluteal
    D. Rectus femoris
    E. Vastus lateralis

18-34. Which is the preferred site for an intramuscular injection in children?

    A. Deltoid
    B. Dorsogluteal
    C. Ventrogluteal
    D. Rectus femoris
    E. Vastus lateralis

18-35. Which of the following is a modification of an IM injection that is used to prevent irritation to the subcutaneous tissues?

    A. A-track method
    B. K-track method
    C. Z-track method
    D. M-track method
    E. L-track method

18-36. Which size needle would you use for an intramuscular injection?

    A. 3/8-inch length, 21 gauge
    B. 1/2-inch length, 25 gauge
    C. 5/8-inch length, 23 gauge
    D. 1 1/2-inch length, 21 gauge
    E. 1 1/2-inch length, 25 gauge

18-37. What is the reason for aspirating the plunger when administering an injection?

    A. Demonstrate amount injected
    B. Make patient more comfortable
    C. Reduce air bubbles
    D. Check for appearance of blood
    E. To reposition the patient

18-38. Which syringe should you use for allergy testing?

    A. 3 ml syringe
    B. tuberculin syringe
    C. insulin syringe
    D. 5 ml syringe
    E. 2.5 ml syringe

18-39. Why are anticholinergics used preoperatively?

    A. To increase gastrointestinal peristalsis
    B. To dilate the pupils
    C. To lower intraocular pressure
    D. To dry secretions and prevent hypotension and bradycardia
    E. To increase gastric secretions and prevent muscle cramps and constipation

18-40. What is the generic name for Benadryl?

    A. Salicyclic acid
    B. Isoretinoin
    C. Lindane
    D. Nystatin
    E. Diphenhydramine

ANSWERS

18-1. The correct answer is A. The FDA was established in 1930 as part of the U.S. Department of Health and Human Services (DHHS). The FDA has various responsibilities, among those are to enforce provisions of the 1938 Federal Food, Drug, and Cosmetic Act. Essentially, this act established more specific regulations to prevent tampering with drugs, foods, and cosmetics.

18-2. The correct answer is B. First, the FDA provides no regulations about who can write prescriptions. Second, it is a fallacy that only physicians can write prescriptions. Legislation allows licensed physicians, licensed nurse practitioners, registered certified physician assistants, clinical pharmacists, dentists, and veterinarians to write prescriptions for their specific field of work, within limitations.

18-3. The correct answer is B. The DEA was established in 1970 to enforce provisions of the Controlled Substances Act in order to control medicines/drugs that were being abused by society.

18-4. The correct answer is A. This act organized drugs into five levels according to their degree of danger. Schedule I has the highest abuse potential and includes drugs not even approved for medical use in the United States. Schedule V has the lowest abuse potential and consists primarily of preparations used in cough medicines.

18-5. The correct answer is D. The generic or common name is assigned to every drug. It is never capitalized. Generally, the generic name is the same as the official name, which is the name as it appears in the official reference.

18-6. The correct answer is C. A pharmaceutical company identifies its product by the trade name, which is always capitalized. It is copyrighted and used exclusively by that company. The generic name is the common name assigned to each drug. When 17 years have passed and the pharmaceutical company's original patent on the drug has expired, other companies may begin to combine the same chemicals from that specific generic product for marketing. The drugs may differ in color, cost, and ingredients that are used to hold the drug together. They may not differ in the actual content of the drug.

18-7. The correct answer is D. Contraindicated means that a drug should *not* be given for a particular condition or in a specific population, in this case, pregnancy.

18-8. The correct answer is E. Adverse reactions or side effects are common in many medications. Photosensitivity is increased reaction to sunlight. Tinnitus is a ringing in the ears.

18-9. The correct answer is E. Metabolism and excretion depend on variables such as age, weight, and sex. Additionally, it has been proven that the more positive the patient feels about the medication he or she is taking, the more positive the physical response.

18-10. The correct answer is C. The loading dose refers to the initial high dose used to quickly elevate the level of drug in the body; it is often followed by a series of lower maintenance doses.

18-11. The correct answer is D. Contaminated needles are never recapped, but are discarded uncapped in a sharps container immediately.

18-12. The correct answer is D. The parenteral route includes giving a drug via any route other than via the gastrointestinal tract. Examples are via injection: IV, IM, subQ, and ID. Other parenteral routes include topical administration and inhalation.

18-13. The correct answer is D. An anaphylactic reaction is a severe, possibly fatal, allergic response to a drug. It can include itching, urticaria (hives), hyperemia (reddened, warm skin), vascular collapse, shock, cyanosis, laryngeal edema, and dyspnea. Treatment can include CPR, epinephrine, corticosteroids, and antihistamine.

18-14. The correct answer is D. A paradoxical effect is an unexpected response to a drug. It is the opposite effect from that expected. For example, if a medicine is intended to cause drowsiness and it causes excitement instead, it is having a paradoxical effect.

18-15. The correct answer is C. Metabolism is the physical and chemical alterations that a substance undergoes in the body. The liver is the primary site of this process.

18-16. The correct answer is D. Pharmacokinetics refers to the four processes that drugs must undergo in the body: absorption, distribution, metabolism, and excretion.

18-17. The correct answer is D. Although it is possible for some drugs to be eliminated through perspiration, feces, bile, breast milk, or exhaled through the lungs, *most* drugs are excreted by the kidneys.

18-18. The correct answer is E. The intravenous route is the quickest: drugs enter the bloodstream immediately.

18-19. The correct answer is E. PRN means whenever necessary. DC means discontinue. SL means sublingual. NPO means nothing by mouth. BID means twice a day.

18-20. The correct answer is E. Medication orders contain six parts: date, patient's name, medication name, dosage, route of administration, and frequency of administration. Medication orders should always be written and signed by the health care worker. In an emergency, a verbal order may be given, but a signed order must follow within 24 hours.

18-21. The correct answer is D. The gauge refers to the diameter of the needle lumen. Needle gauges vary from 16 (largest diameter lumen) to 27 (smallest diameter lumen).

18-22. The correct answer is B. If Lasix is only available in 40 mg tablets, you must break one in half and administer 1.5 to make 60 mg.

18-23. The correct answer is A. If Phenergan is only available as 25 mg/1 ml, you would need half as much. This means that you would administer only half of the vial.

18-24. The correct answer is A. Guidelines to review before giving medicines are called the six rights of medication administration. This means that the medical assistant should check the following before giving any medicine: right medication, right amount, right time, right route, right patient. Finally, they should provide right documentation after administering medications.

18-25. The correct answer is E. Medical assistants have a responsibility for safe administration of medication. This includes providing patient education, being familiar with the medication before administration (i.e., becoming familiar with the precautions, contraindications, potential side effects, giving the medication accurately, and finally careful observation of the patient after taking the medicine in case of adverse effects). Medical assistants are not responsible for diagnosing the patient with an illness or disease.

18-26. The correct answer is A. An essential duty of the medical assistant is documentation. Every medication given must be recorded on the patient's record. Correct documentation includes dose, time, route, location (of injection), and effectiveness (if the medication is given PRN, like for pain control). The medical assistant must also initial the record after administering the medication. Correct documentation does not include the patient's insurance.

18-27. The correct answer is A. Administration of medication carries moral, ethical, and legal responsibilities. A medical assistant has the responsibility to question an unusual dosage, the incorrect medicine, conflicting interactions, or significant allergies that the patient might have. The manufacturing process of the medicine should not be a concern.

18-28. The correct answer is A. Advantages of giving medication orally include convenience, patient comfort, and economy (because there are fewer equipment costs). Other factors to consider when giving medication orally include slower onset of action (than the parenteral route) and that the rate and degree of absorption will vary with gastrointestinal contents and motility.

18-29. The correct answer is B. The medical assistant should stay with the patient until the medication is swallowed. One should not leave the medication at the bedside unless ordered by the physician. Also, the most important medicines should be given first.

18-30. The correct answer is B. Nasogastric tubes have been put in place for tube feeding or suction. When they are already in place, medications can be administered through the tube. The medication should be given at room temperature. One should make sure that the tube is properly placed in the stomach by two tests—aspirating stomach contents to check for pH and listening for air with a stethoscope. The patient's head should be elevated and the medicine should flow through the tube by gravity. One should flush the tube afterwards with water. The procedure may be stopped with any signs of discomfort.

18-31. The correct answer is D. Intradermal injections are given at a 10- to 15-degree angle.

18-32. The correct answer is E. The gauge is the diameter of the shaft of the needle. For intradermal injections, a thin needle with a small diameter should be used. Gauges of needles are numbered in reverse order. Therefore, a thin needle would have a gauge of 26–27.

18-33. The correct answer is C. The ventrogluteal site is the preferred site for IM injections to adults. The ventrogluteal site, or gluteus medius muscle, is relatively free of major nerves or vessels, thereby making it a choice site. The dorsogluteal site is no longer the choice site because an improperly done injection may cause damage to the sciatic nerve or superior gluteal artery or vein. The deltoid muscle is an option but is a smaller site. An improperly administered injection may damage a variety of nerves and blood vessels in the area.

18-34. The correct answer is E. The preferred site for an IM injection in children is the vastus lateralis, the anterior lateral thigh, part of the quadriceps femoris. These muscles are the most developed in children under the age of 3.

18-35. The correct answer is C. The Z-track method is a type of intramuscular injection that is used when medications are given that contain materials that would cause irritation if they leaked into the subcutaneous tissue through the path made by the needle. The technique involves pulling the skin to one side and inserting the needle at a 90-degree angle. When the skin returns to the normal position, the needle track is sealed off.

18-36. The correct answer is D. Needle length is measured in inches or fractions of inches (1/2, 5/8, 1). Shorter needles are used for intradermal or subcutaneous injections. Longer needles ($1\frac{1}{2}$ and 2 inches) are used for intramuscular injections. Keep in mind that the length of the needle depends on the type of injection and the size of the patient. The gauge is the size of the lumen or hole. The gauge is numbered in reverse order: the thinner needle with the smaller diameter has the larger number (25 for subcutaneous injections) and the thicker needle with a larger opening (18–21) is used for IM injections.

18-37. The correct answer is D. The reason to aspirate the plunger when administering an injection is to make sure that the needle has not entered a blood vessel. If blood does appear, the needle must be withdrawn immediately and a new site should be prepared for injection. If blood does not appear, the medication may continue to be injected.

18-38. The correct answer is B. The tuberculin syringe should be used for allergy testing, tuberculosis testing, and other subcutaneous injections when a small amount of medicine is ordered (e.g., with children).

18-39. The correct answer is D. Anticholinergics are drugs that block the action of the parasympathetic nervous system. They can be used preoperatively to reduce the secretions of the mouth, pharynx, bronchi, and GI tract, as well as reduce gastric activity. Another advantage to using this type of medication preoperatively is to prevent cholinergic effects during surgery like hypotension or bradycardia. Atropine (Atreza) is a cholinergic blocker that is used preoperatively that has the added effect of bronchodilation to reduce the incidence of laryngospasm during general surgery.

18-40. The correct answer is E. Benadryl is an antihistamine. Its generic name is diphenhydramine.

Medical Emergencies and First Aid

Medical assistants are expected to identify and respond to a variety of medical emergency situations that may occur in the physicians office. This chapter outlines both the preparation and action required to be an effective part of the medical team responding to an emergency.

EMERGENCIES

Medical emergencies need immediate clinical assessment, stabilization, and treatment of the patient to prevent morbidity and mortality. The life-threatening nature of these conditions requires that the problem be corrected quickly to stop organ damage and prevent death. Sudden disturbances in cardiac rhythm, cardiogenic shock, cardiopulmonary arrest, and severe allergic reactions are the most serious medical emergencies.

PREPLANNED ACTION

In any medical setting, there should be a preplanned protocol in place. The medical assistant (as well as all of the other health care providers) should know the policies and procedures, their legal implications, how to document incidents correctly, and finally, how to use equipment such as the crash cart and automated external defibrillator.

Policies and Procedures

Emergencies develop quickly and without warning. It is essential that there are policies and procedures in place regarding how to handle them. Typically, there is an office handbook of policies and procedures. The steps in the handbook should be carried out calmly and carefully. Emergency policies may vary from setting to setting, but all have the same goal in mind—risk management. Emergency medical services (EMS) should be activated when additional support is needed.

Legal Implications and Action Documentation

It is important to consider legal implications and documentation. Documentation should be done on all office emergencies. The specifics of an event should be included in a patient's chart. Good Samaritan laws protect from liability any health care workers who offer first aid. Essentially, these laws protect an individual who gives first aid in a reasonable and prudent manner from being sued. Good Samaritan laws vary by state.

Equipment

In addition to supportive measures in medical emergencies, quick therapeutic interventions are essential in most emergencies. Therefore, access to the right equipment to resolve the problem is critical.

Crash Cart

A crash cart holds a selection of drugs and equipment that are most effective and appropriate in these critical situations. Common drugs that can be found on a crash cart are listed in Table 19-1, and equipment found on a crash cart is listed and described in Table 19-2. Table 19-3 lists some general supplies that may be found on a crash cart. The inventory of supplies on a crash cart should be routinely monitored to assure that all supplies are replaced and medications are not expired.

Automated External Defibrillator

An automated external defibrillator (AED) is a portable electronic device used in cases of life-threatening cardiac arrhythmias that have led to cardiac arrest. If the victim does not have a pulse, the AED should be used. The AED shocks the heart to restore a more normal heart rhythm. Automated external defibrillators are designed to be easy to use and are becoming increasingly common in public places. When used quickly (within the first 5 minutes of an event), AEDs have been shown to dramatically increase the survival rate of victims suffering from cardiac arrest. Medical assistants should be trained in the use of the AED.

Table 19-1 Common Drugs on a Crash Cart

Drug	Indication/Use
Aspirin	Fever, heart attack
Atropine	Slow heartbeat
Bretylium tosylate (Bretylol)	Ventricular fibrillation
Calcium chloride	Cardiac resuscitation when weak or inadequate contractions return following defibrillation
Dextrose	Insulin hypoglycemia
Diazepam (Valium)	Anxiety
Diphenhydramine (Benadryl)	Allergic reaction (antihistamine)
Dopamine	Low blood pressure
Epinephrine	Low blood pressure
Furosemide (Lasix)	Edema
Glucagon	Insulin reaction
Insulin	Diabetic hyperglycemia
Isoproterenol (Isuprel)	Cardiac arrest
Lidocaine	Local anesthetic; IV for cardiac arrhythmia
Magnesium sulfate	Anti-arrhythmic
Midazolam (Versed)	Preoperative sedation
Nitroglycerin	Chest pain associated with angina
Phenobarbital	Sedative
Verapamil	Tachycardia; angina; hypertension
Xylocaine	Local anesthetic

Table 19-2 Common Equipment on a Crash Cart

Equipment	Indication
Airways (for nasal and oral use)	Help manage airway
Ambu-bag	Breathing bag to assist respiratory ventilation
Bulb syringe	Suction
Central venous catheters	Catheters placed in large central veins (near the heart) so that medications and fluids can reach the heart quickly
Defibrillator	Electrical device with two paddles to shock the heart back to normal—sometimes kept by itself
Endotracheal tubes	Allows for airway management and mechanical ventilation
Oxygen tank (with mask and cannula)	Delivers increased oxygen

Table 19-3 General Supplies on a Crash Cart

Supplies
Adhesive tape
Alcohol wipes
Bandage scissors
Bandage material
Blood pressure cuff
Constriction band
Dressing material
Gloves
Hot and cold packs
IV tubing
Needles and syringes
Orange juice (or other sugar substitute)
Penlight
Personal protective equipment
Stethoscope

ASSESSMENT AND TRIAGE

Quick and accurate assessment is critical in emergencies. Triage refers to the process of giving attention to the most severe victims or the most severe injuries in one particular victim. Life-threatening problems need to be identified first. Examples of such situations include airway and breathing problems, severe bleeding, head trauma, poisoning, open chest and abdominal wounds, shock, severe allergic reactions, and second-degree and third-degree burns. During assessment, one should remember to check the victim for a bracelet or ID card with the universal emergency medical identification symbol, which will identify any serious health problems.

If the patient is found unresponsive, always remember the ABCs for assessment and treatment priorities. First, "A" stands for airway: Is the airway open? This is the most important first assessment because if there is an obstruction, breathing is automatically stopped. Try to open the patient's airway by tilting their head back with one hand while lifting up their chin with your other hand. Second, "B" stands for breathing: Is the patient breathing? Assess for movement of the chest and listen for sounds of breathing. If not breathing, pinch the patient's nose closed and give two full breaths into the patient's mouth. If breaths won't go in, reposition the head and try again to give breaths. If still blocked, perform abdominal thrusts (Heimlich maneuver). The last step is "C," which stands for circulation. Check for a carotid pulse by feeling for 5–10 seconds at the side of the patient's neck. If there is a pulse but the patient is not breathing, give rescue breathing at the rate of one breath every 2 seconds.

Table 19-4 Assessment of ABCs

Assessment	Description	Response
Airway	Check to see if victim has an open airway.	Perform head-tilt/chin-lift to ensure an open airway.
Breathing	Look for the chest rising and falling; listen for breathing sounds.	Perform rescue breathing if the patient is not breathing (but has a pulse).
Circulation	Check for pulse.	Perform CPR if the patient does not have a pulse.

If there is no pulse, begin chest compressions (CPR) by performing 30 compressions to every 2 breaths for all patients, regardless of age or size. Table 19-4 outlines how to assess the ABCs.

EMERGENCY PREPAREDNESS

Emergency preparedness includes recognizing an emergency and responding correctly. A medical assistant can have an important role in such events. For example, a medical assistant can give CPR and give first aid. In addition, the medical assistant should know when to call for more help by activating EMS (911 in most areas) or calling poison control, suicide hotlines, or abuse shelters. A medical assistant is also responsible for documenting emergencies and restocking supplies and equipment.

FIRST AID

First aid refers to the immediate care rendered in a medical emergency until advanced care is available. A medical assistant should be able to identify and respond to the following: bleeding/pressure points, burns, cardiac and respiratory arrest, choking, problems related to diabetes, fractures, poisoning, seizures, shock, stroke, syncope, and wounds. Each is described in more detail in the sections that follow.

Bleeding/Pressure Points

Bleeding, also called hemorrhaging, can be external or internal. External bleeding can be seen from the outside of the body. Examples of external bleeding include bleeding from wounds, open fractures, and nosebleeds (epistaxis). Direct pressure should be applied over the wound using a clean and sterile dressing. Additional dressings should be applied on top if blood soaks through. Pressure points also can be used to help control external bleeding. Pressure is applied over the artery closest to the wound, between the injury and the heart. Major pressure points include the temporal artery, the facial artery, the carotid artery, the radial-ulnar artery, the brachial artery, the subclavian artery, and the femoral artery. For example, to control bleeding from a laceration to the upper leg, pressure should be applied to the femoral artery, which is between the injury and the heart.

Internal bleeding cannot be seen overtly. Internal bleeding results from hemorrhage of an organ or tissue internally. Examples include bleeding from the gastrointestinal tract or respiratory tract. Since there are no overt external signs of bleeding, it is essential for the medical assistant to recognize other signs and/or symptoms. Such symptoms are similar to those of shock such as a rapid, weak pulse, low blood pressure, cold, clammy skin, shallow breathing, dilated pupils, and dizziness. EMS should be called while the medical assistant monitors vital signs.

If blood loss is significant (20–40% of a patient's total blood volume), hypovolemic shock can result. With both types of bleeding, vital signs should be monitored, the patient should be kept calm, and additional medical attention should be sought.

Burns

A burn is an injury caused by heat (flames, boiling water), sun (solar radiation), chemicals, or electricity. Burns are classified according to their depth or the layers of skin involved. Table 19-5 illustrates

Table 19-5 Burn Classifications

Burn	Description
First degree (Superficial burn)	Superficial damage to epidermis only; superficial sunburn
Second degree (Partial-thickness burn)	Damage to epidermis and dermis; blistered, pink skin
Third degree (Full-thickness burn)	Damage to epidermis, dermis, and subcutaneous tissue, also potential damage to muscle below; charred black-brown skin

the types of burns. Burns are serious because the break in skin may cause infection and loss of fluid; burns can also result in difficulty breathing. EMS should be called in incidents when a victim has trouble breathing, has burns on more than one part of the body, was burned by chemicals or electricity, or has burns on the face, hands, feet, or genitals. Other types of burns usually require medical attention as well. Until medical attention can be sought, the burn should be cooled either by immersion in cold water or with a clean, cool cloth.

The "rule of nines" is used to calculate the percentage of body surface affected by burns in adults. The body is divided into parts based on a multiple of 9. For example, the head is 9%, each arm is 9%, each leg is 18%, the ventral trunk is 18%, and the dorsal trunk is 18%. The burned body parts are added together to determine the percentage of body surface affected.

Cardiac and Respiratory Arrest/CPR

Cardiac and respiratory arrest is also known as cardiopulmonary arrest or circulatory arrest, where there is sudden cessation of normal blood circulation due to the failure of the heart to pump effectively, causing termination of breathing. Various medical emergencies (choking, shock, cardiac emergencies) can lead to cardiac and respiratory arrest. Respiratory arrest alone leads to cardiac arrest, and vice versa. The common name for cardiac arrest is heart attack. CPR or cardiopulmonary resuscitation is required if the victim is both not breathing and does not have a pulse. Time is critical to the survival of the victim. Assessment relies upon the medical assistant's best judgment. For example, if the victim is seen falling or in crisis, 911 should be called first. However, if the victim is found unconscious and CPR is needed, the medical assistant should proceed with 5 cycles of 30 compressions for every 2 breaths prior to activating EMS. CPR represents preliminary care until the victim is able to receive advanced medical treatment. CPR should be performed until EMS arrives and takes over care of the patient.

CPR guidelines are based on the ABCs: airway, breathing, and circulation. The ABCs require that the A must come before B, which must come before C. Thus, the airway must be open in order for breathing to occur, and you must have breath sounds in order for circulation to occur. According to Basic Cardiac Life Support (BCLS) Guidelines, if a victim has a pulse but needs rescue breathing, the medical provider should give one breath every 2 seconds. If the victim does not have a pulse, one should start CPR.

Table 19-6 details the steps involved in rescue breathing, and Table 19-7 details the steps involved in CPR. The new American Heart Association guidelines have simplified CPR delivery. The thinking behind these changes was that CPR was too confusing for a lay person to administer. Streamlined procedures should yield broader use of CPR.

Choking/Heimlich Maneuver

The universal sign for choking is a person clutching his or her throat with both hands. In a conscious adult who can no longer talk or cough, the Heimlich maneuver is used. The Heimlich maneuver uses abdominal thrusts to clear the airway. This is done by standing behind the victim and wrapping your hands around his or her waist. Make a fist with one hand and place the thumb side near the victim's bellybutton. While the other hand is placed over the fist, give upward thrusts into the victim's abdomen. Continue this motion until the victim begins to breathe (cough, talk). If the victim becomes

Table 19-6 Steps in Rescue Breathing

1. Check for responsiveness; if not responsive, call for help (EMS).

2. Roll the patient on their back.

3. Open the airway by tilting the head back and lifting the chin carefully.

4. Look, listen, and feel for breathing.

5. If not breathing, use a face mask (if available) to give two slow breaths.

6. If no face mask, pinch the patient's nose shut, and seal your mouth around the patient's to give two slow breaths.

7. Check the carotid pulse for 5–10 seconds.

8. If there is a pulse but no breathing, continue to give a breath every 2 seconds in all patients (adults, children, and infants) Note: New American Heart Association guidelines have simplified rescue breathing procedures with all patients receiving one breath every 2 seconds.

9. If no breath and no pulse, give CPR.

unconscious, lower him or her to the ground on their back. Do a finger sweep to attempt to remove any obstruction. Perform a head tilt and chin lift and give two slow breaths. If the breaths still do not go in, continue to give abdominal thrusts by straddling the victim. Give five abdominal thrusts, then a finger sweep, and then two slow breaths until the object becomes dislodged or air goes into the victim. Rescue breathing is used if the victim is not breathing but has a pulse. CPR is used if the victim is both not breathing and does not have a pulse.

Diabetic Coma/Insulin Shock

Diabetic emergencies are due to either too much or too little blood sugar. Table 19-8 gives a brief description of each.

Fractures

Fractures are breaks in the bone. They can be life-threatening if they rupture an artery, cause severe infection, or interrupt breathing. An x-ray is the best way to assess damage to a bone. The various types of fractures are listed in Table 19-9.

First aid for fractures is rest (minimize movement), ice, and elevation (to reduce pain and swelling). Call EMS in certain serious circumstances: severely broken bone(s); breaks to the head, neck, or back; and breaks that cause the victim trouble breathing.

In incidents where you must move the victim, use splints to immobilize the injury. The body part should be splinted in the position in which it was found. Splint the injured area and the joints above and below the injured area. Splints may be soft (made from towels or blankets) or rigid (cardboard, metal strips). You may also use another body part, such as by splinting an injured arm to a chest; this is called an anatomic splint. Apply ice and raise the injured part, if possible, to reduce swelling. If necessary, cover the wound with a sterile dressing.

Poisoning

Poisoning occurs when a toxic substance is taken into the body. Poisoning can occur by ingestion, inhalation, absorption, or injection. Signs of ingested poisons are gastrointestinal-related, such as nausea, vomiting, diarrhea, and abdominal pain, along with difficulty breathing, changes in consciousness, seizures, or burns around the lips or tongue or on the skin. Signs of inhaled poisons are pale or blue skin. Signs of absorbed poisons are integumentary-related, such as rash, swelling, and/or breathing difficulty. Signs of injection poisoning are related to the poison. Drug abuse and insect stings are both common causes of injection poisoning. Insect stings are particularly dangerous in the allergic patient and can lead to anaphylactic shock. In this situation, an antihistamine should be administered as soon as possible. If you suspect poisoning, call the poison control center and/or EMS immediately. Remove the source of poison if possible (such as carbon monoxide in inhaled poisoning). As a medical assistant,

Table 19-7 Steps in CPR

1. Determine that the patient is not breathing and has no pulse.

2. Follow the steps from Table 19-6 for rescue breathing (two successful breaths have been given and there is still no pulse).

3. Locate the compression site:

   In adults and children: Locate the xiphoid notch, place hands about 2 inches above notch.

   In infants: One finger width below nipple line.

4. Perform compressions:

   Adults: Two hands stacked

   Children: Heel of one hand

   Infants: Two or three fingers

   The rate of compressions per minute should be 100. Compression depth should be:

   Adults: 1.5–2 inches

   Children: 1–1.5 inches

   Infants: 0.5–1 inch

5. Compress the patient's chest and then give rescue breaths. The ratio of compressions to breaths should be:

   Adults:30:2

   Children:30:2

   Infants:30:2

   Note: New American Heart Association guidelines have simplified CPR procedures with all patients receiving the same ratio of compressions to breaths.

   However, if doing 2-man CPR, the ratio of compressions to breaths should be:

   Adults: 30:2

   Children 15:2

   Infants 15:2

6. Continue compressions for 1 minute and then recheck for breathing and pulse for 5–10 seconds.

7. Continue CPR.

8. Stop CPR only in the following circumstances:

   - The patient recovers.
   - EMS or other trained help arrives or you are replaced by another person who knows CPR.
   - The scene becomes unsafe.
   - You are too exhausted to continue.
   - Physician directed (do not resuscitate).

Table 19-8 Diabetic Emergencies

Diabetic Emergency	Description
Diabetic ketoacidosis (can lead to diabetic coma)	Caused by extremely high blood sugar; treatment is prompt administration of insulin; patient may have rapid respirations and fruity acetone breath.
Insulin shock	Caused by extremely low blood sugar (and/or an excess of insulin); treatment is prompt administration of juice/sugar.

Table 19-9 Fractures

Fractures	Description
Closed (simple)	Broken bone but *no* open wound in the skin.
Colles'	A fracture of the wrist (the distal radius); occurs when falling with an outstretched arm.
Comminuted	Bone is crushed into small pieces.
Compound	Broken bone *with* an open wound in the skin.
Compression	A spontaneous fracture in which the bone is pressed together (typically seen in osteoporosis of the spine).
Greenstick	Bone is bent or partially broken; occurs in children.
Impacted	Broken ends of the bone are forced into each other.
Oblique	Fracture occurs at an angle.
Open (compound)	Broken bone *with* an open wound in the skin.
Pathologic	Bone breaks because of a disease process (e.g., cancer).
Simple (closed)	Broken bone but *no* open wound in the skin.
Spiral	Bone breaks in a twisting motion (sports injury).
Stress	Small break in a bone because of chronic, excessive overuse (e.g., running).
Transverse	Bone breaks straight across the bone.

do not try to give the victim anything to eat or drink, or to induce vomiting unless told to by the poison control experts. Monitor airway, breathing, and circulation in the acute circumstance.

Seizures

A seizure is a sudden convulsive episode caused by an electrical problem in the brain. With a seizure, a victim may have change in sensations (auras such as strange tastes, smells, sounds, or even hallucinations), body movements (uncontrolled muscular contractions), or awareness (loss of consciousness). A seizure may be caused by anything that disrupts normal brain structure and function, such as head trauma, stroke, drugs, electrolyte and glucose abnormalities, and structural abnormalities of the brain.

Epilepsy is the condition of having recurrent seizures. A patient with epilepsy requires ongoing treatment with antiepileptics.

There are various types of seizures, as described in Table 19-10. Treatment is supportive and not intended to stop the seizure or restrain the patient. Never put anything in the victim's mouth or hold the victim down while he or she is seizing.

Shock

Shock is an emergency state in which the body does not receive enough oxygen for the cells to function. This may ultimately lead to cellular death, organ failure, and whole body failure/death. Symptoms of shock include the four Ps: pallor (paleness), perspiration (clammy, sweaty skin), pulse (weak, rapid, or irregular), and pulmonary difficulty (increased respiratory rate). Loss of consciousness may occur. Several types of shock exist; these are described in Table 19-11, along with the best course of immediate action. In most cases of shock, the best course of action is to activate EMS and check the victim's airway, breathing, and circulation. While waiting for EMS, a victim should be kept as comfortable as possible—lay flat and keep warm. A victim's legs can be elevated to increase blood return to the heart if there is no head, neck, back, leg, or hip injuries.

Table 19-10 Seizures

Seizure	Description	Treatment
Generalized tonic clonic seizure (grand mal seizure)	Convulsions with brief loss of consciousness for 1–2 minutes; when it ends, the patient's muscles relax and he or she may lose bladder control, have a headache, and fall asleep.	Protect victim from injury (cushion head, move sharp objects). If person vomits, clear mouth. Keep track of duration and symptoms that occur. Call EMS for further help. Have the victim rest until EMS arrives.
Absence seizure (petit mal seizure)	No convulsion occurs—a person stares off into space for a few seconds; may be seen with lip smacking, chewing, repeated blinking, or hand movements; when it ends, a person is unaware that the seizure has occurred; more commonly seen in children.	Prevent accidental injury that may occur during the seizure. Seek additional medical treatment.
Febrile seizure	Caused by a high fever; mostly seen in infants and small children; convulsions usually last 1–2 minutes; generally, these are harmless long term.	Bring down the fever. Apply washcloths rinsed in luke-warm water. Seek additional medical attention.

Table 19-11 Types of Shock

Shock	Cause	Action
Anaphylactic	Shock caused by severe allergic reaction that may result in respiratory distress	Activate EMS. Check ABCs.
Cardiogenic	Shock caused by inadequate heart function	Activate EMS. Check ABCs.
Hypovolemic	Shock resulting from low blood volume (hemorrhage or severe dehydration)	Activate EMS. Check ABCs.
Insulin	Shock caused by extremely low blood sugar	Give juice or sugar. Activate EMS. Check ABCs.
Neurogenic	Shock caused by trauma to the brain or spinal cord	Activate EMS. Check ABCs.
Septic	Shock caused by systemic infection (often bacterial)	Activate EMS. Check ABCs.

Stroke

The common term for a cerebral vascular accident is stroke. A cerebral vascular accident results from depriving brain cells of oxygen. Ischemia of brain tissue occurs by either: (1) occlusion of a blood vessel in the brain, or (2) rupture of a blood vessel. Occlusion of cerebral vasculature can be the result of plaque formation, emboli, or thrombosis. Rupture of a blood vessel may be the result of an aneurysm. Both types of stroke cause cell death. A victim's stroke symptoms are related to the location in which the stroke occurs. Symptoms vary and are typically one-sided. Such symptoms include numbness or paralysis in the face, arm, or leg; loss of vision; mental confusion; slurred speech; and difficulty swallowing.

A transient ischemic attack (TIA) is a "mini-stroke" and forewarns of a potential stroke to come. Victims who experience a TIA have symptoms of a stroke that resolve quickly. Most TIAs occur rapidly and last less than 5 minutes.

Immediate emergency care is important in a victim experiencing a stroke. EMS should be activated for rapid transport to the hospital. If thrombolytic drugs are given within a certain time frame, permanent brain injury can be avoided.

Syncope

Another term for syncope is fainting. There are many causes of syncope, but they all result in a sudden decrease in blood pressure or oxygen and a brief loss of consciousness. Before fainting, a person usually feels nauseous, weak, dizzy, or cold. Help the person to sit down with his or her head between the knees to increase blood flow to the brain. Those people who do faint will usually wake up quickly after collapsing. Immediate management is to let the victim recover while lying flat. This includes raising the legs and monitoring airway, breathing, and circulation. With the legs raised, a patient's head is at the same level as the heart, which helps restore blood flow to the brain. Long-term treatment is to determine and treat the cause of the syncope. Often syncope is caused by a vasovagal nerve response. Table 19-12 describes some of the common causes of syncope.

Wounds

Typically wounds are classified as either open or closed. A closed wound has no break in the skin; examples are contusions and hematomas. An open wound is a break in the skin; examples include abrasions, avulsions, incisions, lacerations, and puncture wounds. The different types of wounds are described in Table 19-13. Remember the mnemonic *RICE* to treat closed wounds: rest, ice, compression, and elevation. Open wounds are more serious in that there is risk of infection (including tetanus). Open wounds may also require suturing. A wound that is bleeding heavily needs to be treated immediately. Pressure should be applied directly to the wound to try to stop the bleeding. Once bleeding stops, the wound can be cleaned gently with antiseptic soap and water to get all debris or dirt out. An antibiotic ointment can be applied before wrapping the wound firmly in a dressing or bandage. It is important not to cut off circulation. For this reason, tourniquets are no longer used. Constriction bands may be used instead and is applied tightly enough to stop the bleeding but not so tight to cut off blood flow completely. When using a constriction band, check to make sure a pulse is still felt distally.

Table 19-12 Causes of Syncope

Syncope	Description
Cardiac	Caused by an irregular cardiac rhythm (tachyarrhythmias, bradyarrhythmias, heart block) or organic heart disease (myocardial infarction, aortic stenosis).
Neurologic	Caused by a neurologic condition (seizure, stroke, TIA).
Postural	Caused by a sudden change in body position; blood pressure may drop suddenly when a person stands up too quickly (orthostatic hypotension).
Vasovagal	Caused by events that stimulate the vagus nerve—urination, coughing, defecation, anticipation of pain, emotional distress; the vagus nerve is part of the parasympathetic nervous system, which experiences overstimulation at the same time that there is withdrawal of the sympathetic nervous system.

Table 19-13 Types of Wounds

Wounds	Description
Abrasion	Scraping of the skin, typically very superficial
Avulsion	A portion of skin is torn—partial or total Partial avulsion = a portion of skin remaining as a "flap" Total avulsion = skin is completely torn off, causing excessive bleeding
Contusion (bruise)	Bleeding under the skin, causing discoloration (black and blue) and swelling
Incision (cut)	A smooth edge split in the skin caused by a sharp object
Hematoma	Bleeding and excess fluid and swelling underneath the skin
Laceration	A jagged-edge cut caused by a sharp object
Puncture	The skin is pierced by a sharp object (needle, nail)

QUESTIONS

19-1. Which of the following statements is true regarding the role of the medical assistant?

    A. If a medical assistant is at an emergency, there is no need to call EMS.

    B. A medical assistant can decide when to stop giving CPR.

    C. Good Samaritan laws do not protect medical assistants.

    D. A medical assistant's role does not include documentation.

    E. A medical assistant can give first aid as well as CPR.

19-2. When is the Heimlich maneuver performed?

    A. To help transport a patient who cannot walk

    B. In the case of anaphylactic shock

    C. To dislodge an object obstructing the airway

    D. To aid in the treatment of a puncture wound

    E. To induce vomiting after ingestion of poison

19-3. A patient comes into the emergency clinic after eating shellfish. She is now flushed and having trouble breathing. Which of the following medications should you have available?

    A. Ipecac

    B. Oxygen

    C. Dextrose

    D. Insulin

    E. Epinephrine

19-4. The "rule of nines" is used in the treatment and management of

    A. sepsis.

    B. strokes.

    C. burns.

    D. diabetic emergencies.

    E. fractures.

19-5. A patient arrives at the emergency clinic short of breath with slightly blue nailbeds and lips. What treatment is the best choice of management for the patient?

    A. Give CPR.

    B. Induce vomiting.

    C. Take a temperature.

    D. Administer oxygen.

    E. Give electroshock wave therapy.

19-6. A fracture in which the bone protrudes through the skin is called a(n) _____fracture.

    A. Colles'

    B. convoluted

    C. greenstick

    D. closed

    E. open

19-7. Prior to administering CPR, what are the first three things to assess?

    A. Vital signs, breathing, and compressions

    B. Airway, breathing, and circulation

    C. Temperature, pain, and consciousness

    D. Alertness, breathing, and circulation

    E. Skin tone, bleeding, and circulation

19-8. According to Basic Cardiac Life Support (BCLS) Guidelines, if a victim has a pulse but needs rescue breathing, the medical provider should give one breath every _____ second(s).

   A. 1
   B. 2
   C. 3
   D. 4
   E. 5

19-9. If you witness a victim fall from a window, which is the most appropriate FIRST response?

   A. Activate EMS.
   B. Ask others what caused the event
   C. Run to help the victim
   D. Run to find a physician.
   E. Comfort the other people watching

19-10. You might find all of the following medications on a crash cart EXCEPT

   A. atropine.
   B. furosemide (Lasix).
   C. epinephrine.
   D. amoxicillin.
   E. dextrose.

19-11. To control bleeding from a laceration to the upper leg, direct pressure should be placed over which of the following pulse points?

   A. Dorsalis pedis
   B. Carotid
   C. Brachial
   D. Radial
   E. Femoral

19-12. Which is the preferred position for the patient who faints and is lying on the ground?

   A. Lying on the side
   B. Sitting up
   C. Head and shoulders propped up, legs flat
   D. Head and shoulders flat, legs raised
   E. Propped up with a pillow under the head

19-13. You discover an unresponsive person lying on the ground. Assuming EMS has been activated, which of the following needs to be assessed first?

   A. Does the patient have a pulse?
   B. Is the patient breathing?
   C. Is the airway open?
   D. Is the patient bleeding?
   E. Is the patient able to communicate what happened?

19-14. What is the purpose of the Good Samaritan laws?

   A. To treat trauma patients first
   B. To call the victim's family immediately
   C. To allow for good communication between the provider and patient
   D. To prevent the spread of hepatitis B
   E. To protect an individual who gives first aid from being sued

19-15. Which of the following burns does not require immediate attention?

    A. Victim has trouble breathing.
    B. Victim was in the hot sun all day.
    C. Victim has burns on face, hands, feet, or genitals.
    D. Victim was burned by chemicals.
    E. Victim has burns on multiple body parts.

19-16. When caring for a person having a seizure, all of the following are good steps to take EXCEPT

    A. hold victim down to restrain from convulsing.
    B. remove any dangerous objects in the vicinity to prevent injury.
    C. do not put anything in the victim's mouth.
    D. cushion the patient's head.
    E. if victim vomits, clear mouth by rolling head to side.

19-17. With which of the following conditions will the patient have rapid respirations and fruity acetone breath, along with extremely high blood sugar?

    A. Insulin shock
    B. Diabetic ketoacidosis
    C. Diabetes mellitus type II
    D. Gestational diabetes
    E. Diabetic neuropathy

19-18. All of the following are appropriate reasons for stopping CPR EXCEPT

    A. the victim does not respond and dies.
    B. EMS arrives and takes over care.
    C. the scene becomes unsafe.
    D. the victim recovers.
    E. you are too exhausted to continue.

19-19. Which artery is used to check the pulse when performing CPR?

    A. Brachial
    B. Ulnar
    C. Radial
    D. Femoral
    E. Carotid

19-20. In adult CPR, what is the ratio of compressions to breaths?

    A. 5:1
    B. 20:1
    C. 10:2
    D. 30:2
    E. 15:2

19-21. Which group is most at risk for poisoning?

    A. Children ages 1–5
    B. Teenagers
    C. Young adults ages 20–30
    D. Adults ages 30–40
    E. Adults ages 40–50

19-22. What is the first step to take in *any* poisoning?

    A. Call the manufacturer.
    B. Give water.
    C. Give ipecac.
    D. Contact the local poison control center.
    E. Call a physician.

ANSWERS

19-1. The correct answer is E. A medical assistant has an important role in emergencies. For example, a medical assistant can give CPR and give first aid (for bleeding/pressure points, burns, cardiac and respiratory arrest, choking, problems related to diabetes, fractures, poisoning, seizures, shock, stroke, syncope, and wounds). In addition, the medical assistant should know when to call for more help by activating EMS (911 in most areas) or calling poison control, suicide hotlines, or abuse shelters. A medical assistant is also responsible for documenting emergencies and restocking supplies and equipment.

19-2. The correct answer is C. The Heimlich maneuver is performed to dislodge an object obstructing an airway. When using the Heimlich maneuver, the patient is still conscious but cannot speak. If the patient becomes unconscious, lower him or her to the ground on their back. Do a finger sweep to attempt to remove any obstruction. Perform a head tilt and chin lift and give two slow breaths. If the breaths still do not go in, continue to give abdominal thrusts by straddling the victim. Give five abdominal thrusts, then a finger sweep, and then two slow breaths until the object becomes dislodged or air goes into the victim.

19-3. The correct answer is E. This patient is experiencing anaphylactic shock. Anaphylaxis is a life-threatening medical emergency because of rapid constriction of the airway. Administration of epinephrine (adrenaline) prevents worsening of the airway constriction, stimulates the heart to continue beating, and may save the victim's life.

19-4. The correct answer is C. The "rule of nines" is used in the treatment and management of burns. The body is divided into parts divisible by 9. For example, the head is 9%, each arm is 9%, each leg is 18%, the ventral trunk is 18%, and the dorsal trunk is 18%. The affected body parts are added together to determine the percentage of body burned.

19-5. The correct answer is D. This patient is suffering from cyanosis, which is a physical sign rather than a diagnosis. It is characterized by bluish discoloration of the skin and mucus membranes. Treatment of cyanosis is based on identifying and treating its cause, and restoring normal flow of oxygenated blood.

19-6. The correct answer is E. An open or compound fracture is a fracture in which the bone protrudes through the skin. Do *not* try to reposition or move the bone. Treatment protocol includes immobilizing with a splint, covering the wound with a sterile dressing, and arranging transportation to the hospital. A convoluted fracture is one that is broken in many pieces. A greenstick fracture is an incomplete fracture, meaning that the bone does not completely break. These are most common in children. In a closed fracture, the bone does not puncture the skin.

19-7. The correct answer is B. CPR guidelines are based on the ABCs: airway, breathing, and circulation.

19-8. The correct answer is B. According to Basic Cardiac Life Support (BCLS) Guidelines, if a victim has a pulse but needs rescue breathing, the medical provider should give one breath every 2 seconds. If the victim does not have a pulse, one should start CPR.

19-9. The correct answer is A. One of the most important roles of the medical assistant is to recognize emergencies and to respond appropriately. If the victim is seen falling or in crisis, 911 should be called first. However, if the victim is found unconscious and CPR is needed, the medical assistant should proceed with 5 cycles of 30 compressions for every 2 breaths prior to activating EMS.

19-10. The correct answer is D. A selection of drugs that are most effective and appropriate in emergency situations are kept in a special cart known as a crash cart in all hospital departments responsible for patient care. Amoxicillin is an antibiotic in the penicillin group of drugs. It is not included on crash carts. Among those drugs that are included on crash carts are atropine, bretylium tosylate, calcium chloride, dextrose, diazepam, diphenhydramine (Benadryl), dopamine, epinephrine, furosemide (Lasix), hetastarch (Hespan), isoproterenol (Isuprel), lidocaine, magnesium sulfate, and midazolam (Versed).

19-11. The correct answer is E. Direct pressure should be placed over the femoral artery to control bleeding to the upper leg. The femoral artery is between the injury (the upper leg) and the heart.

19-12. The correct answer is D. When a patient faints, if already lying down, position them on their back and raise their feet higher than their head. In this position, a patient's head is at the same level as the heart, which helps restore blood flow to the brain. If he or she is sitting, carefully support them in a bent position, with their head between their knees.

19-13. The correct answer is C. Always remember the ABCs for assessment and treatment priorities. Is the airway open? This is the most important first assessment because if there is an obstruction, breathing is automatically stopped. Try to open the victim's airway by tilting their head back with one hand while lifting up their chin with your other hand. Second, is the patient breathing? Assess for movement of the chest and listen for sounds of breathing. If not breathing, pinch the victim's nose closed and give two full breaths into the victim's mouth. If breaths won't go in, reposition the head and try again to give breaths. If still blocked, perform abdominal thrusts (Heimlich maneuver). Finally, check circulation. Check for a carotid pulse by feeling for 5–10 seconds at the side of victim's neck.

19-14. The correct answer is E. Good Samaritan laws protect from liability any health care workers who offer first aid. Essentially, these laws protect an individual who gives first aid in a reasonable and prudent manner from being sued. Good Samaritan laws vary by state.

19-15. The correct answer is B. EMS should be called in incidents when a victim has trouble breathing, has burns on more than one part of the body, was burned by chemicals or electricity, or has burns on the face, hands, feet, or genitals.

19-16. The correct answer is A. Treatment of seizures is supportive and not intended to stop the seizure or restrain the patient. Never put anything in the victim's mouth or hold the victim down while seizing.

19-17. The correct answer is B. Diabetic ketoacidosis is caused by extremely high blood sugar. A patient may have rapid respirations and fruity acetone breath. Treatment is prompt administration of insulin because this condition can lead to diabetic coma.

19-18. The correct answer is A. CPR should be stopped only for the following reasons: the victim recovers, EMS or other trained help arrives or you are replaced by another person who knows CPR, the scene becomes unsafe, you are too exhausted to continue, or the physician directs it (do not resuscitate). It is not appropriate to stop CPR if the victim is not responding.

19-19. The correct answer is E. The carotid artery is used when checking the pulse before and during CPR. The radial artery is not as reliable because the body will shut down blood flow to the extremities.

19-20. The correct answer is D. In adult CPR, you give 30 compressions for every 2 breaths. Children and infants also should receive the same ratio of 30 compressions for every 2 breaths. New American Heart Association guidelines have simplified CPR procedures with all patients receiving the same ratio of compressions to breaths.

19-21. The correct answer is A. The group most at risk for poisoning is children ages 1–5. This is because they are most at risk for ingestion of substances while not under careful supervision.

19-22. The correct answer is D. The first step to take in any poisoning is to contact the local poison control center. Callers should be prepared to give details regarding the poison and the age, weight, and health status of the individual who took the poison.

Nutrition

An understanding of basic principles of nutrition and special dietary needs are an important part of the medical assistant's duties. Often, it is the medical assistant who will be responsible for explaining dietary guidelines to the patient. Nutrition is all about the study of food and how our bodies use food as fuel for growth and daily activities.

The macronutrients, or "big" nutrients, include proteins, carbohydrates, and fats. They provide energy, which is measured in kilocalories. (Often called "Calories" and written with a capital C. One Calorie actually is equivalent to 1000 calories so to be technically correct, one should use the capital C when referring to food. However, people do use the two interchangeably.) You will find the macronutrients in Table 20-1. Water and fiber may also be included as macronutrients, although they do not provide energy directly.

There may be a question or two on the exam about energy yield from nutrients. You can figure out the number of calories in any food when you know the grams of carbohydrates, proteins, and fats. Table 20-2 illustrates the energy yield of macronutrients.

As an example, the energy yield for a slice of bread that has 8 grams of carbohydrates, 3 grams of protein, and 2 grams of fat is:

8 grams carbohydrates × 4 calories/gram = 32 calories
+ 3 grams protein × 4 calories/gram = 12 calories
+ 2 grams fat × 9 calories/gram = 18 calories
Total calories = 62

The micronutrients, or "little" nutrients, are the vitamins and minerals that we need to be healthy. Table 20-3 lists the micronutrients that are water-soluble. Because these vitamins are water-soluble, they do not commonly build up in the body to cause toxicity. However, they are not stored in the body and must be supplied regularly. Table 20-4 lists the fat-soluble micronutrients. Deficiencies of fat-soluble vitamins may be the result of malabsorption syndromes. Cystic fibrosis and celiac sprue are two examples of malabsorption syndromes. Toxicity of fat-soluble vitamins is more common than for water-soluble vitamins because they accumulate in fat.

Minerals are another type of micronutrient. Minerals are necessary for the normal functioning of the body's cells. The body needs large quantities of calcium, chloride, magnesium, phosphate, potassium, and sodium. These minerals are called macrominerals.

The body needs small quantities of chromium, copper, fluoride, iodine, iron, manganese, molybdenum, selenium, and zinc. These minerals are called trace minerals. All trace minerals are harmful if too much is ingested.

Some minerals—especially the macrominerals—are important as electrolytes. The body uses electrolytes to help regulate nerve and muscle function and to maintain acid-base and fluid balance. Table 20-5 lists some of the important macrominerals.

Table 20-1 Macronutrients

Nutrient	Building Units	Important Notes
Carbohydrates	Monosaccharides	Carbohydrates are our main source of energy. Excess carbohydrates are stored as glycogen in the liver. Glycogen can be broken down in times of hunger.
Proteins	Amino acids	Proteins are essential to growth and repair of muscle and other body tissues. Proteins are needed to construct enzymes, hormones, antibodies, and other important body proteins. The human body can synthesize most amino acids; however, nine need to be provided in the diet. These nine amino acids are known as essential amino acids.
Fats	Fats can actually be broken down into different forms: *Saturated fats:* Derived primarily from animal sources, such as beef, and hard at room temperature. Saturated fats are the type you generally would like to avoid. *Unsaturated fats:* Can be further divided into monounsaturated and polyunsaturated fat. Generally, unsaturated fats come from plant sources such as canola oil, olive oil, and similar products. Monounsaturated fats should replace saturated fats whenever possible. *Omega-3 fatty acids:* Fat found in fish oils and some dietary sources such as flax seeds and walnuts; thought to be very beneficial to cardiovascular health. *Cholesterol:* Fat found in the blood; it is a reflection of dietary fat intake. There are two types: LDL (low-density lipoprotein), also known as the "bad" cholesterol, because increased amounts contribute to heart disease and atherosclerosis, and HDL (high-density lipoprotein), also known as the "good" cholesterol, because increased amounts actually lower levels of LDL in the bloodstream, which is good for cardiovascular health. *Triglycerides:* Fat that circulates in the blood with HDL and LDL; composed of three fatty acids and glycerol. High levels are associated with atherosclerosis.	Fat is actually an essential nutrient, and a very small amount is needed on a daily basis to maintain normal body function. The body needs about 15 grams of fat a day, or the equivalent of 1 teaspoon of fat. Americans generally take in about 5 tablespoons of fat a day, or about 75 grams. *Mnemonic:* **HDL** is **H**ealthy. **LDL** is **L**ousy.

(continues)

Table 20-1 Macronutrients (Continued)

Nutrient	Building Units	Important Notes
Fiber	Indigestible but edible portion of our diet	Fiber is essential for the health of our digestive system, providing bulk and stimulation for the intestines. Dietary fiber may be used to treat and prevent constipation, hemorrhoids, diverticular disease, and irritable bowel syndrome.
Water	H_2O—hydrogen and oxygen ions	The most abundant inorganic compound in the body is water. Water contributes to about 65% of an individual's body weight and performs various functions in the body. Water intake is controlled by thirst, with the thirst center located in the hypothalamus.

The MyPyramid food guide, shown in Figure 20-1, is one way for people to understand how to eat healthy. A balanced diet is one that includes all the food groups of the food pyramid. The U.S. Department of Agriculture (USDA) changed the food pyramid in 2005 because it wanted to convey a better example of how to eat healthier. This new food pyramid addresses flaws in the original USDA food pyramid and offers up-to-date information, allowing people to better follow guidelines concerning what they should eat.

A poor diet can have an impact on our health and cause various deficiency diseases. The following are some of the common ones that may be seen on the exam:

- *Scurvy:* Scurvy results from lack of vitamin C. Because vitamin C is necessary for collagen synthesis, scurvy findings include swollen gums, bruising, anemia, and poor wound healing.
- *Beriberi:* Beriberi is the lack of vitamin B_1, and is characterized by cardiac and nervous system pathology. Beriberi is seen in severe alcoholism with malnutrition. Wernicke-Korsakoff syndrome is a neurological disorder that can result from beriberi. This syndrome is a combination of Wernicke's encephalopathy and Korsakoff's psychosis.
- *Kwashiorkor:* This condition results from protein malnutrition; the clinical picture is of a small child with a swollen belly
- *Marasmus:* This condition results from overall malnutrition and lack of all macronutrients, which results in tissue wasting; the clinical picture is of a thin, starving child.

A poor diet also contributes to the following health-threatening conditions:

- Obesity
- High cholesterol
- High blood pressure

Table 20-2 Energy Yield of Macronutrients (per gram)

Nutrient	Calories per Gram
Carbohydrate	4
Protein	4
Fat	9
Alcohol	7

Table 20-3 Micronutrients: Water-Soluble Vitamins

Vitamin	Also Known As	Important Notes and Related Diseases
B_1	Thiamine	Deficiency causes beriberi and Wernicke-Korsakoff syndrome. These diseases, characterized by cardiac and nervous system pathology, are seen in severe alcoholism with malnutrition. *Mnemonic:* **Ber1Ber1**
B_2	Riboflavin	Deficiency causes sores at the corners of the mouth (cheilosis) and corneal vascularization.
B_3	Niacin	Deficiency causes pellagra, which is characterized by diarrhea, dermatitis, and dementia. Pellagra is an endemic disease in Africa, Mexico, Indonesia, and China.
B_6	Pyridoxine	Deficiency causes convulsions and hyperirritability.
B_{12}	Cobalamin	Deficiency causes pernicious anemia and neurologic disorders. Pernicious anemia is a condition in which red blood cells do not divide normally and are too large due to a lack of vitamin B_{12} in the body. Typically, this condition results from the impaired ability to absorb B_{12} because of a lack of intrinsic factor. Intrinsic factor is produced by the parietal cells of the stomach. It is necessary for the absorption of vitamin B_{12} later on in the terminal ileum.
C	Ascorbic acid	Deficiency causes scurvy. Because vitamin C is necessary for collagen synthesis, scurvy findings include swollen gums, bruising, anemia, and poor wound healing. *Mnemonic: British sailors used to carry limes to prevent s***Curvy***. Hence, the sailors were called "limeys."*
Folate	Folic acid	Folic acid is essential for cell growth and the reproduction of RBCs. It is found in green leafy vegetables. Because folic acid is not stored very long in our bodies, supplemental folic acid in early pregnancy reduces neural tube defects (spina bifida). *Mnemonic: Eat ***Foliage*** for ***Folic*** acid and think about the ***Fetus***.*

Table 20-4 Micronutrients: Fat-Soluble Vitamins

Vitamin	Also Known As	Important Notes and Related Diseases
A	Retinol	Vitamin A is for vision. Deficiency causes night blindness and dry skin. *Mnemonic: Think ***Retin-A*** (used topically for acne) and carrots are good for your eyes.*
D		Vitamin D is for bone calcification. Drinking milk fortified with vitamin D is important for strong bones. Deficiency causes rickets (bending of the bones) in children and osteomalacia (soft bones) in adults.
E		Vitamin E is an antioxidant that protects the RBCs from hemolysis. Deficiency may cause anemia. *Mnemonic: ***E*** is for ***Erythrocytes***.*
K		Vitamin K is necessary for the formation of blood clotting factors. Deficiency causes hemorrhage. *Mnemonic: ***K*** is for ***Koagulation***.*

Table 20-5 Important Macrominerals

Mineral	Symbol	Important Notes and Related Diseases
Calcium	Ca	Calcium (along with vitamin D) is for bone calcification. Deficiency causes osteoporosis (porous bones).
Chloride	Cl	Chloride is important as an electrolyte and helps maintain acid-base balance.
Copper	Cu	Copper is a component of many enzymes and helps with iron absorption and hemoglobin (RBC) formation. Wilson's disease is an autosomal recessive disease and causes excessive copper accumulation in the liver or brain. It can be fatal unless copper is restricted.
Fluoride	Fl	Fluoride is required for healthy teeth. *Mnemonic:* **FL**oss *your teeth.*
Iodine	I	Iodine is required for the formation of thyroid hormone. Deficiency can cause goiter (enlarged thyroid gland), hypothyroidism in adults, and cretinism in children. *Mnemonic: Salt is commonly made with iodine because people tend to add salt to food.*
Iron	Fe	Iron is an important component of muscle cells and of hemoglobin (enables red blood cells to carry oxygen and deliver it to the body's tissues). Iron-deficiency anemia is common.
Magnesium	Mg	Magnesium helps build strong bones and teeth. It also activates certain enzymes and helps regulate the heartbeat.
Phosphorus	P	Phosphorus is required for the formation of bone and teeth and for energy production. It is also used to form nucleic acids, including DNA (deoxyribonucleic acid). Disorders include demineralization of the bone and fatigue.
Potassium	K	Potassium is required for normal nerve and muscle function and is involved in electrolyte balance. Potassium helps to regulate the heartbeat. Disorders include hyperkalemia (high blood potassium) and hypokalemia (low blood potassium).
Sodium	Na	Sodium helps the body maintain a normal electrolyte and fluid balance. It is required for normal nerve and muscle function. Restriction is needed for hypertensive patients and congestive heart failure patients.
Zinc	Zn	Zinc is required for healthy skin, healing of wounds, and growth. Deficiency can cause dwarfism.

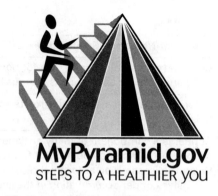

Figure 20-1 The USDA's MyPyramid Food Guide

Source: http://www.mypyramid.gov/downloads/MiniPoster.pdf

Table 20-6 Dietary Restrictions and Diseases

Diet	Related Diseases
Reduced purine	Gout
Reduced sodium	Hypertension, congestive heart failure
Reduced cholesterol	Cardiovascular disease, high cholesterol, obesity, gallbladder disease
Increased folic acid	Pregnancy
Increased calcium and vitamin D	Osteoporosis, rickets, osteomalacia
Increased fiber	Constipation, diseases of the colon
Increased iron	Iron-deficiency anemia
Increased sodium	Addison's disease
Increased potassium	Patients on diuretics
Bland food	Ulcers, gastritis

In addition, a poor diet contributes to chronic systemic diseases, including the following:

- Cardiovascular disease
- Diabetes
- Osteoporosis

Certain dietary restrictions need to be followed in many diseases. Table 20-6 illustrates some dietary restrictions and diseases. There may be questions about these conditions on the exam.

QUESTIONS

20-1. The term *metabolism* is best defined as

    A. the sum of energy produced by all the chemical reactions and mechanical work of the body.
    B. a measure of carbohydrate utilization.
    C. the number of calories it takes to keep from shivering on a cold day.
    D. the length of time it takes to digest and absorb fats.
    E. the percentage of muscle mass a person has.

20-2. Which vitamin requires intrinsic factor in order to be absorbed?

    A. K
    B. E

C. C
D. B$_{12}$
E. A

20-3. Carbohydrates are stored as _____ in the liver.

    A. glycogen
    B. saturated fat
    C. protein
    D. ATP
    E. DNA

20-4. Glycogen is formed in the liver:

    A. during a starvation period.
    B. after eating.
    C. before eating.
    D. in diabetic patients only.
    E. in obese patients only.

20-5. Which of the following releases energy to power cellular processes?

    A. Bases
    B. Acids
    C. Proteins
    D. ATP
    E. DNA

20-6. The building blocks of proteins are

    A. monosaccharides.
    B. nucleic acids.
    C. enzymes.
    D. fatty acids.
    E. amino acids.

20-7. The building blocks of carbohydrates are

    A. monosaccharides.
    B. nucleic acids.
    C. enzymes.
    D. fatty acids.
    E. amino acids.

20-8. The rate of cellular chemical reactions is increased by special proteins called

    A. monosaccharides.
    B. nucleic acids.
    C. enzymes.
    D. fatty acids.
    E. amino acids.

20-9. Inorganic elements such as potassium, sodium, and calcium are classified as

    A. monosaccharides.
    B. nucleic acids.
    C. enzymes.
    D. carbohydrates.
    E. minerals.

20-10. The most abundant inorganic compound in the body is

    A. sodium chloride.
    B. calcium phosphate.
    C. water.
    D. magnesium.
    E. sulfur.

20-11. How many kilocalories is one gram of carbohydrate?

    A. 4 kilocalories
    B. 7 kilocalories
    C. 8 kilocalories
    D. 9 kilocalories
    E. 10 kilocalories

20-12. A deficiency of Vitamin D in children can result in

    A. osteoporosis.
    B. cretinism.
    C. beriberi.
    D. osteomalacia.
    E. rickets.

20-13. Which condition can be caused by a lack of iodine?

    A. Cretinism
    B. Scurvy
    C. Kwashiorkor
    D. Osteoporosis
    E. Beriberi

20-14. Scurvy can be the result of a deficiency of vitamin

    A. A.
    B. C.
    C. D.
    D. E.
    E. K.

20-15. Which of the following vitamins is recommended in pregnancy in order to prevent neural tube defects?

    A. Biotin
    B. Riboflavin
    C. Thiamine
    D. Folic acid
    E. Pantothenic acid

20-16. A person with hypertension should decrease their intake of

    A. calcium.
    B. phosphorus.
    C. iodine.
    D. potassium.
    E. sodium.

20-17. A person with gout should decrease their intake of

  A. salt.
  B. fat.
  C. glycogen.
  D. purine.
  E. fiber.

20-18. Which vitamin is essential in order to prevent night blindness?

  A. A
  B. K
  C. E
  D. B
  E. D

20-19. Which vitamin is essential for proper blood clotting?

  A. A
  B. K
  C. E
  D. B
  E. D

20-20. Which disease results from severe alcoholism with malnutrition and lack of Thiamine (vitamin B_1)?

  A. Pellagra
  B. Osteoporosis
  C. Wernicke-Korsakoff
  D. Kwashiorkor
  E. Marasmus

20-21. Who established the dietary guidelines to help Americans make healthy food choices?

  A. MA
  B. FDA
  C. USDA
  D. CDC
  E. AAMA

ANSWERS

20-1. The correct answer is A. The term *metabolism* is best defined as the sum of energy produced by all the chemical reactions and mechanical work of the body.

20-2. The correct answer is D. Vitamin B_{12} requires intrinsic factor in order to be absorbed later on in the terminal ileum. Intrinsic factor is produced by the parietal cells of the stomach.

20-3. The correct answer is A. Carbohydrates are stored as glycogen in the liver. Glycogen can be broken down in times of hunger.

20-4. The correct answer is B. Glycogen is formed in the liver after eating. Glycogen is a polysaccharide that can be readily converted to glucose as needed by the body to satisfy its energy needs.

20-5. The correct answer is D. ATP or adenosine triphosphate is the major energy currency of the cell. When the third phosphate group of ATP is removed by hydrolysis, a substantial amount of free energy is released.

20-6. The correct answer is E. The building blocks of proteins are amino acids. The human body can synthesize most amino acids. However, nine need to be provided in the diet. These nine amino acids are known as essential amino acids.

20-7. The correct answer is A. The building units of carbohydrates are monosaccharides or simple sugars. Monosaccharides form disaccharides, which then form polysaccharides or complex carbohydrates.

20-8. The correct answer is C. Enzymes are special proteins that speed up chemical reactions.

20-9. The correct answer is E. Inorganic elements such as potassium, sodium, and calcium are classified as minerals. They (particularly potassium and sodium) can also be thought of as electrolytes when they dissolve in water and become charged ions.

20-10. The correct answer is C. The most abundant inorganic compound in the body is water. Water contributes to about 65% of an individual's body weight and performs various functions in the body. Water intake is controlled by thirst, with the thirst center located in the hypothalamus.

20-11. The correct answer is A. One gram of carbohydrate is 4 Calories or kilocalories.

20-12. The correct answer is E. Vitamin D is required for bone calcification. Drinking milk fortified with Vitamin D is important for strong bones. Deficiency causes rickets (bending of the bones) in children and osteomalacia (soft bones) in adults.

20-13. The correct answer is A. A lack of iodine can cause cretinism, a condition of severely stunted physical and mental growth. Iodine is required for the formation of thyroid hormone. It has affected many people worldwide and continues to be a major public health problem in many countries.

20-14. The correct answer is B. Scurvy can be the result of a deficiency of Vitamin C (ascorbic acid). Because Vitamin C is necessary for collagen synthesis, Scurvy findings include swollen gums, bruising, anemia, and poor wound healing. British sailors used to carry limes to prevent scurvy. Hence, the sailors were called "limeys."

20-15. The correct answer is D. Folic acid or folate is recommended in pregnancy in order to prevent neural tube defects (Spina Bifida). Repeated studies have shown that women who get 0.4 milligrams daily prior to conception and during early pregnancy reduce the risk that their baby will be born with a serious neural tube defect.

20-16. The correct answer is E. A person with hypertension should decrease their intake of sodium (salt). Sodium aids in fluid balance so a diet low in salt can help to lower blood pressure.

20-17. The correct answer is D. A person with gout should decrease their intake of purine. Excess uric acid in the body causes gout. Uric acid results from the breakdown of purines. Foods rich in purine (an amino acid) are organ meats like liver and kidney and alcohol.

20-18. The correct answer is A. Vitamin A is required for good vision. Deficiency causes night blindness. Beta-carotene is the molecule that gives carrots, sweet potatoes, squash, and other yellow or orange vegetables their orange color. Beta-carotene is an important precursor of vitamin A in the human diet. Hence, the expression carrots make you able to see in the dark.

20-19. The correct answer is B. Vitamin K is necessary for formation of blood clotting factors. *Pneumonic: K is for Koagulation.* Deficiency causes hemorrhage.

20-20. The correct answer is C. Severe alcoholism with malnutrition and lack of Thiamine (Vitamin B_1) result in Wernicke-Korsakoff syndrome, characterized by cardiac and nervous system pathology.

20-21. The correct answer is C. The U.S. Department of Agriculture (USDA) established the dietary guidelines as The Food Guide Pyramid to help Americans make healthy food choices.

Index